MANUAL OF
Neurologic Emergencies

MANUAL OF
Neurologic
Emergencies

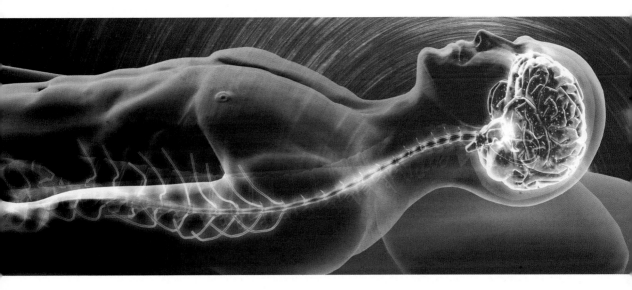

Andy S. Jagoda, MD

Professor and Chair Emeritus of Emergency Medicine
Icahn School of Medicine at Mount Sinai
New York, New York

Christopher A. Lewandowski, MD

Clinical Professor of Emergency Medicine
School of Medicine—Wayne State University
Executive Vice Chair
Department of Emergency Medicine
Henry Ford Hospital
Detroit, Michigan

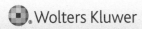 Wolters Kluwer

Philadelphia · Baltimore · New York · London
Buenos Aires · Hong Kong · Sydney · Tokyo

Series Editor:

Ron M. Walls, MD

Acquisitions Editor: Keith Donnellan
Senior Development Editor: Ashley Fischer
Editorial Coordinator: Vinoth Ezhumalai
Marketing Manager: Kirsten Watrud
Production Project Manager: Sadie Buckallew
Design Coordinator: Stephen Druding
Manufacturing Coordinator: Beth Welsh
Prepress Vendor: S4Carlisle Publishing Services

9 8 7 6 5 4 3 2 1

Printed in Singapore

Library of Congress Cataloging-in-Publication Data

ISBN-13: 978-1-975142-78-0

ISBN-10: 1-975142-78-0

Library of Congress Control Number: 2021914824

---

shop.lww.com

MKO721

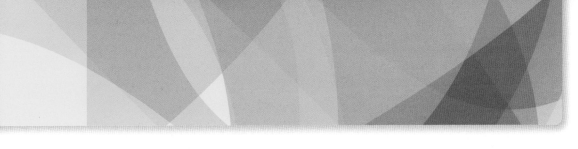

Contributors

Ethan Abbott, DO
Assistant Professor
Department of Emergency Medicine
Icahn School of Medicine at Mount Sinai
Physician
Department of Emergency Medicine
Mount Sinai Health System
New York, New York

Charles M. Andrews, MD
Associate Professor
Departments of Emergency Medicine, Neurology
and Neurosurgery
Medical University of South Carolina
Associate Professor
Departments of Neurosurgery, Neurology and
Emergency Medicine
Medical University of South Carolina Health
Charleston, South Carolina

E. Megan Callan, MD
Fellow, Neurocritical Care
Medical University of South Carolina
Charleston, South Carolina

Amy D. Costigan, MD
Assistant Professor
Department of Emergency Medicine
University of Massachusetts Medical School
Emergency Physician
Department of Emergency Medicine
University of Massachusetts Medical Center
Worcester, Massachusetts

Jonathan A. Edlow, MD
Professor
Department of Emergency Medicine
Harvard Medical School
Attending Physician
Department of Emergency Medicine
Beth Israel Deaconess Medical Center
Boston, Massachusetts

Daniel Eraso, MD
Assistant Professor of Emergency Medicine
University of Florida College of
Medicine–Jacksonville
Jacksonville, Florida

Steven A. Godwin, MD, FACEP
Professor and Chair
Department of Emergency Medicine
Assistant Dean for Simulation Education
University of Florida College of
Medicine–Jacksonville
Jacksonville, Florida

Scott A. Goldberg, MD, MPH
Assistant Professor
Department of Emergency Medicine
Harvard Medical School
Director of Emergency Medical Services
Department of Emergency Medicine
Brigham and Women's Hospital
Boston, Massachusetts

Andy S. Jagoda, MD
Professor and Chair Emeritus of Emergency
Medicine
Icahn School of Medicine at Mount Sinai
New York, New York

Alex Janke, MD
Resident in Emergency Medicine
Yale School of Medicine
New Haven, Connecticut

Corlin Jewell, MD
Resident in Emergency Medicine
University of Wisconsin
Madison, Wisconsin

George Kramer
Research Assistant in Emergency Medicine
Icahn School of Medicine at Mount Sinai
New York, New York

Cappi Lay, MD
Assistant Professor
Departments of Neurosurgery and Emergency
Medicine
Icahn School of Medicine at Mount Sinai
Director, Neurosciences Intensive Care Unit
Departments of Neurosurgery and Emergency
Medicine
Mount Sinai Hospital
New York, New York

Christopher A. Lewandowski, MD
Clinical Professor of Emergency Medicine
School of Medicine–Wayne State University
Executive Vice Chair
Department of Emergency Medicine
Henry Ford Hospital
Detroit, Michigan

Joseph B. Miller, MD, MS
Clinical Associate Professor
Department of Emergency Medicine
School of Medicine–Wayne State University
Residency Director
Departments of Emergency Medicine and Internal
*   Medicine*
Henry Ford Health System
Detroit, Michigan

Ashley Norse, MD
Associate Professor
Department of Emergency Medicine
University of Florida College of
*   Medicine–Jacksonville*
Associate Chair of Operations
Department of Emergency Medicine
UF Health Jacksonville
Jacksonville, Florida

Angela Hua, MD, FACEP
Associate Professor
Donald's Barbara Zucker School of Medicine at
*   Hofstra/Nestwell*
Hempstead, New York
Faculty
Department of Emergency Medicine
Long Island Jewish Medical Center
New Hyde Park, New York

Lauren M. Post, MD
Evans, Georgia

Elaine Rabin, MD
Associate Professor
Department of Emergency Medicine
Icahn School of Medicine at Mount Sinai
Attending Physician and Residency Director
Department of Emergency Medicine
Mount Sinai Hospital
New York, New York

Christopher Reverte, MD
Assistant Professor
Department of Emergency Medicine
Icahn School of Medicine at Mount Sinai
Mount Sinai Morningside and Mount Sinai West
New York, New York

Jeremy Rose, MD
Assistant Professor of Emergency Medicine
Icahn School of Medicine at Mount Sinai
New York, New York

Andrew N. Russman, DO, MA
Assistant Professor
Medicine (Neurology)
Cleveland Clinic Lerner College of Medicine
Head, Cleveland Clinic Stroke Program
Cerebrovascular Center, Neurological Institute
Cleveland Clinic
Cleveland, Ohio

Benjamin H. Schnapp, MD, MEd
Assistant Professor
Department of Emergency Medicine
University of Wisconsin School of Medicine and
*   Public Health*
Associate Residency Program Director
Emergency Physician
UWHealth
Madison, Wisconsin

Matthew S. Siket, MD, MS, FACEP
Associate Professor
Departments of Surgery and Neurological Sciences
Division of Emergency Medicine
The Robert Larner, M.D. College of Medicine at the
*   University of Vermont*
Associate Program Director
University of Vermont Emergency Medicine
*   Residency Program*
The University of Vermont Medical Center
Burlington, Vermont

Brian Silver, MD
Professor and Chair of Neurology
Department of Neurology
University of Massachusetts Medical School
Worcester, Massachusetts

Edward P. Sloan, MD
Professor Emeritus of Emergency Medicine
University of Illinois College of Medicine
Chicago, Illinois

Rebecca Elizabeth Traub, MD
Associate Professor
Department of Neurology
University of North Carolina School of Medicine
Chapel Hill, North Carolina

Melissa Villars, MD
Resident in Emergency Medicine
Icahn School of Medicine at Mount Sinai
New York, New York

Charles R. Wira III, MD
Associate Professor
Department of Emergency Medicine
Yale Acute Stroke Program
Department of Neurology
Board Certified Internal and Emergency Medicine
Yale School of Medicine
New Haven, Connecticut

Preface

Five to 10% of emergency department visits are for a primary neurologic complaint. Fortunately, the majority of these presentations are not associated with a life-threatening condition—but an important subset is. Early recognition and treatment of these conditions can be the difference between a good, functional outcome and permanent disability or death. State-of-the-art care that delivers quality and safety requires a commitment to both clinical and system-based excellence.

Failure to perform an adequate clinical evaluation and to develop a differential diagnosis are consistently identified as factors linked to bad outcomes. Most neurologic emergencies present with a complaint and not a diagnosis; these complaints are often nonspecific and the clinician must be able to carefully gather the historical and physical examination data needed to generate a differential diagnosis that will then direct diagnostic testing. Based on the evaluation, diagnostic considerations are narrowed and help with risk stratification and informed decision-making with the patient. Front-line providers must be facile in their diagnostic and communication skills or risk failing to meet their patients' needs. Subtle findings of posterior circulation strokes, idiopathic intercranial hypertension, cerebral venous thrombosis, nonconvulsive seizure, and epidural abscess are just a few of the processes that have historically been missed on first visits to clinicians, often as the result of failed systematic evaluations and/or bias in approaching the patient's complaint.

Time-sensitive treatments have raised the bar for the front-line clinician and have underscored the maxim "time is brain." Stroke, status epilepticus, traumatic brain injury, and meningoencephalitis are examples where delay in treatment may have catastrophic consequences. Therefore, over the past 25 years the diagnosis and treatment of many neurologic emergencies have moved upstream to recruit the skills of prehospital providers and emergency physicians. Indeed, from the beginnings of thrombolytic trials for stroke, it became clear that leadership and involvement from emergency providers were fundamental to successful trials and to successful patient care, not just for stroke but for all entities requiring neuroresuscitation. This trial demonstrated the importance of teams and systems of care to ensure optimal outcomes. The impact of emphasizing upstream care became evident with the creation of the National Institutes of Health (NIH)-funded research networks including SPOTRIUS and NETT, which historically laid the foundation for the modern management of many neurologic complaints.

Availability of advanced diagnostic testing, laboratory, and neuroimaging has offered new opportunities for facilitated diagnostics and treatments. Biomarkers for neurologic injury, bedside electroencephalogram (EEG), computed tomography (CT) angiography, CT perfusion/diffusion scanning, and magnetic resonance imaging (MRI), have all become more available and their value highlighted by functional outcomes that only until recently would be considered miraculous. Of course, many tests and interventions come at an upfront cost in time and resources, which underscores the importance of judicious use of resources with a clear understanding of when and where they are best used. However, when used correctly, the downstream cost savings more than compensates and from a population health perspective highlights the need for coordinated multidisciplinary, integrated care that is based on the best available evidence.

We embarked in editing this book driven by our passion for improving patient care. We have over 80 years of combined clinical experience and bring our own personal experience with family and friends who have had strokes, complex regional pain syndrome, nonconvulsive seizures, and traumatic brain injury. We have seen the good, and sometimes the not so good, that is driven by the expertise of the clinician who first cares for a patient. With this background, Section I of this book was designed to ensure that the fundamentals of evaluating the patient with a neurologic complaint were covered to ensure that the tools are provided to generate a differential diagnosis, knowing that if a disease does not appear on the list it is unlikely the diagnosis will be made! Section II of the books drills down on specific complaints providing a framework for vectoring care delivery and interventions based on the best available evidence. Hopefully, we have been successful in designing a user-friendly, easy-to-access guide that both the reader and patient will benefit from. Good outcomes depend on a clinician's ability to gather and collate history and physical and diagnostic information. Communication with consultants and patients as well as clear management and follow-up strategies are often pivotal to the outcome. Awareness and application of established practice guidelines/clinical policies and best practice advisories all contribute to the remarkable advances made in caring for the patient with a neurologic complaint.

Andy S. Jagoda, MD
Christopher A. Lewandowski, MD

Contents

Section I

Approach to the Patient

Neuroanatomy: The Basics

Amy D. Costigan

Brian Silver

A solid foundational understanding of neuroanatomy is critical to the recognition and management of neurologic emergencies. This chapter discusses the most important anatomic structures involved in emergent neurologic disease processes and injuries. Subsequent chapters will build on these concepts and how they apply to the physical exam, neuroimaging, and to specific neurologic emergency conditions. Neuroanatomy encompasses all structures of the nervous system and can be divided into two main categories: the central nervous system and the peripheral nervous system. The main components of the central nervous system, including the brain, spinal cord, vasculature, and dural spaces, are presented as well as the somatic and autonomic components of the peripheral nervous system.

CENTRAL NERVOUS SYSTEM

The central nervous system consists of the brain and the spinal cord. The brain is, essentially, the command center for the entire human body. It is a large and complex organ that controls and regulates virtually every action of the human body, including thought, emotion, vision, speech, breathing, and movement. The brain is estimated to contain 100 billion neurons (with approximately 10-20 billion in the cerebral cortex and 55-70 billion in the cerebellum) and an additional 100 glial cells to support neuronal function. The number of synapses in the brain is approximately 100 trillion, representing 1000 synapses per neuron. The brain has three main parts: the cerebrum, the cerebellum, and the brainstem. Although the brain makes up only 2% of total body weight, it receives 20% of the body's cardiac output. The brain depends on this constant blood flow for nutrition and function because it does not store any fuel.

Cerebrum

The cerebrum is the largest portion of the brain and is composed of the right and left hemispheres that are separated by the longitudinal fissure. The cerebral hemispheres are covered by a thin outer layer of gray matter, called the cerebral cortex, which contains billions of neurons to control essential functions such as consciousness, language, memory, and attention. White matter lies below the cerebral cortex and is made up of myelinated tracts that distribute information between brain regions. In general, the left hemisphere is the "dominant" hemisphere in most people and controls language and speech. The right hemisphere is important in the interpretation of visual and spatial information. Tracts that control motor and sensory function mostly (approximately 95%) cross in the lower medulla to the contralateral arm and leg. Therefore, the right hemisphere controls the left hemibody, and the left hemisphere controls the right hemibody. The two hemispheres are connected by a large bundle of nerve fibers, called the corpus callosum, as well as smaller commissures, including the anterior commissure, posterior commissure, and fornix. These are important because they transfer and coordinate information between the two hemispheres.

The cortex folds into peaks, called gyri, and grooves, called sulci, allowing for a larger surface area of brain to fit within the skull. Larger sulci and gyri separate the cerebral hemispheres into four distinct areas, called the frontal, temporal, parietal, and occipital lobes (**Figure 1.1**). Each area has different, although sometimes overlapping, functions.

The frontal lobe is the most anterior portion of the brain and is separated from the parietal lobe by the central sulcus and from the temporal lobe by the lateral sulcus (Sylvian fissure) (Figure 1.1). The frontal lobe controls personality, behavior, speech, body movement, concentration, and intelligence. A clinically important portion of the inferior frontal lobe is called Broca area, which is in the dominant hemisphere and is integral in language processing (**Figure 1.2**). Strokes or damage to this area will cause expressive aphasia, also known as Broca aphasia. This results in impairment in the production of speech but a preservation of the understanding of spoken and written language. Control of gaze is also mediated through the frontal eye fields. Abnormal excitation of one frontal field, such as in a lateralized seizure, will result in gaze away from the excitatory focus and toward the jerking limbs. Destruction of the frontal eye fields, as in a stroke, will result in gaze toward the destruction and away from the hemiparesis. In clinical scenarios where the eyes appear to be deviated toward hemiparetic limbs, consideration of a seizure should also be undertaken with careful examination of the eyes to look for subtle nystagmoid jerking, which confirms the diagnosis.

The temporal lobe, which is separated from the frontal and parietal lobes by the lateral sulcus, also has a language component, called Wernicke area (Figure 1.2). The ability to understand written and spoken language is controlled by this area. Damage to the superior temporal lobe causes a type of receptive aphasia, called Wernicke aphasia. Because patients have difficulty understanding language, they may produce speech that has no meaning and can colloquially be referred to as "word salad." Broca and Wernicke area are connected via a bundle called the arcuate fasciculus (Figure 1.2). The temporal lobe also helps controls memory, hearing, and organization.

The parietal lobe is positioned above the temporal lobe and behind the frontal lobe and central sulcus (Figure 1.1). It has important functions, including the integration of sensory information and visual and spatial processing.

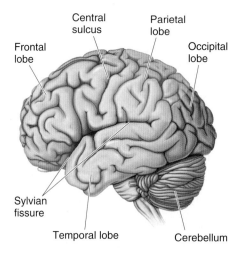

Figure 1.1: The lobes of the cerebrum. Notice the deep Sylvian fissure, dividing the frontal lobe from the temporal lobe, and the central sulcus, dividing the frontal lobe from the parietal lobe. The occipital lobe lies at the back of the brain. These landmarks can be found on all human brains. From Bear MF, Connors BW, Paradiso MA. Neuroscience: past, present, and future. In: Bear MF, Connors BW, Paradiso MA, eds. *Neuroscience: Exploring the Brain.* 4th ed. Wolters Kluwer; 2016:3-22. Figure 1.8.

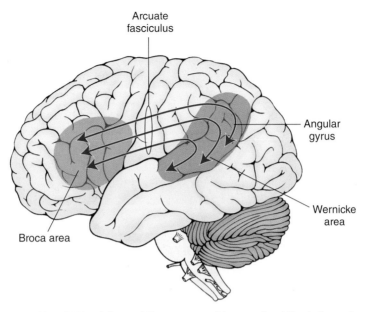

Figure 1.2: Relationship of Wernicke and Broca areas. Diagram is of the left cerebral hemisphere indicating the loci of Broca motor speech area and Wernicke area. There are reciprocal connections between the two regions, which pass in a bundle called the arcuate fasciculus. From Siegel A, Sapru HN. The thalamus and cerebral cortex. In: Siegel A, Sapru HN, eds. *Essential Neuroscience.* 3rd ed. Wolters Kluwer; 2015:462-489. Figure 25.19.

Finally, the occipital lobe is the visual processing center of the brain and is located posteriorly behind the parietal lobe and temporal lobe (Figure 1.1). It contains the primary visual cortex as well as other functional visual areas. Damage to the occipital lobe can cause visual field cuts, visual hallucinations, or even blindness. The calcarine fissure divides the occipital cortex into superior and inferior portions. Damage to the occipital cortex above the calcarine fissure produces lower visual field defects, whereas injury to the occipital cortex below the calcarine fissure produces upper visual field defects. Like motor control, representation of the left visual field (of both eyes) is in the right occipital cortex and that of the right visual field (of both eyes) in the left occipital cortex. Thus, for example, a right occipital injury below the calcarine cortex will produce a left upper visual field defect in both eyes (**Figure 1.3**).

Subcortical Structures

Deep below the cerebral cortex lie the subcortical structures, which include the diencephalon, pituitary gland, limbic structures, and the basal ganglia. These essential structures are integral in memory, hormone production, and emotion.

The diencephalon, the brain between the cerebrum and the brainstem, is found deep within the cerebrum and consists of the thalamus, epithalamus, subthalamus, and hypothalamus. The thalamus is a sensory integration center that has connections to many areas of the brain as well as the reticular activating system, which regulates arousal and sleep-wake transitions. Damage to the anterior thalamus, particularly if bilateral in the setting of deep venous sinus thrombosis, can produce disruption in awareness or even coma. This diagnosis should be considered as a possibility in someone presenting with sudden unresponsiveness, particularly if there is no obvious cardiac or toxic cause. The epithalamus consists mostly of the pineal gland and helps secrete melatonin for circadian rhythms. The subthalamus is involved in the integration of somatic motor function. The hypothalamus is a small structure that connects to the pituitary gland via the infundibular stalk. It contains several small nuclei and is an important control center for the autonomic nervous system and endocrine system, including body temperature, hunger, thirst, fatigue, and sleep.

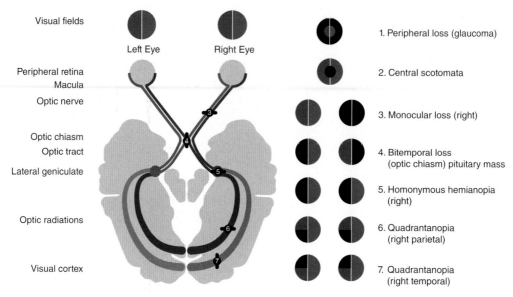

Figure 1.3: Visual field defect. Courtesy of Christopher Lewandowski.

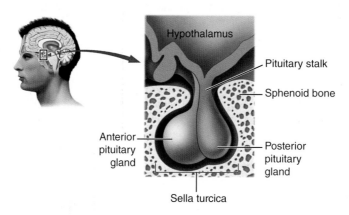

Figure 1.4: The pituitary gland. The posterior pituitary gland is neural tissue; the anterior pituitary gland is endocrine epithelial tissue. From McConnell TH, Hull KL. Metabolism and endocrine control. In: McConnell TH, Hull KL, eds. *Human Form, Human Function: Essentials of Anatomy & Physiology*. Wolters Kluwer; 2011:588-631. Figure 15.17.

Pituitary Gland

The pituitary gland is an endocrine gland that is located off the bottom of the hypothalamus (**Figure 1.4**). Although it is only about the size of a pea, it secretes hormones that have a vast array of important functions such as growth, metabolism, temperature regulation, and pain relief. It helps regulate thyroid and kidney function as well as sex, pregnancy, child birth, and breastfeeding.

The Limbic System

The limbic system is a set of brain structures located next to the thalamus and beneath the medial temporal lobe (**Figure 1.5**). It has many important functions, including emotion, motivation, memory, and behavior. Acute alteration in personality may be caused by processes affecting the limbic system, such as limbic encephalitis, an autoimmune disorder that can produce a rapid onset neuropsychiatric disorder. Two important structures in the limbic system are the hippocampus and amygdala. The hippocampus is involved in the processing of spatial memory and learning. The

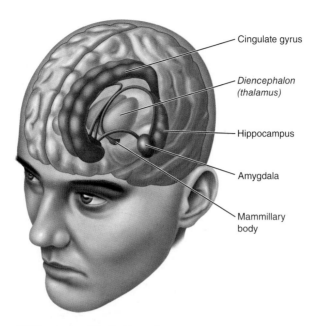

(A) Structures of the limbic system

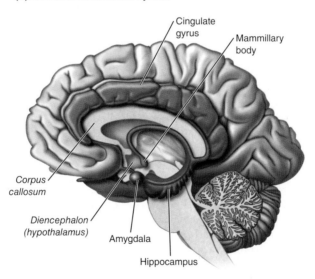

(B) Sagittal view

Figure 1.5: Limbic system. A, The limbic system consists of structures in the cerebral hemispheres that play important roles in emotion. B, The limbic system, viewed in a sagittal brain section. From McConnell TH, Hull KL. Nervous system. In: McConnell TH, Hull KL, eds. *Human Form, Human Function: Essentials of Anatomy & Physiology.* Wolters Kluwer; 2011:280-327. Figure 8.10.

amygdala is the deepest part of the limbic system and is involved in cognitive processes such as memory, attention, emotion, and social processing.

Basal Ganglia
The basal ganglia (**Figure 1.6**) are a group of subcortical nuclei at the base of the forebrain and the top of the midbrain. They consist of striatum (caudate nucleus, putamen, nucleus accumbens, and olfactory tubercle), globus pallidus, ventral pallidum, substantia nigra, and subthalamic nucleus.

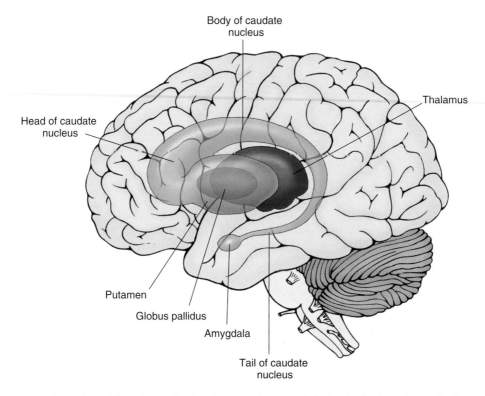

Body of caudate
nucleus

Thalamus

Head of caudate
nucleus

Putamen

Globus pallidus

Amygdala

Tail of caudate
nucleus

Figure 1.6: Location of basal ganglia (sagittal section, medial view). The basal ganglia, located deep within the cerebral hemispheres, consist of the caudate, putamen, and globus pallidus in the cerebrum; the substantia nigra in the midbrain; and the subthalamic nucleus in the diencephalon. The basal ganglia are important in motor control; they facilitate desired movements and inhibit undesired movements. From Siegel A, Sapru HN. The forebrain. In: Siegel A, Sapru HN, eds. *Essential Neuroscience*. 3rd ed. Wolters Kluwer; 2015:197-215. Figure 12.11.

The basal ganglia are important in the control of voluntary motor movements, eye movements, cognition, emotion, and learning. Some disorders of behavior control and movement are rooted in the basal ganglia, including Parkinson and Huntington. Acute injuries of the basal ganglia, for example, to the subthalamic nucleus, can produce unusual syndromes such as uncontrolled ballistic movements of the contralateral limb. The basal ganglia also play a large role in addiction physiology.

The Cerebellum

The cerebellum is a vital structure that gives human beings motor control and coordination. It is attached to the bottom of the brain and lies underneath the cerebral hemispheres in the posterior cranial fossa. It consists of a much more tightly folded cortex than the cerebrum and gives the appearance of parallel folds. Like the cerebrum, the cerebellum is divided into two hemispheres. Between these is a midline section called the vermis (**Figure 1.7**). The cerebellum is connected to the rest of the brain and spinal cord via three pairs of cerebellar peduncles, called the superior, middle, and inferior cerebellar peduncles. The superior cerebellar peduncles connect efferent fibers to the cerebral cortex. The middle cerebellar peduncle connects to the pons, and the inferior cerebellar peduncle receives signals from the vestibular nuclei, spinal cord, and tegmentum. When patients have damage to the cerebellum, they typically exhibit *ipsilateral* decreased motor control. Although they may be able to accomplish gross motor tasks, they have issues with precision and coordination. Patients with cerebellar lesions may exhibit ataxia, ocular skew deviation, poor coordination, dysmetria, dysdiadochokinesia, or a tendency to fall toward the side of the lesion.

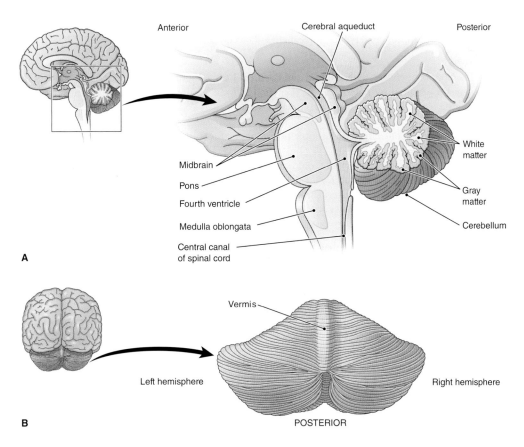

Figure 1.7: The brainstem and cerebellum. A, Midsagittal section (*Note:* The brainstem has three divisions: the midbrain, pons, and medulla oblongata. The white matter of the cerebellum is in a treelike pattern). B, Posterior view of the cerebellum (*Note:* The cerebellum is divided into two hemispheres). From Cohen BJ. The sensory system. In: Cohen BJ, ed. *Memmler's Structure and Function of the Human Body.* 10th ed. Wolters Kluwer; 2013:188-209. Figure 9.8.

The Brainstem

The most posterior portion of the brain that is continuous with the spinal cord is called the brainstem. It consists of three main parts: the midbrain, the pons, and the medulla oblongata (see Figure 1.7). The brainstem transmits motor and sensory information between the brain and the body. Ascending sensory tracts and descending motor tracts are located here, and ten of the body's cranial nerves also emerge from the brainstem. It also integrates crucial information for cardiovascular control, respiratory control, pain, alertness, and consciousness.

Midbrain

The rostral most portion of the brainstem is called the midbrain and is separated into four structures called the tectum, cerebral aqueduct, tegmentum, and cerebral peduncles. The tectum is located on the dorsal side of the midbrain and is responsible for reflexes to auditory and visual stimuli. The cerebral aqueduct is part of the ventricular system and drains cerebrospinal fluid from the third ventricle to the fourth ventricle. Cranial nerve nuclei for the oculomotor nerve (III) and trochlear nerve (IV) are located on the ventral side of the gray matter surrounding the cerebral aqueduct. The midbrain tegmentum is ventral to the cerebral aqueduct and communicates with the cerebellum via the superior cerebellar peduncles. The tegmentum contains a large network of neural synapses and nuclei with white matter tracts. The cerebral peduncles form lobes ventrally to the tegmentum and contain additional white matter tracts. Syndromes such as the top of the basilar syndrome caused by a distal basilar artery occlusion, around the level of the midbrain, will produce a variety of syndromes, including alternating hemiparesis, visual hallucinations, and coma. Mortality is approximately 80% if recanalization is not achieved.

Pons

The pons lies between the midbrain and the medulla (see Figure 1.7). The pons helps control sleep as well as respiratory rate. It can be separated into the basilar part of the pons ventrally and the pontine tegmentum. Posteriorly, it contains the cerebellar peduncles, which connect the pons and the cerebellum and midbrain. Because it acts as a connection point between these different areas, damage to the pons can cause issues with autonomic functions, movement, sensory problems, dysfunction in arousal, and coma. The pons contains several cranial nerve nuclei, including trigeminal nerve (V), abducens nerve (VI), facial nerve (VII), and vestibulocochlear nerve (VIII). Because the nerve roots to the face exit above the decussation, strokes affecting the pons can result in ipsilateral facial weakness and contralateral arm and leg weakness. A brainstem stroke should be considered if there is clear facial weakness on the side opposite to limb weakness.

Medulla

The medulla is a long cone-shaped structure that is responsible for several autonomic functions, including heart rate, blood pressure, breathing, vomiting, and sleep. The upper open part of the medulla forms the fourth ventricle, and the lower closed portion surrounds the central canal of the spinal cord. Several white matter tracts synapse in the medulla. The nuclei for cranial nerves IX to XII are also present here.

THE ARTERIAL VASCULAR SYSTEM

A continuous supply of arterial blood flow is vital for the brain because it does not have any energy or fuel stores of its own. The arterial blood supply to the brain is a made up of a complex series of vessels that ultimately anastomose in a ring called the circle of Willis (**Figure 1.8**). The arterial blood is supplied by two main pairs of arteries: the bilateral internal carotid arteries and the bilateral vertebral arteries. The internal carotid arteries supply the anterior circulation to the cerebrum, whereas the vertebral arteries join to form the basilar artery and supply the posterior circulation to the cerebellum and brainstem. The circle of Willis creates a connection at the base of the skull between the anterior and the posterior circulatory systems of the brain.

The anterior circulation of the brain begins at the bilateral internal carotid arteries, which first branch with the ophthalmic artery and then branch into the anterior cerebral artery (ACA) and the much larger middle cerebral artery (MCA). The anterior cerebral arteries supply blood to the entire midline of the cerebral hemispheres (**Figure 1.9**). They connect with their contralateral counterpart via the anterior communicating artery (A Comm) to complete the anterior ring of the circle of Willis (Figure 1.8). Strokes in the anterior cerebral artery are less common; acute isolated or predominant contralateral lower extremity motor deficits should raise suspicion of this kind of stroke. This is illustrated in **Figure 1.10,** which shows the motor homunculus of the cerebral cortex. The homunculus ("little man") is a famous graphical representation of a man lying within the brain and diagrams the areas of the body controlled by each region. It demonstrates how the midline cerebral hemisphere, which is supplied by the ACA, primarily controls the lower extremity.

The middle cerebral artery (MCA) courses into the lateral sulcus and perfuses most of the lateral surface of the cerebral cortex (Figure 1.9). It is divided into four segments (M1-M4). Owing to the direct flow of blood from the internal carotid artery and the large amount of cerebrum supplied by the MCA, this artery accounts for the most common territory in the cerebrum affected by acute stroke. Neurologic deficits vary depending on the extent and hemisphere, but they include aphasia (typically left hemisphere), neglect (most often in right hemisphere strokes but can occur less commonly with left hemisphere strokes), hemianopia, contralateral hemiparesis, or contralateral hemisensory loss. The MCA is the main artery typically amenable to mechanical thrombectomy for large vessel occlusion during acute stroke.

The posterior circulation originates in the bilateral vertebral arteries, which enter the skull through the foramen magnum. The posterior inferior cerebellar artery (PICA) branches off the vertebral artery to supply the posterior and inferior cerebellum. The two vertebral arteries join to form the basilar artery, which is responsible for supplying the pons, cerebellum, and inner ear

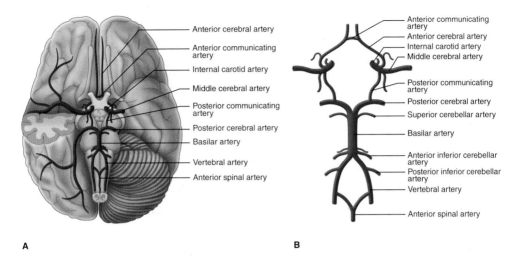

A   **B**

Figure 1.8: Circle of Willis (arterial blood supply to the brain). A, The circle of Willis seen from below the brain. B, Schematic of the circle of Willis. From Ciechanowski M, Mower-Wade D, McLeskey SW. Anatomy and physiology of the nervous system. In: Morton PG, Fontaine DK, eds. *Critical Care Nursing*. 10th ed. Wolters Kluwer; 2013:691-722. Figure 32.8.

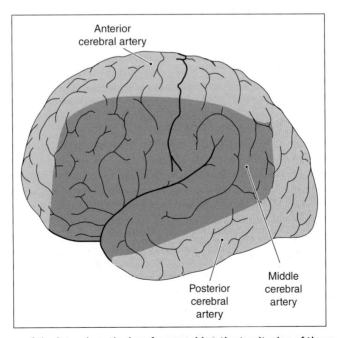

Figure 1.9: Diagram of the lateral cortical surface marking the territories of three cortical arteries. From Bhatnagar S. Cerebrovascular system. In: Bhatnagar S, ed. *Neuroscience for the Study of Communicative Disorders*. 5th ed. Wolters Kluwer; 2018:181-206. Figure 7.4B.

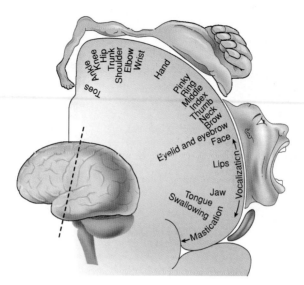

Figure 1.10: The homunculus of the motor strip. From Drislane F. The approach to weakness. In: Drislane F, ed. *Blueprints Neurology.* 5th ed. Wolters Kluwer; 2019:40-48. Figure 5.4.

via the anterior inferior cerebellar artery (AICA), pontine arteries, the superior cerebellar artery, and the internal auditory artery. The differential diagnosis for acute unilateral hearing loss should include an AICA territory infarction, particularly if there is associated dizziness and/or dysmetria. The basilar artery terminates when it divides into the two posterior cerebral arteries (PCA). These two vessels supply the inferior and posterior cerebrum and are joined by the posterior communicating artery (P Comm) to complete the posterior ring of the circle of Willis (Figure 1.8).

Posterior cerebral artery strokes can present as hemianopia and hemisensory loss. Strokes in the basilar artery most commonly present as ischemia in the pons, and patients can have paresis, ataxia, weakness of bulbar muscles, and oculomotor gaze palsies. "Locked-in syndrome" is a result of a large ventral pontine stroke that mimics coma or persistent vegetative state. The key diagnostic feature is preservation of eye or eyelid movements through which an affected individual can respond affirmatively or negatively to questions. Basilar artery occlusion should be strongly considered in any patient presenting with sudden onset coma.

The border zone areas supplied by the very distal portions of the middle, anterior, and posterior cerebral arteries are particularly vulnerable to a type of stroke called watershed stroke. Sudden drops in blood pressure, particularly in the setting of fixed proximal artery narrowing, will result in ischemic strokes in these areas. These border zone areas are also sensitive to episodes of significant hypoperfusion during global hypoxemic events. An important concept, particularly in the setting of acute ischemic stroke, is the effect of collateral blood supply. Collateral blood supply comes from arteries that meet at the ends of the arteries that have blood flow diminished, as might occur during acute arterial occlusion, that is, acute ischemic stroke. With good collateral supply, the time to permanent tissue loss is extended, whereas the opposite is true with poor collateral blood supply. Examples of collateral blood supply are the branches of the external carotid artery providing supplemental blood flow to distal branches of the middle cerebral artery. The quality of collateral blood supply is affected by genetics, age, and physical fitness.

THE VENOUS VASCULAR SYSTEM

Unlike veins in other parts of the body, the venous system of the brain has an independent course from the arterial system. There are both superficial and deep components to the venous vascular system (**Figure 1.11**). The superficial system is composed of the venous sinuses that are located on the surface of the cerebrum and have walls that are composed of dura matter. The major dural venous sinus, called the superior sagittal sinus, runs in a sagittal direction under

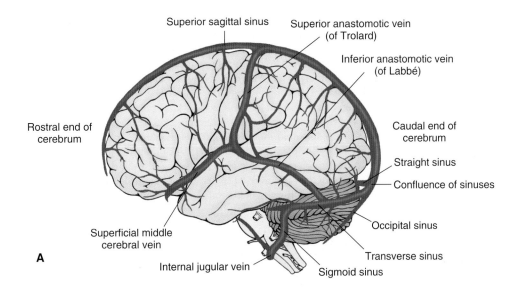

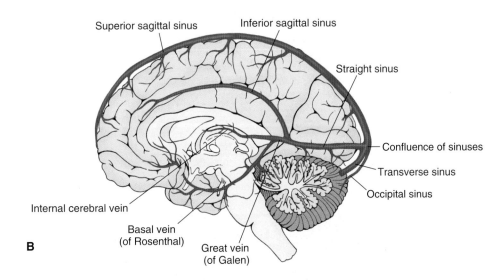

Figure 1.11: Major dural sinuses and veins. A, Major dural sinuses shown here include the superior sagittal, straight, occipital, transverse, and sigmoid sinuses. The superior sagittal, straight, transverse, and occipital sinuses join at the confluence of sinuses. Major veins include the superficial middle cerebral vein, the superior anastomotic vein of Trolard, and the inferior anastomotic vein of Labbé. B, Major dural sinuses shown here include the superior sagittal, inferior sagittal, straight, occipital, and transverse sinuses and their confluence. Major veins shown here include the great vein of Galen, the basal vein of Rosenthal, and the internal cerebral vein. From Siegel S, Sapru HN. Blood supply of the central nervous system. In: Siegel S, Sapru HN, eds. *Essential Neuroscience*. 4th ed. Wolters Kluwer; 2019:538-552. Figure 26.6.

the midline and then into an area called the confluence of sinuses. After this, two transverse sinuses bifurcate and travel laterally into the sigmoid sinuses. These then go on to form the bilateral jugular veins and into the superior vena cava. Cerebral venous sinus thrombosis is a neurologic emergency that occurs when clot forms within the venous sinus and can present with headache, neurologic deficits, and seizure. It most commonly occurs in the superior sagittal sinus.

The deep venous drainage system has several veins that join at the midbrain to form the vein of Galen or great cerebral vein (see Pediatric Issues section) and into the internal cerebral vein. This connects to the inferior sagittal sinus, forms the straight sinus, and then joins the superficial venous system at the confluence of sinuses, as described previously. Thrombosis in the deep venous system, a medical emergency with high risk of mortality, causes behavioral issues such as delirium, amnesia, mutism as well as bilateral thalamic lesions. Imaging cues that suggest the diagnosis are swollen thalami bilaterally on head CT scan.

The cavernous sinus is a clinically important dural venous sinus that is found in the bilateral middle cranial fossa next to the sphenoid bone. The internal carotid artery travels through the cavernous sinus as well as several important cranial nerves, including the abducens nerve (CN VI), oculomotor nerve (CN III), trochlear nerve (CN IV), as well as the ophthalmic and maxillary branches of the trigeminal nerve (CN V) (**Figure 1.12**). Because of its close location to the paranasal sinuses, orbit, and meninges as well as the absence of valves in the veins draining to and from the

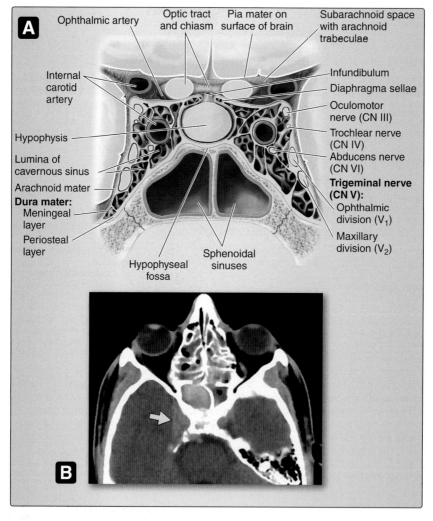

Figure 1.12: Cavernous sinus thrombosis. A, Coronal cross section through cavernous sinus. B, Axial CT scan demonstrating expansion and abnormal hyperdensity (*arrow*) in right cavernous sinus due to the presence of dense thrombosis. From Harrell KM, Dudek RW. Head and cranial nerves. In: Harrell KM, Dudek RW, eds. *Lippincott® Illustrated Reviews: Anatomy*. Wolters Kluwer; 2019:323-412.

cavernous sinus, infection can spread to this area, causing cavernous sinus thrombosis or infection. In addition, carotico-cavernous fistula can occur between the ICA and the cavernous sinus owing to trauma or aneurysm rupture.

THE VENTRICULAR SYSTEM

The ventricular system of the brain is a network of communicating spaces within the brain parenchyma filled with cerebrospinal fluid (CSF) (**Figure 1.13**). A special structure in the walls of the ventricles called choroid plexus produces the clear CSF, which protects and cushions the brain and

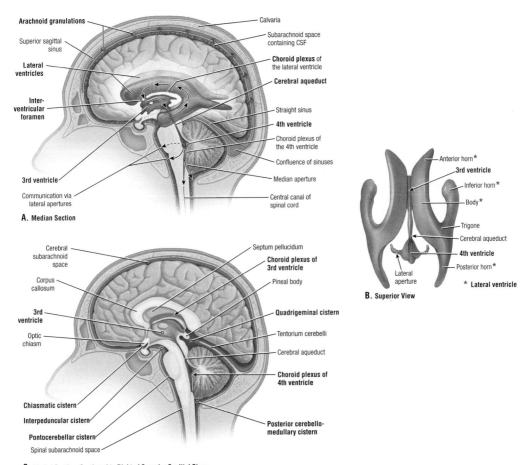

Figure 1.13: Ventricular system, A, Circulation of cerebrospinal fluid (CSF). B, Ventricles: lateral, third, and fourth. C, Subarachnoid cisterns. The ventricular system consists of two lateral ventricles located in the cerebral hemispheres, a 3rd ventricle located between the right and left halves of the diencephalon, and a 4th ventricle located in the posterior parts of the pons and medulla. CSF secreted by choroid plexus in the ventricles drains via the interventricular foramen from the lateral to the 3rd ventricle, via the cerebral aqueduct from the 3rd to the 4th ventricle, and via median and lateral apertures into the subarachnoid space. CSF is absorbed by arachnoid granulations into the venous sinuses (especially the superior sagittal sinus). Hydrocephalus. Overproduction of CSF, obstruction of its flow, or interference with its absorption results in an excess of CSF in the ventricles and enlargement of the head, a condition known as hydrocephalus. Excess CSF dilates the ventricles; thins the brain; and, in infants, separates the bones of the calvaria because the sutures and fontanelles are still open. From Moore KL, Dalley AF II, Agur AMR. Head. In: Moore KL, Dalley AF II, Agur AMR, eds. *Clinically Oriented Anatomy*. 8th ed. Wolters Kluwer; 2018:829-989. Figure 8.37.

spinal cord. The four ventricles of the brain include the left and right lateral ventricles, the third ventricle, and the fourth ventricle. These spaces are connected by several foramina, or openings. CSF flows from the two lateral ventricles within the cerebral hemispheres, through the interventricular foramina (foramen of Monro) into the third ventricle. It then flows into the fourth ventricle via the cerebral aqueduct of Sylvius and then passes through the middle foramen of Magendie (median aperture) and two lateral foramena of Luschka (lateral apertures). CSF then enters the subarachnoid space, flows around the superior sagittal sinus and is absorbed into the venous system via arachnoid granulations. CSF can also flow down around the spinal cord in the subarachnoid space to the lumbar cisterns and around the cauda equina. This large cistern below L2 is the space where a lumbar puncture is generally performed.

An important anatomic consideration within the ventricular system is the narrowness of the cerebral aqueduct (Figure 1.13). This is clinically significant because it can easily become blocked by blood after a hemorrhagic stroke. CSF is continuously produced, so the blockage leads to increased pressure within the lateral ventricles of the brain, causing hydrocephalus. This emergency may require a ventriculostomy, or entry hole, into the ventricles to allow accumulated CSF to drain through a temporary catheter or shunt.

Another serious cause of obstructive hydrocephalus is the development of a colloidal cyst, which is a gelatinous tumor found just posterior to the foramen of Monro (intraventricular foramen) in the third ventricle. As it grows, it can cause obstructive hydrocephalus and increased intracranial pressure. Patients experiencing symptoms of colloid cysts can have headache, vertigo, memory issues, double vision, syncope, and rarely sudden death.

MENINGES AND DURAL SPACES

The brain and spinal cord are covered in three layers, called meninges, which serve as protection to the central nervous system. The three layers include the dura mater, arachnoid mater, and the pia mater (**Figure 1.14**).

The dura mater is the thick and durable outermost membrane that lies adjacent to the skull and vertebrae. An epidural hematoma results from bleeding that occurs between the dura mater and the skull. This is typically caused by injury to the temporal bone and bleeding from the middle meningeal artery that runs through this space. Epidural hematoma can also occur within the spinal canal.

The middle layer of the meninges is the arachnoid mater. It is a thin, transparent membrane of fibrous tissue with a spider web appearance (hence the name). A subdural hematoma is the result of hemorrhage between the dural and the arachnoid mater.

The final layer of the meninges is called the pia mater, which consists of a very thin and delicate membrane that firmly adheres to the surface of the brain and spinal cord and is impermeable to fluid. The space between the arachnoid and the pia mater is called the subarachnoid space, which is filled with cerebrospinal fluid; a subarachnoid hemorrhage is bleeding in this area. The subarachnoid space extends down the spinal cord. Because the space is filled with CSF, occult subarachnoid bleeding can be detected with lumbar puncture into the subarachnoid space of the spinal canal.

SPINAL CORD

The spinal cord begins at the base of the skull and ends at L1 vertebral body. Inferior to this, the spinal canal consists of a bundle of lumbar, sacral, and coccygeal nerve roots, called the cauda equina. The spinal cord is divided into four sections, called cervical, thoracic, lumbar, and sacral (**Figure 1.15**). It is further separated into thirty-one spinal cord segments with anterior (ventral) and dorsal (posterior) spinal nerve routes. Ventral nerve roots control motor and dorsal nerve roots control sensation (see **Figure 1.16**). They join on each side of the cord, exit through the neuroforamina, and form spinal peripheral nerves; see further on.

The spinal cord ends at the first or second lumbar vertebral bodies with a tapered end, called the conus medullaris. The filum terminale is a thin layer of tissue that connects from the conus medullaris to the base of the coccyx. Injuries below the level of L2 affect the cauda equina ("horse's tail" in Latin) nerve roots and can cause the surgical emergency of cauda equina syndrome (low back pain, perianal sensory loss, loss of bowel or bladder control).

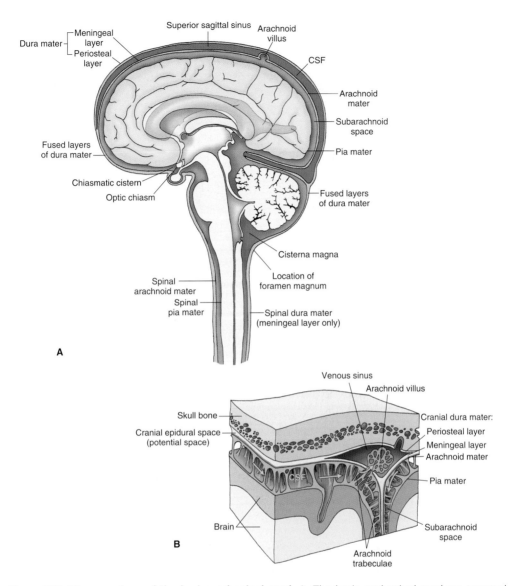

Figure 1.14: The coverings of the brain and spinal cord. A, The brain and spinal cord are covered with three membranes: dura, arachnoid, and pia mater. The periosteal and meningeal layers of the dura are separate at the dural sinuses (e.g., superior sagittal sinus). At other places, the dura consists of fused periosteal and meningeal layers. The space between the arachnoid and pial membranes is called the subarachnoid space. The subarachnoid space is enlarged at some places (e.g., cisterna magna and chiasmatic cistern). Small tufts of arachnoidal tissue (arachnoid villi) project into the dural venous sinuses. Other structures are shown for orientation purposes. B, Magnified view of the dura, arachnoid, and pia maters. CSF, cerebrospinal fluid. From Siegel S, Sapru HN. Meninges and cerebrospinal fluid. In: Siegel S, Sapru HN, eds. *Essential Neuroscience*. 4th ed. Wolters Kluwer; 2019:39-52. Figure 3.1.

The spinal cord is separated cross-sectionally into gray matter surrounded by white matter tracts. The butterfly-shaped central gray matter contains neural cell bodies and synapses, and it is separated into dorsal and ventral horns (Figure 1.16). The dorsal horn is the area that modulates sensory information, including pain, temperature, proprioception, vibration, and touch. The ventral horn is composed of nuclei that control motor. These are the areas at which the motor and sensory ganglia exit to form the spinal nerves (Figure 1.16).

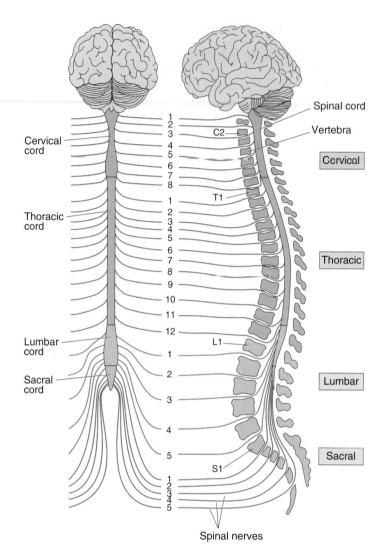

Figure 1.15: Segmental organization of the spinal cord. The spinal cord is divided into cervical, thoracic, lumbar, and sacral divisions (*left*). The cross-sectional view (*right*) shows the spinal cord within the vertebral column. Spinal nerves are named for the level of the spinal cord from which they exit and are numbered in order from rostral to caudal. From Bear MF, Connors BW, Paradiso MA. The somatic sensory system. In: Bear MF, Connors BW, Paradiso MA, eds. *Neuroscience: Exploring the Brain.* 4th ed. Wolters Kluwer; 2016:415-452. Figure 12.11.

The white matter tracts contain ascending and descending fiber pathways that transmit sensory information to the brain and motor information to the rest of the body. These tracts cross to the contralateral side at different areas within the spinal cord. Understanding where they cross helps recognize pathology.

The spinothalamic tract is an afferent pathway that transmits pain and temperature sensation from the body to the brain. After it enters the dorsal horn, this pathway crosses over to the opposite side of the cord within one or two spinal cord segments and ascends on the opposite side to the thalamus and the cerebral cortex. For this reason, a lesion in this tract will result in loss of pain and temperature sensation contralaterally below the level of the lesion and ipsilaterally at the level of the lesion.

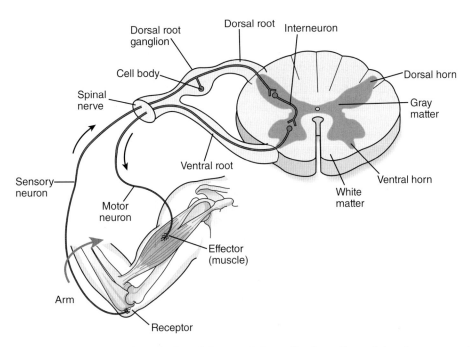

Figure 1.16: Organization in the spinal cord. Sensory information from the peripheral nervous system (PNS) enters into the dorsal side (dorsal horn) of the spinal cord and motor commands exit out the ventral horn. White matter consists of myelinated axons from the ascending and descending tracts of neurons. Gray matter consists of cell bodies and houses the synaptic connections among neurons. The ganglion houses the cell bodies of the sensory neurons outside of the spinal cord, which differ from the motor neuron cell bodies which are in the spinal cord. From Ives JC. Neural mechanisms in planning and initiating movement. In: Ives JC, ed. *Motor Behavior*. Wolters Kluwer; 2014:12-36. Figure 2.8.

The afferent pathway for proprioception, stereogenesis, and vibration begins on the same side of the spinal cord that it enters and does not cross over until the junction between the spinal cord and the brainstem. This pathway is called fasciculus gracilis in the lower spinal cord and fasciculus cuneatus in the upper spinal cord and are collectively called the posterior columns. They synapse just prior to crossing contralaterally at the nucleus gracilis and nucleus cuneatus. Because it does not cross until much higher up, the lesion in the posterior column will cause decreased proprioception, stereogenesis, and vibratory sensation ipsilateral to the level of the lesion.

The pathway for light touch has ipsilateral and contralateral components. Some parts remain uncrossed until the level of the brainstem, whereas others cross over at lower levels. For this reason, unilateral spinal cord lesions typically have preservation of light touch sensation.

The previously mentioned sensory pathways all cross over and eventually terminate in the thalamus and then on to the cerebral cortex. Therefore, strokes in the sensory area of the cerebral cortex may result in contralateral deficits of all the modalities, including pain, temperature, proprioception, stereogenesis, vibratory sense, and light touch.

The spinocerebellar pathway is the tract that controls unconscious proprioception. Distinct from the other sensory pathways, the spinocerebellar tract never crosses the midline. It terminates in the ipsilateral cerebellum. Therefore, lesions to the cerebellum typically have ipsilateral symptoms.

The corticospinal tract is the main motor white matter tract and extends from the motor area of the cerebral cortex, down the brainstem, crosses at the junction of the brainstem and spinal cord, and synapses in the anterior horn of the gray matter. It then leaves the cord via the motor ganglion. Motor neurons above the level of the synapse between the cerebral cortex and the anterior horn are called upper motor neurons, and those below this level are called lower motor neurons. Upper motor neuron lesions cause spastic paralysis and hyperreflexia, whereas lower motor neuron lesions cause flaccid paralysis, fasciculations, atrophy, and hyporeflexia. Compressive lesions approaching the spinal cord from the side will result in the Brown-Sequard syndrome, where there is ipsilateral motor, vibratory, and position sensation impairment below the level of the lesion, whereas contralaterally pinprick and temperature sensation are impaired, so-called dissociated sensory impairment, an important diagnostic clue as to lesion location.

SPINAL CORD VASCULATURE

The anterior 2/3 of the spinal cord are supplied by the anterior spinal artery, whereas the posterior 1/3 of the spinal cord is supplied by the two posterior arteries (**Figure 1.17**). For this reason, infarction affecting the anterior spinal artery, as may occur in severe hypotension following aortic dissection, a patient may have paraplegia below the level of the infarction with impaired pinprick and touch sensation and preserved position and vibration sensation. This clinical phenomenon is an important clinical tool that can guide therapy, for example, consideration of reverse Trendelenburg to provide increased flow to the hypoperfused artery. The anterior spinal artery comes from the vertebral arteries at the foramen magnum, along the center of the anterior spinal cord in the anterior median sulcus, to the conus medullaris. Deeper structures of the cord are supplied by the many sulcal arteries that branch from the anterior spinal artery and enter the spinal cord. The periphery of the cord is supplied by branches that form the peripheral arterial plexus.

The posterior spinal arteries come from the vertebral arteries and travel down the cord in the posterior lateral sulci and supply the gray matter of the cord. The two posterior spinal arteries frequently connect with each other as well as with the peripheral and posterolateral plexus. The anterior and posterior spinal arteries connect to each other at the level of the conus medullaris. Blood supply to the spinal cord is supported by many radicular arteries.

The venous system of the spinal cord is composed of the anterior and posterior veins that drain into smaller radicular veins, into the intravertebral and paravertebral plexus, and then into the azygous and pelvic venous systems.

PERIPHERAL NERVOUS SYSTEM

The peripheral nervous system is the part of the nervous system outside of the brain and spinal cord. It is composed of cranial nerves, spinal nerves, ganglia, peripheral nerves, and neuromuscular junctions. The peripheral nervous system is further separated into two distinct components: the somatic nervous system and the autonomic nervous system (**Figure 1.18**).

Somatic Nervous System

The role of the somatic nervous system is voluntary control of movement and perception of sensation. The somatic nervous system is bidirectional, with signals both leaving and entering the central nervous system. Efferent motor nerves are responsible for relaying signals for muscle contraction from the central nervous system to the skeletal muscles of the body. Afferent sensory nerves conduct sensory signals from the body back to the central nervous system. The somatic nervous system consists of 12 cranial nerves that transmit information to and from the brain and 31 spinal nerves that carry information into and out of the spinal cord.

CRANIAL NERVES

Humans have twelve pairs of cranial nerves, which are numbered from a rostral to a caudal position. These are the olfactory nerve (I), optic nerve (II), oculomotor nerve (III), trochlear nerve (IV), trigeminal nerve (V), abducens nerve (VI), facial nerve (VII), vestibulocochlear nerve (VIII), glossopharyngeal nerve (IX), vagus nerve (X), accessory nerve (XI), and hypoglossal nerve (XII). Cranial nerves I and II arise from nuclei in the cerebrum, whereas the remainder arise from nuclei in the brainstem (**Figure 1.19**).

Olfactory Nerve (I)

As indicated by its title, the olfactory nerve conveys the sense of smell. It is a sensory nerve that begins with olfactory receptor neurons in the mucosa of the nasal cavity. When these are stimulated, the signal moves through the olfactory nerve, passing through the cribriform plate of the ethmoid

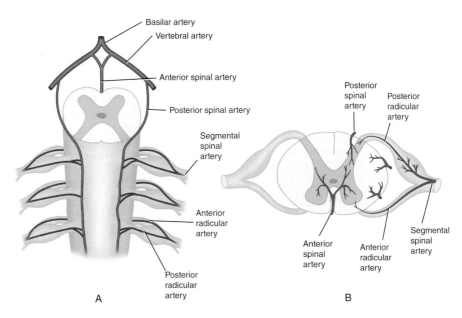

Figure 1.17: A, Arterial supply of the spinal cord showing the formation of two posterior spinal arteries and one anterior spinal artery. B, Transverse section of the spinal cord showing the segmental spinal arteries and the radicular arteries. From Splittgerber R. Blood supply of the brain and spinal cord. In: Splittgerber R, ed. *Snell's Clinical Neuroanatomy*. 8th ed. Wolters Kluwer; 2019:464-487. Figure 17.7.

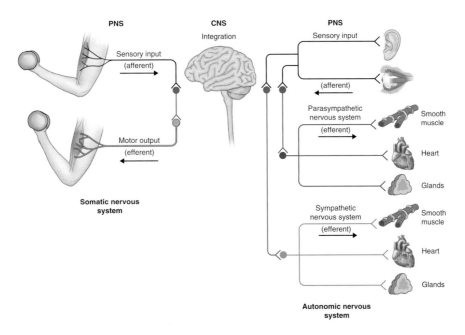

Figure 1.18: Major divisions of the nervous system. The nervous system can be divided anatomically into the central (brain and spinal cord) nervous system (CNS) and the peripheral (sensory organs and nerves) nervous system (PNS). The nervous system can be functionally divided into the somatic nervous system and the autonomic nervous system (ANS). The somatic nervous system leads to contraction of muscle fibers through efferent (motor) neurons. The autonomic nervous system controls the heart, glands, and hollow organs and is essential in maintaining homeostasis. From Plowman S, Smith D. Neuromuscular aspects of movement. In: Plowman S, Smith D, eds. *Exercise Physiology for Health Fitness and Performance*. 5th ed. Wolters Kluwer; 2018:611-646. Figure 20.1.

Base of Brain
(Cranial Nerves)

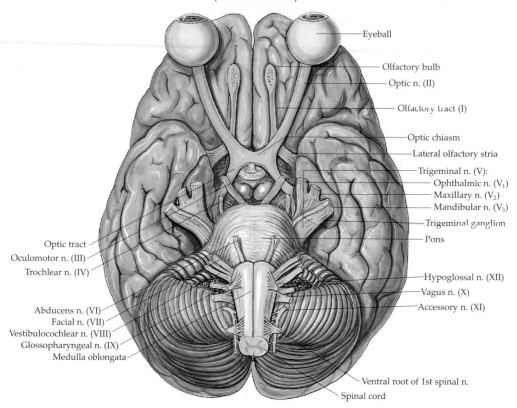

Figure 1.19: **Base of brain (cranial nerves).** Brain Anatomical Chart. From the Anatomical Chart Company, The Brain. Wolters Kluwer, 2000, with permission.

bone, and into the olfactory bulb of the cerebrum. Logically, damage to the olfactory nerve can cause reduced ability to smell and taste.

Optic Nerve (II)

The optic nerve is essential in transmitting visual information from the retina of the eye to the brain. It begins in the optic disc, leaves the orbit via the optic foramen, and meets its bilateral counterpart at the optic chiasm. The medial fibers decussate, or cross, at this area. The optic nerve then continues as the optic tract and terminates in several brain nuclei, including the lateral geniculate nucleus, pretectal nuclei, superior colliculus, and the occipital cortex. Lesions to the optic nerve can cause varying visual deficits, depending on the location of the injury or event.

Oculomotor (III)

The oculomotor nerve works together with the trochlear (IV) and abducens (VI) nerves to control eye movement. The oculomotor nerve originates from the oculomotor nucleus in the pre-aqueductal gray matter of the cerebral aqueduct. It travels out of the cavernous sinus, through the superior orbital fissure, and into the orbit of the eye. Once it enters the orbit, it branches into a superior and inferior division. The superior division supplies motor fibers to the superior rectus and levator palpebrae superioris muscles of the eye, and the inferior division controls the inferior rectus, medial rectus, and inferior oblique muscles. It also gives off parasympathetic roots to the ciliary ganglion to control pupillary constriction and accommodation. Damage to the oculomotor nerve will cause an oculomotor nerve palsy. Patients will have diplopia, ptosis, and a "down and out" positioning of the ipsilateral eye. Patients may also have mydriasis. Diabetic third nerve palsy will result in pupil sparing third nerve palsies because the damage occurs within the core of the nerve, whereas a compressing posterior communicating artery aneurysm will involve the pupil because the initial damage is at the mantle of the nerve, where pupillary control is located.

Trochlear (IV)

The trochlear nerve only innervates a single eye muscle, called the superior oblique muscle. It originates in the trochlear nucleus, runs through the cavernous sinus, and enters the orbit through the superior oblique fissure. Damage to the trochlear nerve will cause inability to move the eye downward owing to impairment of the superior oblique muscle. The trochlear nerve is unique in that it crosses within the brainstem before emerging. Therefore, an injury to the trochlear nucleus will result in contralateral superior oblique muscle palsy, whereas injury to the nerve itself will cause ipsilateral symptoms.

Abducens (VI) Nerves

The abducens nerve functions to abduct the eye by controlling the lateral rectus muscle. The abducens nucleus is located on the floor of the fourth ventricle in the pons. Like CN V and VI, it exits the via the cavernous sinus and enters the orbit through the superior orbital fissure. Damage to the abducens nerve, or a sixth cranial nerve palsy, will cause the patient to be unable to turn the affected eye outward.

Trigeminal Nerve (V)

The trigeminal nerve is responsible for sensation and motor control of the face. It has three branches called the ophthalmic (V1), maxillary (V2), and mandibular (V3). The ophthalmic and maxillary divisions are sensory nerves while the mandibular branch is both sensory and motor. The branches converge to form the trigeminal ganglion and then enter the brainstem at the level of the pons and synapse along the ipsilateral trigeminal nucleus before crossing to the contralateral side. The motor root emerges from the pons at the same area and passes through the trigeminal ganglion out towards peripheral muscles. The ophthalmic branch travels through the cavernous sinus, into the superior orbital fissure, and into the orbit. It carries sensory information from the scalp, upper eyelid, external eye, sinuses, and nose. The maxillary branch (V2) exits through the foramen rotundum in the sphenoid bone to innervate the mid face. The mandibular branch (V3) exits through the foramen ovale of the sphenoid bone and innervates sensation to lower face and helps muscles of mastication. Damage to the trigeminal nerve can cause deficits in sensation to the face. Trigeminal neuralgia is a chronic pain disorder of the face affecting the trigeminal nerve.

Facial Nerve (VII)

The facial nerve controls muscles of facial expression as well as helps with perception of taste from the front two thirds of the tongue. The cell bodies for the taste component nerves of the facial nerve originate in the geniculate ganglion and the motor cell bodies are in the facial motor nucleus. The facial nerve enters the temporal bone through the internal auditory canal and then exits through the stylomastoid foramen. Lesions of the facial nerve can result in a facial palsy such as Bell palsy.

Vestibulocochlear Nerve (VIII)

The nucleus for the vestibulocochlear nerve originates in the pons and like the facial nerve, the vestibulocochlear nerve enters the internal auditory canal in the temporal bone. The vestibulocochlear nerve, however, does not exit the temporal bone and instead innervates the organs that are located within the temporal bone. It transmits sensation from the vestibules and semicircular canals of the inner ear and helps with balance. It also assists with hearing by transmitting information from the cochlea. Damage to the vestibulocochlear nerve may cause vertigo or deafness.

Glossopharyngeal Nerve (IX)

The glossopharyngeal nerve is a mixed nerve that controls sensory information to the oropharynx and back of the tongue, motor to the stylopharyngeus muscle, and parasympathetic input to the parotid gland. This nerve exits the brainstem from the sides of the upper medulla, leaves the skull through the jugular foramen and enters the neck. Injury to the glossopharyngeal nerve can cause issues with gag reflex.

Vagus Nerve (X)

The vagus nerve is vital in its function of innervating the neck and supplying parasympathetic tone to the organs of the torso. It emerges from or converges on four nuclei in the medulla: dorsal nucleus of vagus nerve, nucleus ambiguus, solitary nucleus, and spinal trigeminal nucleus. Like the glossopharyngeal nerve, the vagus nerve also leaves the skull through the jugular foramen and down to the neck, chest, and abdomen. Damage to the vagus nerve may cause autonomic instability, hoarse voice, or swallowing problems.

Accessory Nerve (XI)

The accessory nerve controls the sternocleidomastoid and trapezius muscles of the neck and shoulder. The fibers of the accessory nerve originate in the spinal accessory nucleus of the upper spinal cord at the junction between the medulla and the spinal cord. They then enter the skull through the foramen magnum, travels along the wall of the skull, and then exits through the jugular foramen and into the neck. It is the only cranial nerve that both enters and exits the skull during its course. Damage to this nerve results in difficulty shrugging the shoulder, turning the neck, or in a winged appearance to the scapula.

Hypoglossal Nerve (XII)

The hypoglossal nerve is a motor nerve that controls the muscles of the tongue. It arises in the hypoglossal nucleus in the medulla, exits the skull through the hypoglossal canal in the occipital bone, enters the neck, and then up to the tongue. Damage to this nerve may lead to tongue weakness, difficulties with speech and swallowing, and inability to fully stick out the tongue.

SPINAL NERVES

Spinal nerves carry motor, sensory, and autonomic information between the spinal cord and the body. There are 31 pairs of spinal nerves on each side of the vertebral column. An important point to understand is that the spinal cord is not the same length as the spinal column. Therefore, the spinal and vertebral levels do not always correlate perfectly with each other.

The spinal cord levels and nerve roots are separated into the cervical, thoracic, lumbar, and sacral/coccygeal regions. There are eight paired cervical nerves, 12 paired thoracic nerves, and five paired lumbar nerves, five paired sacral nerves, and one pair of coccygeal nerves (Figure 1.15). The cervical segments innervate the diaphragm and upper arm. The thoracic segments form the intercostal nerves and innervate the associated dermatomes and abdominal wall musculature, the heart, and abdominal organs. The lumbosacral segments innervate the lower extremity, buttocks, and anal regions.

Spinal nerves are composed of a combination of fibers from the dorsal and ventral nerve roots of the spinal cord. The ventral (efferent) root carries motor information from the brain and the dorsal (afferent) root carries sensory information to the spinal cord. Each spinal nerve is bilateral and exits the spinal column through intervertebral foramen that exist between vertebrae. The only exception to this is the first spinal nerve (C1). This exits between the occipital bone and the atlas. All cervical nerves exit above their corresponding vertebrae except C8 which exits below the C7 vertebrae. All spinal nerves below this level exit underneath their corresponding vertebrae (Figure 1.15**).** The area of skin innervated by a specific spinal nerve is called a dermatome (**Figure 1.20**).

Spinal nerves extend to the periphery where they join at four different places called nerve plexuses to form systemic nerves. These include the cervical plexus, brachial plexus, lumbar plexus, and sacral plexus.

Cervical Plexus

The cervical plexus is composed of anterior rami of the first four cervical spinal nerves and supplies innervation to the posterior head and neck and the diaphragm (**Figure 1.21**). It is located underneath the sternocleidomastoid muscle in the neck. It has two branches called cutaneous and muscular. The cutaneous branch of the cervical plexus is composed of four additional branches: the lesser occipital, the great auricular nerve, transverse cervical nerve, and supraclavicular nerves. The muscular branch contains the ansa cervicalis, the segmental branches, and the phrenic nerve which innervates the diaphragm and pericardium.

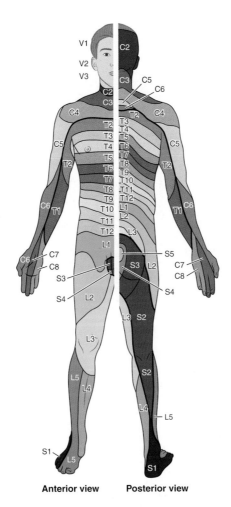

Anterior view   Posterior view

Figure 1.20: Anterior and posterior views of the dermatomes. Although dermatomes are shown as distinct segments, in reality, there is overlap between any two adjacent dermatomes. The sensory innervation of the face does not involve dermatomes but instead is carried by cranial nerve (CN) V; V1 (ophthalmic division), V2 (maxillary division), and V3 (mandibular division). From Moore KL, Dalley AF II, Agur AMR. Overview and basic concepts. In: Moore KL, Dalley AF II, Agur AMR, eds. *Clinically Oriented Anatomy*. 8th ed. Wolters Kluwer; 2018:1-70. Figure 1.36.

Brachial Plexus

The brachial plexus is formed by the anterior rami of C5-T1 and extends through the neck, over the first rib and in the axilla. It supplies motor and sensory information to the chest and upper extremity. It is composed of five nerve roots which merge to form three trunks labeled superior, middle, middle and inferior. The trunks each divide into anterior and posterior divisions which then regroup to form posterior, lateral, and medial cords. Most nerves branches come off the cords, but some branch from the roots or trunk. See **Figure 1.22** for nerve branches and locations.

Lumbar Plexus

The lumbar plexus is formed by the anterior rami of T12-L4 spinal nerves and is in the psoas muscle (**Figure 1.23**). It mainly provides motor and sensory function to the anterior thigh. The lumbar plexus separates into several branches including the iliohypogastric, ilioinguinal, genitofemoral, lateral femoral cutaneous, obturator, and femoral nerves.

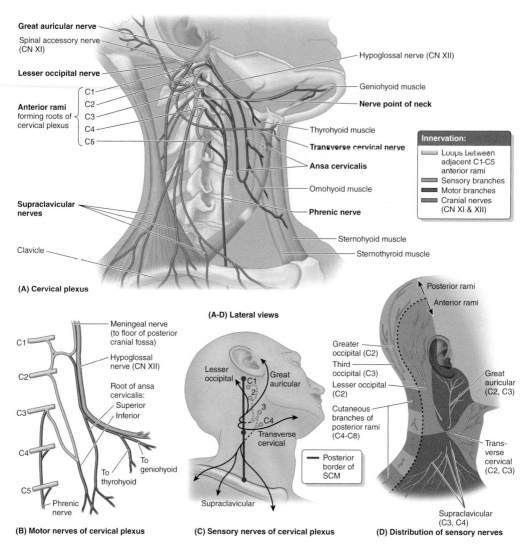

Figure 1.21: Cervical plexus of nerves. A-C. The plexus consists of nerve loops formed between the adjacent anterior rami of the first four cervical nerves and the receiving gray rami communicantes from the superior cervical sympathetic ganglion (not shown here) (Fig. 9.25A). Motor (B) and sensory nerves (C) arise from the loops of the plexus. The ansa cervicalis (A, B) is a second-level loop, the superior limb of which arises from the loop between the C1 and the C2 vertebrae but travels initially with the hypoglossal nerve (CN XII), which is not part of the cervical plexus. D, The areas of skin innervated by the sensory (cutaneous) nerves of the cervical plexus (derived from anterior rami) and by the posterior rami of cervical spinal nerves are shown. From Moore KL, Dalley AF II, Agur AMR. Neck. In: Moore KL, Dalley AF II, Agur AMR, eds. *Clinically Oriented Anatomy*. 8th ed. Wolters Kluwer; 2018:990-1060. Figure 9.14.

Sacral Plexus

The sacral plexus is formed by L4-S4 spinal nerves (**Figure 1.24**). Because the lumbar and sacral plexuses both contain L4, they are sometimes referred together as the lumbosacral plexus. The sacral plexus provides motor and sensory nerves to the posterior thigh, the lower leg, foot, and some of the pelvis. The sacral plexus nerves unite at the greater sciatic foramen to form the sciatic nerve. This splits on the back of the thigh into the tibial and common fibular nerves. Nerves arising from the sacral plexus include the superior and inferior gluteal, posterior cutaneous femoral, piriformis, obturator internus, quadratus femoris, sciatic, common fibular, tibial, pudendal, and coccygeal.

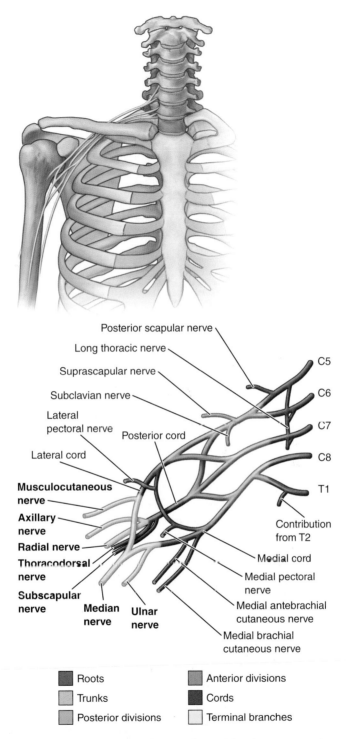

Figure 1.22: **Brachial plexus.** The brachial plexus is formed by the segmental nerves C5-T1. From Anderson MK. Cervical and thoracic spinal conditions. In: Anderson MK, ed. *Foundations of Athletic Training*. 6th ed. Wolters Kluwer; 2017:742-779. Figure 21.9.

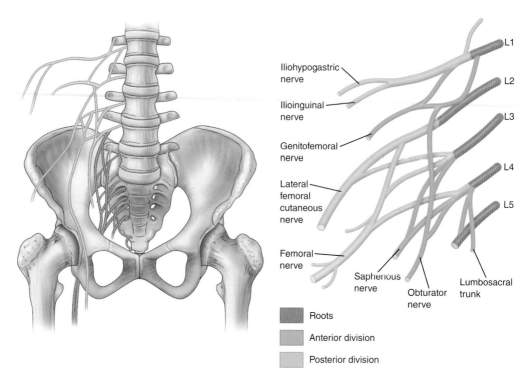

Figure 1.23: Lumbar plexus. The lumbar plexus is formed by the segmental nerves T12 through L5. The lower portion of the plexus merges with the upper portion of the sacral plexus to form the lumbosacral trunk. From Anderson MK. Lumbar spinal conditions. In: Anderson MK, ed. *Foundations of Athletic Training.* 6th ed. Wolters Kluwer; 2017:780-824. Figure 22.4.

The distal peripheral nerves in all limbs comprise a distinct system that can be preferentially affected by certain diseases. Acute weakness that is associated with absence of reflexes should prompt consideration of acute inflammatory demyelinating polyneuropathy (Guillain-Barré syndrome). Patients with this disorder may present in respiratory distress and have autonomic failure resulting in severe bradycardia or tachycardia or severe hypotension or hypertension, resulting in cardiopulmonary arrest.

NEUROMUSCULAR JUNCTION AND MUSCLE

Acetylcholine is released from the presynaptic axon on the nerve to the postsynaptic receptor on the muscle (**Figure 1.25**). Impairment in delivery of the acetylcholine (Eaton-Lambert syndrome) or uptake of acetylcholine at the postsynaptic receptor (Myasthenia Gravis) can produce proximal muscle weakness, which varies over the course of the day. In emergency settings, a myasthenic crisis can present with acute severe weakness requiring intubation. A history of a recent surgery (which is a trigger for some cases of myasthenia gravis) or fluctuating motor symptoms over the course of the day can be a clue to the diagnosis.

Muscle disorders can similarly present with proximal muscle weakness. Depending on the cause, manifestations can include weakness associated with rash (dermatomyositis) or weakness precipitated by exertional activities (enzymatic disorders).

AUTONOMIC NERVOUS SYSTEM

The autonomic nervous system functions to regulate glands, smooth muscles, and cardiac muscle. It is divided into the sympathetic and parasympathetic nervous systems (Figure 1.18). The

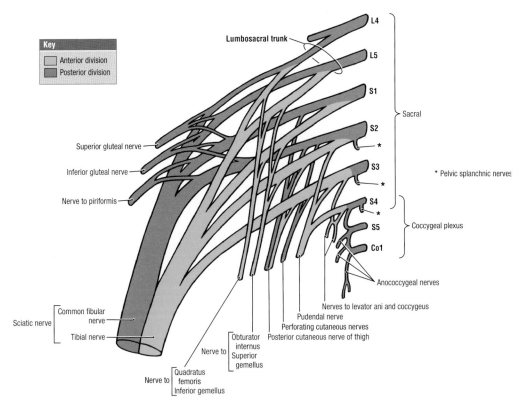

Figure 1.24: Sacral and coccygeal nerve plexuses. Branches of anterior and posterior divisions of sacral and coccygeal plexuses. From Agur AMR, Dalley II AF. Pelvis and perineum. In: Agur AMR, Dalley II AF, eds. *Grant's Atlas of Anatomy*. 15th ed. Wolters Kluwer; 2021:391-470. Figure 5.13b.

sympathetic nervous system is primarily responsible for regulation of hemostasis including pupil diameter, gut motility, sweat secretion, heart contraction, vasoconstriction of blood vessels and urinary output. Its biggest responsibility, however, is the "flight or fight" response. The parasympathetic nervous system is responsible for conserving energy while the body is at rest. Sometimes it is referred to as "feed or breed."

Sympathetic Nervous System: Two types of neurons are involved in the sympathetic nervous system: preganglionic and postganglionic. Preganglionic neurons originate in the interomediolateral columns at T1 to L2 of the spinal cord. Sympathetic nerve fibers leave the spinal cord, synapse with either a prevertebral chain of sympathetic ganglia or preveretebral ganglion plexus. When they synapse in this area, the preganglionic neurons release the neurotransmitter called acetylcholine. This activates nicotinic acetylcholine receptors on the postganglionic neurons which then release norepinephrine. This activates adrenergic receptors on the peripheral tissue causing effects of the sympathetic system. There are three exceptions to this: postganglionic neurons of sweat glands release acetylcholine, chromaffin cells of the adrenal medulla release norepinephrine and epinephrine, and the postganglionic nerves in the kidney release dopamine.

Parasympathetic system originates from the spinal cords at levels S2-S4 as well as cranial nerves III, VII, IX, and X. Like sympathetic fibers, parasympathetic nerve fibers also synapse with cholinergic acetylcholine containing prevertebral ganglia. While the final synapse for sympathetic nerve fibers contains norepinephrine, the second synapse for the parasympathetic nervous system contains acetylcholine.

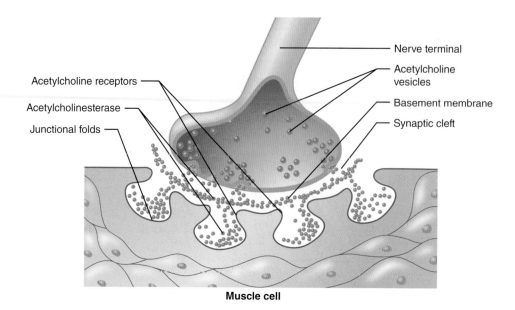

Acetylcholine receptors

Acetylcholinesterase

Junctional folds

Nerve terminal

Acetylcholine vesicles

Basement membrane

Synaptic cleft

Muscle cell

Figure 1.25: Neuromuscular junction. Structure of the neuromuscular junction. From Donati F. Neuromuscular blocking agents. In: Barash PG, Cullen BF, Stoelting RK, et al., eds. *Clinical Anesthesia*. 7th ed. Wolters Kluwer; 2013:527. Figure 20.5.

PEDIATRIC ISSUES

- A vein of Galen "aneurysm" is a rare cause of heart failure in the neonatal population. As discussed, the vein of Galen drains blood from the inferior sagittal sinus to the straight sinus. When a congenital vascular malformation occurs in the vein of Galen, it causes a persistent alternative pathway for venous blood and essentially causes an AV shunt from the carotid and vertebrobasilar systems of the midbrain to the vein of Galen. High flow of blood causes venous dilation and this high rate of blood flow is transmitted the heart thus causing heart failure.
- Obstetrical brachial plexus injuries occur in as many as 0.4% of deliveries. They usually result from shoulder dystocia, use of mechanical extraction, or macrosomia. It occurs with lateral traction on the affected arm during delivery and infants can present with flaccid paresis of the arm.

TIPS AND PEARLS

- Broca area is in the frontal lobe and lesions to this area causes expressive aphasia. Wernicke area is in the temporal lobe and lesions to this area cause receptive aphasia.
- The cerebellum is crucial in motor control and coordination. Lesions to the cerebellum typically have ipsilateral symptoms while lesions to the cerebrum have contralateral symptoms.
- Venous circulation to the brain does not follow the same pathway as the arterial system. It is composed of superficial and deep systems which converge at the confluence of sinuses.
- The three layers of covering of the brain and spinal cord are called dura mater, subarachnoid mater, and pia mater. Blood accumulation in these spaces are referred to as epidural, subdural, and subarachnoid hemorrhages.
- The dorsal horn of the spinal cord controls sensation and the ventral horn controls motor.
- Lesions in the spinal cord affecting motor tracts will be ipsilateral because the motor tracts do not cross until the level of the brainstem. Sensory tracts will cross at varying levels causing some contralateral and ipsilateral symptoms depending on the specific tract.

- Upper motor neuron lesions cause spastic paralysis and hyperreflexia while lower motor neuron lesions cause flaccid paralysis, fasciculations, atrophy, and hyporeflexia.
- The arterial blood supply to the spinal cord is composed of an anterior spinal artery and two posterior spinal arteries.
- There are 12 cranial nerves that are named after their function or location. The trochlear nerve is unique in that it is the only cranial nerve that crosses in the brainstem before emerging.
- There are 31 spinal nerves that provide motor and sensation to the periphery. C1-C7 emerge above the vertebral level while C8 and below emerge below their vertebral level.
- Spinal nerves combine to form nerve plexuses, for example, the cervical, brachial, lumbar, and sacral plexuses.
- The sympathetic nervous system is responsible for "fight or flight" while the parasympathetic nervous system is responsible for "feed and breed."

SUMMARY

A clear understanding of basic neurological anatomy is needed for recognition and diagnosis of neurologic emergencies. No area of the nervous system can be understood in isolation. To localize and treat pathology, one must not only recognize the anatomy of the specific organ, but also its complex inter-connections with other parts of the nervous system. Confident knowledge in functional anatomy will allow clinicians to quickly, efficiently, and appropriately diagnose and manage emergent neurologic conditions.

The Neurologic Examination

Jean Khoury

Andrew N. Russman

The neurologic examination is the essential tool to localize clinical findings within the nervous system, to develop a differential diagnosis, and to guide management. Early recognition of neurologic diseases is important because of the frequent association between time and clinical outcomes. The need for efficiency may result in the need for a focused evaluation before completion of a more detailed neurologic examination.

The history generally directs the clinician toward certain diagnoses. Evaluating mental status, the cranial nerves (CNs), motor and sensory function, reflexes, coordination, and gait will further narrow the differential. Observing the patient's gaze direction and noting other cortical functions (speech, neglect, apraxias, agnosias) are often diagnostic, whereas ongoing monitoring is often needed to recognize full expression of the patient's condition.

It is one thing to examine a patient when they are cooperating, but it becomes quite complex when they are lethargic, obtunded, or comatose. In these situations, the goal of the examiner is to look for specific signs that will help localize the lesion to provide targeted care. For example, a blown pupil will identify impending herniation, whereas abnormal breathing patterns and vital signs may suggest brainstem involvement and increased intracranial pressure (ICP).

The neurologic examination will guide the management of a patient with a neurologic emergency, including diagnostic testing, emergent treatments (ie, thrombolysis and thrombectomy for ischemic stroke), and specialty consultation.

MENTAL STATUS EXAMINATION

Consciousness

A common neurologic presentation in the emergency department (ED) is altered mental status. When a patient's mental status is poor, the major concern is for an intracranial process causing brainstem dysfunction or elevated ICP and damage to the reticular activating system.

Describing the state of consciousness in words that qualify the degree of responsiveness is the first step of the assessment. Somnolence is a state where the patient can respond to voice; lethargy (and obtundation) is when they can respond to moderate (ie, repetitive tactile) stimuli, but quickly drift back to sleep; stupor is when they respond to vigorous repetitive stimuli (noxious stimuli); and coma is when there is absence of a response to any type of stimuli (unarousable unresponsiveness). Peripheral noxious stimuli (such as nail bed pressure) are used to elicit an eye-opening response and the central painful stimuli (such as trapezius twist, supraorbital pressure, and jaw margin pressure) are used to elicit a motor response.

The Glasgow Coma Scale (GCS) is a simple tool used to assess the degree of the obtundation; a single score is of limited value, underscoring the importance of regular, repeat assessments. It is a good prognostic test for patients with traumatic causes of altered mentation; it has less prognostic value in nontraumatic conditions, but provides a tool for monitoring responsiveness. The GCS includes eye-opening and verbal and motor response to different types of stimuli (we recommend pressure to the nail bed, followed by pressure to the supraorbital notch if needed); see **Table 2.1**. The maximum score is 15; 8 or less reflects a potential for cardiopulmonary compromise and the need for close monitoring.

Cognition

Assessing cognition is rarely an emergency unless the change was recent. Screening for nonacute cognitive impairment using detailed assessment scales is not practical in the emergency setting, although especially in the elderly patient, it has an evolving role for proper disposition.

The main cognitive functions that are routinely assessed include orientation, memory, executive function, attention, and language. Orientation is classically tested by asking the patient to say the date and place; orientation to situation should be assessed as well by asking why they are in the hospital. Short-term memory can be evaluated by giving three words to memorize and prompting the patient about the words later during the encounter (delayed recall). Executive function can be assessed by asking the patient a series of questions (ie, "What number would you dial if there was a serious emergency?"), commands (ie, "Show me how you would make that call with this phone"), and to perform a series of motor tasks (ie, the three-step Luria test). Attention can be tested by asking the patient to repeat a sequence of numbers backward or spell a word backward.

Language has multiple parts including speech production, comprehension, naming, and repetition, and all of these should be assessed. Speech production can be involved in a lesion affecting the Broca area, which causes expressive (nonfluent) aphasia; the patient is, for the most part, able to follow commands and understand questions, but is unable to produce fluent speech. The patient's

TABLE 2.1	Updated Glasgow Coma Scale (GCS-40)[a]
Eye Opening	
Spontaneous (4 points)	
To speech (3 points)	
To pressure (2 points)	
None (1 point)	
Verbal Response	
Oriented (5 points)	
Confused (4 points)	
Words (3 points)	
Sounds (2 points)	
None (1 point)	
Best Motor Response	
Obeying commands (6 points)	
Localizing (5 points)	
Normal flexion or withdrawal (4 points)	
Abnormal flexion[b] (3 points)	
Extension (2 points)	
None (1 point)	

[a]Classification of injuries: mild (GCS scores 13-15), moderate (GCS scores 9-12), or severe (GCS scores ™ 8).
[b]Abnormal flexion is described as a slow stereotyped flexion at the elbow with the forearm across the chest, with clenched fist and legs extended.

TABLE 2.2 Short Blessed Test (SBT)[a]	
Item	**Weighing Factor**
1. What year is it now?	Multiply by 4 for every error (maximum error = 1)
2. What month is this?	Multiply by 3 for every error (maximum error = 1)
3. Repeat this name and address after me: John Brown, 42 Market Street, Chicago	
4. About what time is it? (within 1 hour)	Multiply by 3 for every error (maximum error = 1)
5. Count backward 20 to 1	Multiply by 2 for every error (maximum error = 2)
6. Say the months in reverse order	Multiply by 2 for every error (maximum error = 2)
7. Repeat the name and address given previously	Multiply by 2 for every error (maximum error = 5)

[a]0-4 = normal cognition; 5-9 = questionable impairment; >10 = impairment consistent with dementia.

sentences are fragmented, nonfluent, and nonsensical, with paraphasias and grammatical errors. Receptive speech is when the lesion involves the Wernicke area and the patient is unable to understand commands and questions, and speech is usually fluent but not contextual. Repetition and naming should be assessed as well.

The patient's capacity in making their own medical decisions should be assessed, especially in critical situations where their mental state could worsen and communication could be impaired. Testing for capacity can be done by any physician, and consists of determining whether a patient is able to understand the present situation, the benefits and risks of therapeutic options, and the consequences of the refusal of a treatment or procedure. They should be able to clearly state their wishes.

The Short Blessed Test (SBT), also called Orientation-Memory-Concentration Test, is a good screening test with a sensitivity of 95% with a cutoff value of >4 for abnormal. A score of 10 or more is consistent with dementia (**Table 2.2**).

CRANIAL NERVE EXAMINATION

When examining a patient with a neurologic complaint, the CN examination helps localize the lesion in the brainstem.

Olfactory Nerve

CN I (olfactory nerve) passes through the cribriform plant and is often involved in lesions at the base of the skull (trauma, tumor, infection). Any involvement of the olfactory bulb or tracts can cause unilateral anosmia. The olfactory cortex receives input from both nerves, and unilateral involvement of the cortex rarely causes any anosmia.

To test this nerve, the patient must be conscious and able to cooperate. One should use subtle smells (ie, coffee) because noxious odors might be carried by the trigeminal nerve. The patient should have their eyes closed and each nostril tested separately.

Optic Nerve

CN II (optic nerve) forms at the retina initially; nasal fibers (temporal visual field) decussate at the optic chiasm and form optic tracts that give optic radiations traveling either to the lateral geniculate body and occipital cortex (vision) or superior colliculus and Edinger-Westphal nucleus (pupillary reflex); see **Figure 2.1**. Visual acuity, visual fields, color perception, and pupillary reflex should all be assessed.

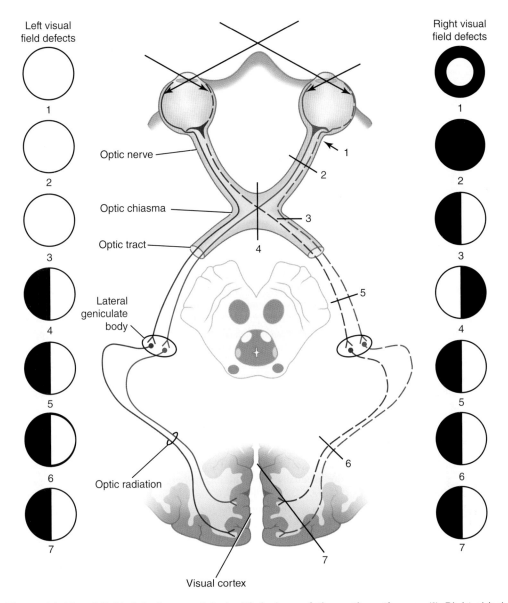

Left visual field defects

Right visual field defects

Optic nerve

Optic chiasma

Optic tract

Lateral geniculate body

Optic radiation

Visual cortex

Figure 2.1: Visual field defects associated with lesions of the optic pathways. (1) Right-sided circumferential blindness due to retrobulbar neuritis. (2) Total blindness of the right eye due to division of the right optic nerve. (3) Right nasal hemianopia due to a partial lesion of the right side of the optic chiasma. (4) Bitemporal hemianopia due to a complete lesion of the optic chiasma. (5) Left temporal hemianopia and right nasal hemianopia due to a lesion of the right optic tract. (6) Left temporal and right nasal hemianopia due to a lesion of the right optic radiation. (7) Left temporal and right nasal hemianopia due to a lesion of the right visual cortex. (From Cranial Nerve Nuclei. In: Splittgerber R. *Snell's Clinical Neuroanatomy.* 8th ed. Philadelphia, PA: Wolters Kluwer; 2019:323-362. Figure 11.24.)

Pupils should be inspected for size, symmetry, and reactivity to light. Asymmetry in pupillary size can be secondary to parasympathetic (CN III, Edinger-Westphal nucleus) involvement, causing the pupil to dilate (mydriasis), or sympathetic involvement, causing the pupil to constrict (myosis). Shape should also be assessed because abnormalities can be caused by ophthalmologic disorders (iris coloboma). Pupillary reflex (constriction) is triggered by light and accommodation, and is carried by the

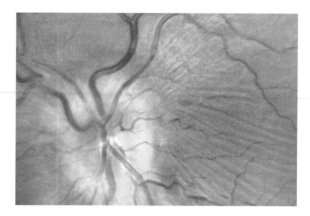

Figure 2.2: Early papilledema. Courtesy of Don C Bienfang, MD. ©2020 UpToDate, Inc. Wolters Kluwer.

optic nerve (afferent pathway) and returns to the circumferential pupillary sphincter by the parasympathetic fibers of the oculomotor nerve, CN III (efferent pathway, nerve fibers from Edinger-Westphal nucleus). Direct and indirect (to the contralateral eye) illumination causes constriction of both pupils (consensual reflex). The optic fibers that are responsible for this reflex pass ultimately to the ipsilateral and contralateral Edinger-Westphal nucleus (parasympathetic nucleus of the oculomotor nuclear complex), which projects axons to the ciliary ganglion (synapse) and then to the ciliary body (accommodation) and pupillary constrictors. Involvement of the optic nerve causes lack of response to light in the ipsilateral eye, but normal consensual response in both eyes when light is shone in the contralateral eye. Patients should be asked to fixate on a distant object to avoid myosis from accommodation. The afferent pupillary defect, or Marcus Gunn sign, is tested via the swinging flashlight test. When the light is on one eye, the pupils constrict initially and then dilate, and when the light moves to the affected eye, the initial constriction is lost, and the pupils continue to dilate. This sign most commonly signals the presence of an ipsilateral optic nerve lesion; it may also occur with homonymous visual loss related to optic tract lesions.

Funduscopic examination is equally important in an emergency setting because it helps identify bilateral papilledema (**Figure 2.2**) , which suggests an increase in ICP. It is ideally performed in a dark room with the patient's pupils dilated, and the patient fixating on a distant object. The examiner should first observe a reddish/orange reflection in the pupil and move closer until they find a vessel that they can track along to the optic disc. The elements of assessment are the disc color, margins, cupping, retinal vessels, and presence of cotton wool spots or neovascularization.

Visual acuity should be assessed after refractive errors are corrected (glasses worn during testing), and each eye separately. If glasses are not available, it should be tested through a pinhole held as close to the eye as possible. Snellen chart is the most used and widely available scale.

Visual fields of each eye are divided by a vertical median into nasal (inner) and temporal (outer) fields, and by a horizontal median into upper and lower fields. Each field has two hemifields and four quadrants. Confrontational testing, one eye at a time, is recommended (ask the patient to cover the other eye). The patient is asked to maintain fixation on the examiner's nose, and fingers are held in each quadrant and then simultaneously in bilateral fields. The patient is asked to count all the fingers they can see. When optic nerve disease is suspected, each eye should be tested for red color detection, which is lost when the optic nerve is compromised as in optic neuritis.

Oculomotor Nerve (III), Trochlear Nerve (IV), and Abducens (VI)

Initially, observe the position of gaze to assess if there is any ophthalmoplegia. An eye that is deviated down and out is suggestive of a CN III lesion. An eye that is deviated inward is suggestive of an abducens nerve lesion. The trochlear nerve (IV) supplies the superior oblique muscle that moves the adducted eye downward; dysfunction of this nerve will cause vertical or torsional diplopia, especially in downgaze. A correctional head tilting to the opposite side of the lesion is suggestive of a trochlear nerve involvement. Examining gaze position in a cooperative patient is usually done by

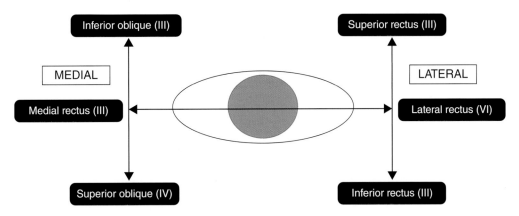

Figure 2.3: Testing of extraocular muscles in the cardinal positions of gaze.

asking them to track the examiner's finger as it moves in all cardinal positions of gaze or in the H shape (**Figure 2.3**). Conjugation should be tested as well because it assesses the function of CN III.

Pursuit and saccades should be assessed when evaluating extraocular movements. The function of pursuit movements is to stabilize the image of a moving object on the foveae, and thus to maintain a continuous clear image of the object as the object changes position. It is a function of the parieto-occipital cortex and cerebellum. It is assessed by observing the patient's eye movements when tracking one's finger, and it is either described as smooth (no interruptions) or choppy. Saccadic movements, originating in the frontal lobe, can be elicited by instructing an individual to look to the right or left (commanded saccades), or to move the eyes to a target (refixation saccades). Abnormal saccades can be hypometric (undershoots), as seen in Parkinsonism, or hypermetric (overshoots), which is typical of cerebellar involvement.

Gaze position is very helpful in localizing the lesion in the cortex and along the brainstem. Conjugate gaze deviation, when both eyes deviate together horizontally, can be due to a destruction or stimulation of the frontal eye fields or a lesion in the pons. A destructive lesion (stroke, tumor) that involves the frontal eye fields will cause a gaze deviation to the same side of the lesion; however, a seizure in that same area will make the eyes go in the opposite direction. A pontine lesion will cause deviation of the eyes contralaterally. Disconjugate gaze deviation is suggestive of an involvement of the brainstem (CN nuclei), CNs, neuromuscular junction, or extraocular muscles rather than of the cortex.

The oculomotor nerve nuclei (CN III) are in the midbrain and have multiple subnuclei. Each subnucleus is responsible for one of the extraocular muscles. Each nucleus receives input from the contralateral abducens nucleus, situated in the pons, through the ipsilateral medial longitudinal fasciculus. CN III has a parasympathetic component that runs in the periphery of the nerve. The parasympathetic nucleus of Edinger-Westphal is in the medial midbrain.

Trigeminal Nerve

The trigeminal nerve or CN V channels all sensory modalities of the face and provides motor input to masticatory muscles. It is tested by assessing sensation to light touch, pinprick, and temperature on the face. Initially, light touch should be tested using superficial friction with fingertips or, ideally, with a cotton wisp. Extinction is a form of hemineglect that is most associated with lesions of the nondominant parietal lobe cortex; it is tested by stimulating both sides simultaneously. Finally, pain sensation is tested using a safety pin and asking the patient to identify if the sensation is sharp (pin) or dull (head) with their eyes closed; the patient is then asked if the sharpness is identical bilaterally.

Weakness of the muscles of mastication can be due to lesions in the upper motor neuron (UMN) pathways synapsing onto the trigeminal (CN V) motor nucleus, in the lower motor neurons (LMNs) of the trigeminal motor nucleus in the pons or as they exit the brainstem to reach the muscles of mastication, in the neuromuscular junction, or in the muscles themselves. Trigeminal motor function is tested by palpating the masseter muscles while the patient clenches the teeth and by asking the patient to open the mouth against resistance. If a pterygoid muscle is weak, the jaw deviates to that side when the mouth is opened.

CN V carries the afferent arm of two major reflexes. The corneal reflex, which is tested mostly in comatose patients using a cotton tip or saline on the cornea, manifests as bilateral eye blinking through CN VII (efferent arm). The jaw jerk reflex or masseter reflex is a stretch reflex used to test the status of a patient's trigeminal nerve (CN V) and to help distinguish an upper cervical cord compression from lesions that are above the foramen magnum. The mandible is tapped just below the lips (at the chin) at a downward angle while the mouth is held slightly open; noticing a brisk mouth closure signifies an abnormal reflex (UMN involvement).

Facial Nerve

CN VII has motor, sensory, and secretory functions. It controls facial musculature and the major muscles that are tested are the orbicularis oculi, orbicularis oris, and frontalis. A branch of CN VII also supplies the stapedius muscle within the middle ear, which reduces the oscillatory range of the tympanic membrane, and, when dysfunctional, the patient may note that sounds seem "louder" than before. It is also responsible for taste sensation in the anterior two-thirds of the tongue (via the chordae tympani nerve), sensation of the soft palate and middle ear, as well as a small amount of cutaneous sensation from the skin in and around the auricle (carried by the nervus intermedius). Finally, the secretory branch supplies the submandibular, sublingual, and lacrimal glands.

Facial nerve palsy can be detected initially by observing for asymmetry in the shape of the mouth, the nasolabial folds, spontaneous expression, and frequency of blinking. The patient should be asked to smile, puff up their cheeks (that the examiner can push on to assess robustness of mouth closure), close their eyes tight, and raise their eyebrows.

Cochlear and Vestibular Nerves

CN VIII has two functions: auditory and vestibular. The cochlear nerve is the portion that is responsible for hearing and can be tested by whispering numbers in one ear as the patient covers the other and asking the patient to repeat the numbers. Another way is to rub fingers together in one ear at a time to produce a rustling sound.

Rinne and Weber tests can help differentiate sensorineural from conductive hearing loss. The Rinne test is performed by placing a vibrating 512 Hz tuning fork on the mastoid process (bone conduction), then asking the patient when they can no longer hear the buzzing, and then move it to the auditory meatus (air conduction). If the patient is able to hear the tuning fork via air conduction (after they were no longer able to hear via bone conduction), it suggests their air conduction is better than bone conduction (Rinne positive), which is seen in normal hearing and sensorineural deafness, whereas conductive deafness has better bone conduction. The Weber test is performed with the same tuning fork placed in the middle of the forehead. The sound should be heard equally in both ears. It will be heard louder in the normal ear in the case of sensorineural deafness and in the affected ear in conductive deafness.

The vestibular nerve transmits sensory information from otolith organs (utricle and saccule) and the three semicircular canals. It has connections to the cerebellum, oculomotor nerves, and anterior horns of the spinal cord. Information from the otolith organs reflects gravity and linear accelerations of the head, whereas the semicircular canals are activated with the rotational movement of the head. Damage to the nerve can cause vertigo, nausea, vomiting. It is tested in symptomatic patients by assessing for nystagmus and oculovestibular reflex.

In normal individuals, head rotation triggers semicircular canals that sense angular acceleration and send a signal to the oculomotor nuclei through the vestibular nerve, moving the eyes contralateral to the head turn, to keep track of a fixed target. Nystagmus is an eye movement occurring when the head is stationary secondary to abnormal stimulation or inhibition of the vestibular apparatus. It has a fast component and slow movement in the opposite direction. The direction of the nystagmus is, by convention, the direction of the fast component. In the setting of a peripheral lesion to the vestibular apparatus, the fast component is away from the involved ear. In central lesions (cerebellum), the fast component is toward the lesion. Testing for gaze-evoked nystagmus is done by having the patient track their finger in all directions of gaze and looking closely for jerky movements of the eyes and describing the direction of the fast and slow components. See **Chapter 10: Dizziness and Vertigo**, for a discussion of maneuvers in the assessment of vertigo and the HINTS (Head Impulse Nystagmus Test of Skew) examination. In benign paroxysmal positional vertigo (BPPV), nystagmus starts after a short latency (seconds), is unidirectional—most often horizontal—with torsional component, fatigues on repeated trial, and is suppressed with prolonged fixation. Central nystagmus is presented at midline gaze, and is multidirectional; the fast component changes direction with changes in gaze or visual fields.

Glossopharyngeal Nerve and Vagal Nerve

Examination of the glossopharyngeal and vagal nerves include testing the gag reflex, asking the patient to swallow or cough, inspecting the soft palate and uvula and evaluating for dysarthria. The clinician should also listen to the patient talk during history taking and assess for hoarseness, dysarthria, and nasal speech. Swallowing can be assessed by giving the patient a glass of water and observing for choking or any subjective complaints. Observe the palatal arches as they contract and the soft palate as it swings up and back to close off the nasopharynx from the oropharynx. Normal palatal arches will constrict and elevate, and the uvula will remain in the midline as it is elevated. With paralysis, there is no elevation or constriction of the affected side, and the uvula deviates to the contralateral side.

Accessory Nerve

CN XI provides motor innervation to two major muscles, which are the trapezius (shoulder elevation) and sternocleidomastoid (SCM, head turn). The examiner should observe the SCM muscles and trapezius for wasting, and then have the patient shrug their shoulder, and turn their head against resistance. The trapezius elevates the ipsilateral shoulder and the SCM turns the head to the contralateral side.

Hypoglossal Nerve

Tongue movement has bilateral representation in both hemispheres in the precentral gyrus, which means that unilateral cortical lesions would generally not cause tongue weakness. Unilateral medial medulla lesions involving the hypoglossal nucleus or nerve would cause ipsilateral tongue weakness and deviation ("lick the lesion"). Slight deviation of the protruded tongue as a solitary finding can usually be disregarded, but a major deviation represents underaction of the hypoglossal nerve and muscle on that side. When examining the tongue, inspect for atrophy, fasciculations, or asymmetry in movement or appearance. The patient should then be asked to stick out their tongue and move it to one side, then the other assessing for tongue position and amplitude of movement. Tongue strength can be assessed objectively by asking the patient to push their tongue on their cheek while the examiner is applying resistance with their thumb.

MOTOR EXAMINATION

The first step in the motor examination is to observe the patient's spontaneous movements, looking if they are favoring one side or the other. It is also useful to identify abnormal movements and if they occur at rest or with motion. Fluctuations and changes in the frequency, amplitude, and pattern of these movements should be assessed during the encounter, as well as whether they are distractible. The trick is to ask the patient questions about other symptoms while observing the involved limb. Distractibility is a major element in favor of functional movement disorders.

Once the patient is undressed, assess the muscles, especially deltoids and quadriceps, for bulk (atrophy or hypertrophy) and fasciculations (twitching of the muscle fibers); LMN disease is suggested if triggered by tapping on the muscles. Comparing both sides to look for asymmetry in muscle size is always useful. Inflammatory myopathies are suggested by tenderness on palpation of the major muscle groups.

Assessing for drift is a sensitive screening test for upper and lower extremity weakness. Pronator drift test is done by asking the patient to extend and raise both arms in front of them as if they were carrying a tray and then by maintaining the arms at the same level for 10 seconds. If there is

TABLE 2.3	Medical Research Council (MRC) Scale for Strength Testing
0/5	No movement
1/5	Barest flicker of movement of the muscle, although not enough to move the structure to which it is attached.
2/5	Voluntary movement that is not sufficient to overcome the force of gravity. For example, the patient would be able to slide their hand across a table, but not lift it from the surface.
3/5	Voluntary movement capable of overcoming gravity, but not any applied resistance. For example, the patient could raise their hand off a table, but not if any additional resistance were applied.
4/5	Voluntary movement capable of overcoming "some" resistance
5/5	Normal strength

upper extremity weakness, the arm will initially pronate and then drift and fall. To test for drift in the lower extremities, the patient should lie prone with their knees flexed at 90 degrees and feet pointing up vertically; the weak leg will drift or drop in about 30 seconds.

Tone is examined by passive mobilization of the joints; ask the patient to relax and then maneuver the limb while carefully keeping the patient comfortable to prevent any resistance. Tone is then qualified as normal, flaccid, rigid, or spastic. Rigidity, seen in extrapyramidal disorders such as Parkinson disease, is non-velocity dependent such that the tone remains increased regardless of how quickly the joint is moved. Spasticity, which is seen with UMN lesions, is velocity dependent and worsens if the examiner moves the joint with increasing speeds. Rigidity can be further described as cogwheel where the movement is interrupted by short stops due to tremor, or lead pipe which is a smooth, steady resistance to passive movement, both seen in extrapyramidal syndromes. Clasp knife "rigidity," which is an indicator of spasticity, is when, after an initial resistance to passive movement of a joint, there is a sudden reduction in tone and the limb moves without resistance through the rest of the movement. Gegenhalten rigidity, also known as paratonia, is seen in catatonia and advanced dementia; the patients exhibit more resistance along the range of the movement and their limbs get fixed in the last position they were in when released.

Next, assessment of strength is done using the Medical Research Council (MRC) scale; see **Table 2.3**. In the emergency setting, examining only the major muscle groups is generally sufficient unless the patient has a specific focal complaint.

SENSORY EXAMINATION

The sensory examination is reliable only when the patient is able to cooperate because it is subject to variability related to suggestibility and emotional experience. It is recommended to perform the examination quickly, after a brief explanation because excessive discussion can cause false-positive findings due to hypervigilance to minor meaningless differences.

A quick screening can be done using light touch (fingertips or cotton wisp); it is not very sensitive, but can detect major sensory loss. It should always be performed bilaterally with comparison between contralateral limbs. Asking the patient if the touch feels the same rather than different is encouraged because it decreases false positives.

Pin prick testing using the needle portion of the safety pin can assess for milder sensory deficits, testing small myelinated and unmyelinated fibers that transmit pain and temperature. Ideally, moving from an area with decreased sensation to a normal area improves perception of a difference. Using a pin is also useful to detect a sensory level below which the patient has loss of sensation, which helps localize lesions in the spinal cord. Identifying a level is best performed on the back, in an ascending manner.

Proprioception can be tested in the upper or lower extremities. The trick is to grab the lateral aspect of the proximal part of the toe or finger with one hand and move the distal phalange up or down and prompting the patient on the position. Romberg test is a good screening tool for impairment of proprioception (posterior columns or peripheral neuropathy); it is done by asking the patient to stand with their feet together and then to close their eyes; if they sway and step outward, it is a positive Romberg. If the patient is unable to stand with their feet together while their eyes are open, it points to a dysfunction in the vestibular or cerebellar systems.

Vibration is tested placing a tuning fork on bony prominences; it is recommended to record the number of seconds for which the vibration is felt. It is not usually performed in the emergency setting, but can be helpful to localize the spinal cord involvement (vibration is impaired with lesion to the posterior columns).

REFLEXES

Deep tendon reflexes (DTRs) are obtained by swinging a reflex hammer and tapping the patient's tendons. It is sometimes difficult to obtain a response, and distracting the patient with a conversation or specific maneuvers such as Jendrassik can help. The latter is performed by asking the patient to clench their teeth, clamp both sets of fingers into a hook-like form, and pull the fingers in opposite directions while the examiner tests lower extremity reflexes. The most tested muscle tendons are the following: ankle (S1-S2), knee (L3-L4), biceps (C5), brachioradialis (C6), and triceps (C7).

Grading the reflex depends on the intensity of the response. If there is no response even with distraction, it is marked zero. If there is a normal response, it is marked 2+. When the reflex is hypoactive and requires a Jendrassik maneuver to be elicited, it should be rated 1+. A 3+ response means that the reflex is brisk with spread along adjacent joints activating nearby reflex arcs, and 4+ is reserved for brisk reflexes with clonus at the joint. Brisk reflexes (3+ and 4+) are indicative of UMN lesions, whereas absent or diminished reflexes are seen with LMN involvement.

Plantar reflex is done to look for signs of UMN involvement. It is done by stroking the lateral border of the patient's foot (plantar surface) with a tongue depressor, in a semicircular pattern, going from the heel to the big toe. The normal response or flexor plantar reflex is flexion of the big toe and flexion with adduction of the other toes. An abnormal response or extensor plantar reflex (Babinski sign) is an extension of the big toe with abduction or fanning of the other toes.

CEREBELLAR MANEUVERS/MOVEMENT AND COORDINATION

Cerebellar lesions affect coordination of motor movements causing ataxia. A lesion involving the hemispheres will cause ipsilateral appendicular or limb ataxia, which will be detected by finger-to-nose and heel-to-shin testing described later. Lesions to the midline portion of the cerebellum (vermis) will cause axial or truncal ataxia, which is usually detected by having the patient ambulate; voice (drunken or staccato) and eye movements can be abnormal as well. Damage to the flocculonodular lobe will cause abnormalities in the vestibular function and will be detected via the vestibulo-ocular reflex (multidirectional nystagmus).

Observing the patient at rest, when sitting, standing, or ambulating can give the examiner clues to a cerebellar dysfunction. With truncal ataxia, there is usually a tendency to lean laterally or fall backward and sometimes forward as well. Gait is wide based and unsteady, with a tendency to lean toward the affected side in unilateral lesions.

Excessive rebound seen with cerebellar lesions is tested first; after having the patient extend their arms in front of them (eg, when evaluating for pronator drift), quick and transient downward pressure is applied to the patient's arms, causing an excessive upward motion after the release followed by a downward motion as the patient recalibrates the movement.

Tremors can be caused by cerebellar lesions; they are usually present with action, with increased amplitude at the end of the movement, and can be observed during finger-to-nose testing and resolves at rest and with posture.

Dysmetria or past-pointing is evaluated during finger-to-nose and heel-to-shin testing. Dysmetria refers to difficulty judging distance to a target and not just missing a target. These findings should be out of proportion to limb weakness. This is done by having the patient touch the examiner's finger, placed at arm's length from the patient, and then their nose repeatedly and rapidly. The heel-to-shin test is performed in a supine patient, by asking them to smoothly take the heel of one foot and move it up and down the shin of the other leg.

Other signs of cerebellar dysfunction include difficulty with rapid alternating movements or dysdiadochokinesis (finger tapping, foot tapping, pronation/supination of the hands), as well as heel-to-toe tandem gait.

FUNCTIONAL NEUROLOGIC EXAMINATION

Functional weakness, which can involve one limb or more, can be differentiated from true paralysis by assessing effort related to function. During strength testing, there is notable contraction of agonist and antagonist muscles simultaneously, which intermittently causes jerky movements of the limb ("give-way" weakness). The limb will initially move as desired, but then collapse with any resistance applied. The trick to detect effort-related weakness is to apply varying resistance force to the limb, starting with a minimal push followed by a gradual increase in power, revealing that the patient's effort to resist varies along the movement. The patient's facial expressions suggest that they are giving their best effort (grunting, frowning, etc.). This pattern of weakness is also seen when there is pain-related limitation of the movement. In true paralysis, the patient applies maximum force throughout the range of motion.

Reflexes are usually within the limits of normal, without pathologic reflexes (no Babinski). Inspection is usually unrevealing; atrophy and fasciculations are absent.

The Hoover sign can help identify functional hemiplegia. The examiner places one hand under the heels of the paralyzed leg and the other on top of the nonparalyzed one. The patient is then asked to raise the nonparalyzed leg, feeling downward pressure by the paralyzed leg, which is unusual with organic weakness. The next step is to place both hands under the patient's heel and ask them to raise the paretic leg, noticing lack of downward pressure from the normal leg (which normally pushes downward to raise the opposite leg).

In a similar maneuver, the examiner tells the patient that they are testing the normal limb, while asking the patient to try to push the knees together and the apparently paralyzed limb will adduct with normal power.

The Babinski trunk-thigh test is another test that can identify functional hemiplegia. In neurologic hemiplegia, when a patient is asked to sit up from a recumbent position with arms crossed, there is an involuntary flexion of the paretic leg (both legs are flexed in paraplegia). In functional weaknesses, the normal leg is flexed and the paralyzed leg remains extended.

When the patient complains of sensory loss to one side of their face, the tuning fork split sign can be used. Vibration spreads bilaterally placed on each side of the frontal bone, and should not be affected with unilateral sensory loss. If the patient is unable to feel the vibration on one side of the forehead, this is very suggestive of a nonneurologic cause.

Gait assessment, which shows a bizarre gait with an irregular pattern of ambulation, with variation in amplitude and appearance, excessive slowness, uneconomic postures, and sudden buckling of the knees without a fall, is considered functional.

Vision loss can be assessed using an optokinetic strip (video of moving black and white strips) and observing for an ocular jerk movement, which, when present, argues against complete blindness. This test should be performed with the "good eye" covered.

Nonepileptic (psychogenic) seizures often present with asynchronous and variable movements that wax and wane with specific findings, including forward pelvic thrusts, arched back, and rolling or looking from side to side. Although more common in epileptic seizures, both tongue biting or incontinence are reported in nonepileptic events. By definition, generalized epileptic seizures have loss of consciousness; an incomplete loss of awareness during the event would be diagnostic of a nonepileptic seizure. Forced eye closure is usually present, whereas in epileptic seizures, the eyes remain open.

TIPS AND PEARLS

- The Cushing reflex (hypertension, bradycardia, and irregular breathing) in obtunded patients suggests an increase in ICP.
- When testing visual fields with finger counting, it is recommended to use one, two, or all five fingers because others are difficult to distinguish.

- Loss of red saturation indicates inflammation in the optic nerve impairment.
- When testing extraocular muscles, the patient should keep their head still as the examiner's finger moves slowly. The moving finger should be positioned far enough in front of the patient so they can see it in all directions of gaze.
- CNs IV and VI are most likely impacted with head injury or mass lesions.
- CN III deficit with pupillary sparing is most likely due to intrinsic disease.
- Nystagmus of central origin is multidirectional, changes direction with gaze, and is worse with fixation of gaze. It appears without latency, persists, and can be purely vertical, usually downbeat, whereas peripheral nystagmus is horizontal and torsional upbeat.
- CN VII nerve can be tested indirectly by performing corneal reflex because it carries the information in the efferent branch of the reflex arc, causing blinking. One should expect isolated contralateral blinking with conjunctival stimulation if CN V is intact and only unilateral ipsilateral facial nerve involvement is suspected.
- With UMN facial weakness above the nucleus located in the pons, the patient has weakness in the lower face (orbicularis oris), but can still wrinkle their forehead and close their eyes. With LMN facial weakness (ie, Bell palsy, pontine stroke), all muscles on the ipsilateral side of the face are affected. Owing to the co-localization of the facial colliculus and abducens nucleus, patients with pontine stroke having LMN facial weakness will have lateral rectus palsy.
- Atrophy, fasciculation, and flaccid tone are seen with peripheral nervous system (PNS) involvement versus spasticity, dystonia, and abnormal movements seen with central nervous system (CNS) lesions.
- Neuromuscular junction disease is characterized by fluctuations, fatigable weakness, normal (sometimes decreased) tone, and normal reflexes.
- Double tactile stimulation of both limbs at a time, after testing each limb separately, can assess for sensory inattention and neglect, which is a parietal lobe function. It is done by asking the patient to close their eyes and prompting them whether right, left, or both limbs are being touched.
- The Brown-Sequard or hemicord syndrome secondary to unilateral spinal cord lesion presents with diminished proprioception, vibration sensation, and weakness on the side of the lesion, and decreased pinprick and temperature sensation on the contralateral side. Testing for pinprick sensation can help identify the level.
- Vibration is tested on the interpharyngeal joint of the big toe or proximal interpharyngeal joint of the thumb. In lower extremities, vibration should be felt for 10 to 12 seconds, whereas for upper extremities, it lasts 16 to 18 seconds.
- When testing reflexes, hold the hammer by the end of the rod and let it fall on the joint in a pendulum swinging motion.
- To test the knee/patellar reflex, the leg should be in passive flexion at the knee, with the examiner's wrist below the knee and the hammer striking the patellar tendon between the tibial tuberosity and inferior border of the patella.
- To test the ankle jerk (Achilles reflex), the leg should be externally rotated and the foot in dorsiflexion at the ankle.
- Keep in mind that 1+ and 3+ reflexes can be seen in normal individuals without neurologic disorder.
- Address the patient's breathing pattern because it helps localize the level of involvement. Cheyne-Stokes respiration or rhythmic waxing and waning of respiratory amplitude can be seen with bilateral hemispheric dysfunction. Central reflex hyperpnea or continuous deep breathing can be seen with bilateral hemispheric, lower midbrain, or upper pons dysfunction. Apneustic respiration with prolonged inspiratory time and pauses is seen in pontine lesions. Ataxic respiration characterized by infrequent irregular breaths can be secondary to lower pons or upper medulla involvement.

Abnormal Vision, Pupils, and Eye Movements

Ashley Norse

CLINICAL CHALLENGE

Eye complaints can be a sign of minor irritation or significant neurologic or systemic diseases such as stroke, multiple sclerosis, or myasthenia gravis. Eye complaints can be the presenting symptom of disease from multiple organ systems ranging from the sequela of uncontrolled hypertension and diabetes to infectious disease and food borne pathogens. Approximately 2% of all emergency department (ED) visits each year are for eye-related complaints, and although life-threatening diagnoses are rare, a disproportionate percentage of serious neurologic diagnoses are made in patients who present to the ED compared to ambulatory clinics.[1,2]

ANATOMY AND PATHOPHYSIOLOGY

To understand the pathology that can affect the eye, it helps to understand eye anatomy and the visual pathway. Light enters the eye through the dome-shaped cornea and traverses the aqueous humor in the anterior chamber. To maintain a constant eye pressure, the eye is continuously producing and draining aqueous humor. Muscles in the iris (the colored part of the eye) dilate or constrict the pupil to control the amount of light entering the posterior chamber of the eye. The lens sits behind the pupil and changes shape to allow the eye to focus on objects that are up close or far away.

The light then enters the posterior chamber and traverses the vitreous, hitting the retina. Photoreceptors in the retina generate signals, rods for dim light (black and white) vision and cones for color and bright light vision. The macula, in the center of the retina, contains the fovea, with the highest concentration of cones, and thus is responsible for our detailed, central vision. The remainder of the retina provides peripheral vision.

The retina sends electrical impulses through the optic nerve to the brain. The visual signals exit via the optic nerve and travel to the optic chiasm where the impulses decussate. Information from the nasal portion of each retina decussate and are interpreted by the opposite side of the brain. The signals continue from the optic chiasm to the lateral geniculate bodies, and on to the occipital lobe via the optic radiations. The Edinger-Westphal nuclei, or oculomotor complexes, are parasympathetic fibers located in the midbrain and responsible for extraocular movements of the eye, accommodation, pupillary constriction, and convergence.

APPROACH

History

The emergency clinician must use key findings in the history to help localize the pathology and direct the physical examination and workup of the patient. Critical components of the history include onset of symptoms, history of trauma, progression of the symptoms, relieving of exacerbating symptoms, whether the symptoms are unilateral or bilateral, and the presence or absence of other neurologic symptoms. Other important associated symptoms include eye redness, photophobia, floaters, sensation of flashes of light (photopsias), and the presence of pain at rest or with eye movement. In the absence of trauma, the presence of pain suggests an inflammatory or infectious process and narrows the differential diagnosis. A history of progressive symptoms raises concern for a compressive lesion, whereas intermittent symptoms, especially if associated with diplopia and ptosis, is concerning for a neuromuscular junction disorder such as myasthenia gravis. Systemic symptoms such as generalized weakness and neurologic symptoms, such as vertigo, dizziness, ataxia, or aphasia, are red flags for critical conditions, for example, stroke, bleed, or other brainstem lesions.

Past medical history should focus on diseases known to cause eye pathology including hypertension and diabetes, and conditions associated with immunocompromise including human immunodeficiency virus (HIV). Hematologic disorders such as sickle cell anemia or multiple myeloma can cause a hyperviscosity syndrome and eye complaints. Family history should include questions about migraine headaches, multiple sclerosis, lupus, and vascular disease.

Abnormal Vision

Abnormal vision complaints will commonly be blurry vision, in actuality, which may result from a simple refractory issue, but can also be due to a corneal abrasion, hyphema, iritis, uveitis, glaucoma, lens dislocation, or stroke. Blurry vision must also be differentiated from floaters that are often due to posterior chamber pathology such as retinal detachment or retinal hemorrhage. Retinal detachment can also present with the complaint of the sensation of a curtain falling over the eye, which results from the retinal pulling away from the choroid and sclera.

Central retinal artery occlusion (CRAO) or central retinal venous occlusion (CRVO) can present with sudden complete unilateral vision loss. In sudden vision loss, it must be determined whether the vision loss is monocular or binocular, and whether it involves the entire visual field or an isolated visual field cut. Important associated visual symptoms include floaters, flashing lights, halos, and distorted color vision. A review of systems should seek extraocular symptoms including jaw or tongue claudication, temporal headache, proximal muscle pain or stiffness (giant cell arteritis), and headaches (ocular migraine).

Diplopia

The differential for diplopia is extensive, and key features of the history are critical to determining the cause (see Table 3.7 later in this chapter). It must be determined whether the diplopia is monocular or binocular. Monocular diplopia is defined as double vision that does not correct when one eye is closed or occluded. Monocular diplopia is usually caused by intraocular pathology, with the most common cause being a refractive error. Lens dislocations (spontaneous or traumatic) can also be a cause of monocular diplopia. Binocular diplopia is double vision that resolves when one eye is closed and is caused by misalignment of the visual axes.

In addition to onset of the diplopia (sudden versus gradual), and the presence or absence of pain, another important question in a patient with diplopia is the directionality of the diplopia. Diplopia can be horizontal with side-by-side images, vertical with the images above and below each other, or torsional. The directionality of the diplopia is equally important as the type of diplopia. Horizontal diplopia, without vertical separation, is often indicative of medial or lateral rectus muscle pathology, whereas torsional or oblique diplopia is more commonly caused by superior or inferior oblique muscle dysfunction or lateral medullary syndrome. Vertical diplopia is often a sign of brainstem pathology; it is also seen in isolated cranial nerve (CN) IV pathology.

The most common cause of diplopia is an isolated CN VI palsy, often from trauma or compression. A sudden onset of binocular diplopia suggests ischemia, whereas a gradual onset suggests a compressive lesion or systemic disease. A fluctuation in symptoms may suggest transient ischemic attacks (TIAs), but neuromuscular disease must be ruled out as well.

Physical Examination

The physical examination should include a complete neurologic examination in addition to the eye examination. The provider should focus on any subtle findings including head positioning, facial asymmetry, CN abnormalities, extremity weakness, and sensory deficits. In patients with complaints of headache and vision changes, the physical examination should also include palpation of the temples for tenderness or nodularity over the course of the temporal artery.

The eye examination typically has nine components (**Table 3.1**): the external eye examination, a visual acuity and visual field examination, a pupil examination, the extraocular muscle examination, a funduscopic examination to view the posterior chamber, a slit lamp examination to look at the anterior chamber, a fluorescein examination, as well as intraocular pressure (IOP) measurements. In addition to these eight components, bedside ultrasound (US) is a valued adjunct that can diagnose papilledema/increased IOP, vitreous hemorrhage, and retinal detachment.

The External Eye Examination

The external eye examination includes an examination of the orbital and periorbital structures, the lids and lashes, as well as the ductal and lacrimal systems. By just looking at the patient, critical physical examination findings such as proptosis, ptosis, lid lag, anisocoria, and head position can be identified.

If there is a history of trauma, inspection for periorbital edema or ecchymosis is important. Subtle finding of proptosis or a sunken orbit may be missed if the provider does not have a high index of suspicion. Shining a light in the unaffected eye can cause pain in the traumatized eye by stimulating a consensual response, indicating traumatic iritis. A patient presenting after trauma to the eye can also have orbital fractures with extraocular muscle entrapment causing diplopia. Trauma patients may also present with a sunken eye due to a complete blowout fracture of the orbit or with a proptotic eye secondary to a retrobulbar hematoma. Patients with retrobulbar hematoma may also have vision loss, a dilated and nonreactive pupil, and elevated ocular pressure. In the absence of trauma, proptosis can be a sign of space-occupying lesions of the orbit or systemic disease, such as thyroid disease.

Erythema and edema of the orbital and periorbital structures are a sign of infection. The conjunctiva should be examined for any signs of infection, inflammation, chemosis, or hemorrhage. A red eye can be a sign of acute iritis, glaucoma, infection, or trauma (**Table 3.3**). Patients with iritis and acute glaucoma will usually have findings of decreased visual acuity and may have abnormal pupillary examinations in addition to a red eye. A hyphema, which is blood in the anterior chamber of the eye (**Figure 3.1**), or a hypopyon, which is pus in the anterior chamber resulting from infection or corneal ulceration (**Figure 3.2**), can often be seen on an external eye examination as well.

TABLE 3.1	Nine Components of the Eye Examination
	Component
I	General inspection
II	VA/VF
III	Pupil examination
IV	EOM examination
V	Funduscopic examination (posterior chamber)
VI	Slit lamp examination (anterior chamber)
VII	Fluorescein examination
VIII	Tonometry (pressure)
IX	US

EOM; Extra-ocular muscle; US, ultrasound; VA/VF, visual acuity/visual field.

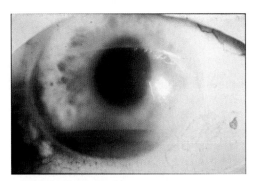

Figure 3.1: Hyphema.

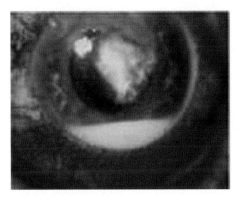

Figure 3.2: Hypopyon.

Visual Acuity and Visual Field Examinations

Testing for visual acuity and visual field deficits are key components of the eye examination. Visual acuity is ideally measured using a Snellen chart at 20 ft; a handheld chart is an alternative. Each eye is measured separately with and without the patient's glasses. If the patient does not have their glasses, a pinhole refractor can be used. If visual acuity corrects with glasses or a pinhole refractor, the problem is a refractory error. If the patient cannot read the eye chart at all, perception of hand motion and light should be assessed.

A test for *red desaturation* is helpful to assess optic nerve function: If color plates are not available, a quick assessment can be performed by asking the patient to cover each eye alternately while looking at a red object and report any relative dullness of the color in one eye. Many patients with optic neuritis will lose some of their color vision in the affected eye, especially red, and are not aware of the loss until tested.

Peripheral visual fields are assessed by confrontation, and central visual fields (eg, in suspected macular degeneration) are assessed using an Amsler grid. Bilateral field cuts localize pathology posterior to the retina and should always be investigated with either computed tomography (CT) or magnetic resonance imaging (MRI). Causes of bilateral field cuts include space-occupying lesions, stroke, bleeds, abscess, encephalitis, migraine, and arteriovenous malformations (**Figure 3.3**).

Pupil Examination

The pupillary examination includes looking for signs of asymmetry or irregularity. Direct and consensual pupillary light responses are examined (**Figure 3.4**) by shining a light in the first eye, which should cause both pupils to constrict equally. The pupillary reaction in the illuminated eye is called the ***direct response***, and the reaction in the other eye is the ***consensual response***. The afferent pupillomotor fibers from the optic nerve undergo hemidecussation in the chiasm, with a second hemidecussation of the pupillomotor fibers in the brainstem, so direct and consensual responses of

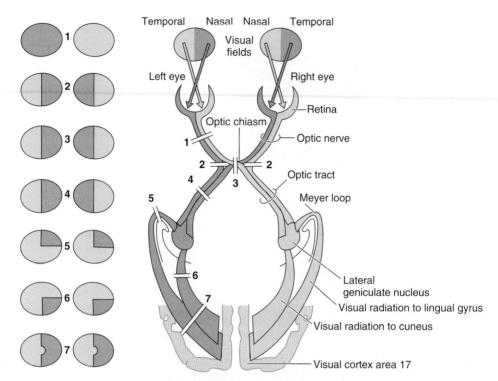

Figure 3.3: The visual pathway from the retina to the visual cortex showing visual field defects.
(1) Ipsilateral blindness. (2) Binasal hemianopia. (3) Bitemporal hemianopia. (4) Right hemianopia. (5) Right upper quadrantanopia. (6) Right lower quadrantanopia. (7) Right hemianopia with macular sparing. From Gould DJ, Brueckner-Collins JK, Fix JD, eds. In: Visual system. High-Yield™: Neuroanatomy (Figure 14.1). 5th ed. Wolters Kluwer; 2016:108-115.

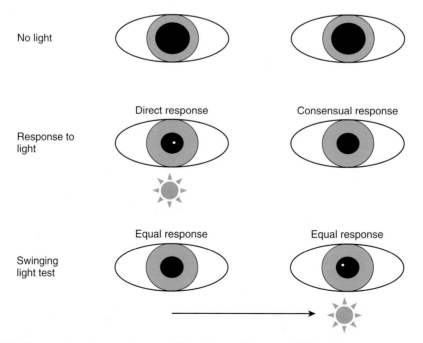

Figure 3.4: Abnormal and normal eye positions in cranial nerve (CN) palsies.

the eyes should be equal. The test should be repeated on the opposite eye. To test for an afferent pupillary defect, the light is again shone in the first eye and then swung to the other eye (swinging flashlight test). If the pupils respond differently to the light stimuli, a retinal or optic nerve disease process is suspected.

A tonic pupil (Adie pupil) has parasympathetic denervation and will not constrict well to light, but typically reacts better to accommodation. It is a common, benign cause of anisocoria, seen more often in females (70% of cases). About 20% of the population has pupil asymmetry of up to 1 mm; however, anisocoria can also be a sign of pathology. Patients who present with a dilated pupil along with a CN III palsy may have an aneurysm at the junction of the posterior communicating artery and the middle cerebral artery. Horner syndrome presents with a constellation of symptoms including a dilated pupil, ptosis, oculosympathetic paralysis, and ipsilateral anhydrosis.

Extraocular Muscle Examination

There are six extraocular muscles of the eye that attach to the sclera. The lateral rectus is innervated by the abducens nerve (CN VI) and is responsible for outward gaze. The superior oblique is innervated by the trochlear nerve (CN IV) and moves the eyes up and outward. The inferior, superior, and medial rectus muscles are all innervated by the oculomotor nerve (CN III) and move the eye in and up. Examination of the extraocular muscles should be performed in the H pattern while holding the head steady, with close observation of both eyes through the full range of motion.

Injury to the lateral rectus muscle or a palsy of CN VI will cause the affected eye to turn inward, and patients will have limited abduction of the affected eye with horizontal diplopia that is worse when looking toward the affected side. Injury to the superior oblique or palsy of CN IV will cause the affected eye to be displaced slightly upward and have vertical or oblique/torsional diplopia. Patients may compensate with a head tilt to the side of the palsy, making an isolated CN IV palsy difficult to diagnosis. Palsy of CN III results in the affected eye turning down and outward. Patients are unable to supraduct, infraduct, or adduct the affected eye. Patients with a complete CN III palsy will also have ptosis and may have a dilated pupil (**Figure 3.5**).

The diplopia that results during range of motion in patients with an ocular myositis or trauma is different from the diplopia seen with a CN palsy. Ocular myositis can be distinguished from CN pathology in that it abruptly restricts eye movement away from the muscle, whereas a CN palsy smoothly and progressively impairs movement toward the weakened muscle. Entrapment of the inferior rectus muscle after trauma to the eye or face prevents the affected eye from tracking with the nonaffected eye, especially on upward gaze.

Funduscopic Examination (Posterior Chamber Examination)

Funduscopy is performed to look for signs of retinal pathology and papilledema (**Figure 3.6**). More details, for example, hemorrhage, exudate, and abnormalities of the optic disc, are visible if the eyes are dilated. Structures of the posterior chamber include the retina, macula, fovea, optic nerve, optic disk, the central retinal artery, the retinal veins, and the vitreous.

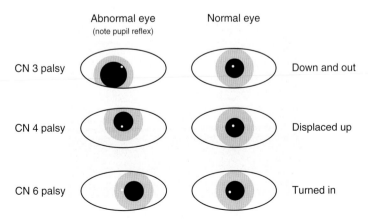

Figure 3.5: Abnormal and normal cranial nerve (CN) palsies.

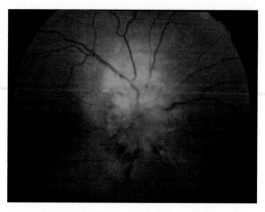

Figure 3.6: Papilledema—note the obscured optic disk margins and hyperemia due to dilated capillaries.

Patients presenting with acute sudden vision loss most often have pathology in the posterior chamber: CRAO, CRVO, retinal detachment, or vitreous hemorrhage. Patients with a CRAO may also have a relative afferent pupillary defect regardless of their visual acuity. Classic ophthalmoscopy signs include retinal edema (ischemic retinal whitening) and a cherry red spot due to underlying normal choroidal circulation (**Figure 3.7**). In the acute phase, segmentation of blood in retinal arterioles, known as box-cars may also be seen. A retinal embolus may be visible in up to 40% of patients.

Patients with a CRVO will have findings of a blurred optic disk margin and areas of ischemia and hemorrhage in the retina (**Figure 3.8**). Patients with a retinal detachment and hemorrhage may present with complaints of floaters or vision loss. A retinal detachment will appear as marked elevation or separation from the surrounding retinal (retinal fold or flap) (**Figure 3.9**). The detachment may appear gray, with dark blood vessels in the folds. The vitreous should also be examined for signs of pigment that looks like dust the color of tobacco (Shafer sign), which is suggestive of a retinal detachment. In retinal hemorrhage that is dispersed, red blood cells can be seen posterior to the lens in the vitreous. In localized retinal hemorrhages, the bleeding will be seen within the area of the retinal involved.

Bedside point-of-care ultrasonography of the eye has become a valuable adjunct in the physical examination of patients with eye complaints, especially in cases of posterior chamber pathology. Retinal detachments and retinal hemorrhage can be rapidly and accurately visualized on ultrasonography of the eye (see "Ocular Ultrasound" section).

Findings in optic nerve pathology will vary on direct ophthalmoscopy. Patients with glaucoma will present with a large optic cup. Patients with optic neuritis frequently will have a normal examination, although the optic nerve may be swollen in some patients (more extensive optic neuritis).

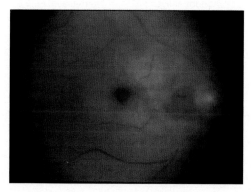

Figure 3.7: Central retinal artery occlusion—retinal edema (ischemic retinal whitening) and a cherry red spot due to underlying normal choroidal circulation.

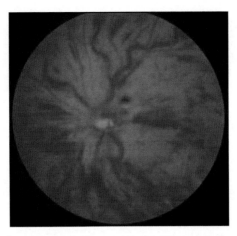

Figure 3.8: Central retinal venous occlusion—note the blurred optic disk margin as well as areas of ischemia and hemorrhage in the retina.

Bilateral optic disc swelling is seen in intracranial hypertension, from idiopathic intracranial hypertension (see Figure 3.6) , cerebral venous sinus thrombosis, or intracranial hemorrhage. Unilateral papilledema is extremely rare and suggests a disease in the eye itself such as a mass/tumor.

Slit Lamp Examination (Anterior Chamber Examination)
The slit lamp examination allows for visualization of the structures of the anterior chamber of the eye including the sclera, conjunctiva, cornea, iris, pupil, lens, and the aqueous humor. Signs of inflammation or infection in the structures of the anterior chamber, known as *cell* and *flares*, are a critical physical examination finding of iritis (traumatic or infectious) or uveitis. The cornea should be examined for injection, chemosis, opacification, discharge, and foreign bodies. The lens should be examined for opacification (cataract) and for positional changes. Subluxation of the lens can occur spontaneously or after trauma, causing vision loss or monocular diplopia. The abnormal lens is apparent on direct visualization or ultrasonography. If a foreign body is suspected, the eyelids should be everted to rule out a retained foreign body under the eyelid. A small hyphema or hypopyon, not seen on external examination, should be visualized on slit lamp.

Patients presenting with painful vision loss, whether sudden or gradual, should have a thorough anterior chamber examination to look for signs of acute narrow-angle glaucoma, iritis, temporal arteritis, optic neuritis, and lens dislocation or subluxation. Patients with acute narrow-angle glaucoma will present with varying complaints ranging from a sudden-onset headache and vomiting to eye pain and sudden painful vision loss. Physical examination usually reveals a red eye with

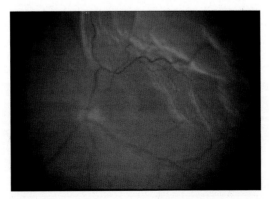

Figure 3.9: Retinal detachment that appears as marked elevation or separation from the surrounding retinal (retinal fold or flap in top right quarter of the retina).

TABLE 3.2	Treatment of Acute Angle-Closure Glaucoma/Increased Intraocular Pressure	
Reduce Aqueous Humor Production		**Increase Outflow**
• Topical β-blocker: timolol 0.5%, 1-2 qtt • Carbonic anhydrase inhibitor: acetazolamide 500 mg IV or po • Systemic osmotic agent: mannitol, 1-2 g/kg IV (use if IOP still elevated after other treatments)		• Topical α-agonist: phenylephrine 1 qtt • Miotics: pilocarpine 1%-2% • Topical steroid: prednisolone acetate 1%, 1 qtt q 15 min ×4, then hourly

IOP, intraocular pressure; IV, intravenous; po, per oral.

perilimbal injection, conjunctival edema, and increased IOP (>50 mm Hg). Patients may also have a dilated, poorly reactive pupil (**Table 3.2**). Experienced providers may be able to see a shallow anterior chamber depth on slit lamp examination or ocular US.

   Iritis (anterior uveitis) may be infectious, traumatic, or the result of a systemic disease or an autoimmune process. It classically presents with eye pain, blurry or decreased vision, and photophobia. Patients may also have a small, constricted pupil on the affected side. Physical examination classically reveals perilimbal redness ("ciliary flush") and cells and flares on slit lamp examination (**Table 3.3**).

Fluorescein Examination

The fluorescein examination involves staining the eye with fluorescein and examining the eye under a cobalt-blue light to look for abnormalities in the cornea, including corneal abrasions, ulcerations, and foreign bodies. The pattern of fluorescence uptake can also diagnose retained foreign bodies and inflammatory and infectious processes such as ultraviolet (UV) keratitis and herpes zoster. A retained foreign body under the upper eyelid may present with the "ice-rink sign" (multiple linear, superficial abrasions with the appearance of skate marks on ice). In cases of a retained foreign body, the slit lamp can also be used to provide magnified visualization and aid in removal. Herpes zoster is diagnosed by the presence of a dendritic lesion on fluorescein examination. UV keratitis, classically seen in welders or in UV exposures, is the most common cause of radiation injury to the eye, and fluorescein staining will show superficial punctate epithelial surface irregularities covering the entire surface of the cornea. Seidel sign, streaming of the aqueous humor through the fluorescein stain, is indicative of a ruptured or perforated globe.

Intraocular Pressure Measurements

IOPs must be documented in patients presenting with eye complaints, which are not relieved by topical anesthetics, to rule out pathology presenting with increased IOP, primarily glaucoma. Baseline IOP measurements should be obtained in patients with a hyphema, hypopyon, or iritis. Topical anesthetics should be applied before measuring IOPs. A suspected ruptured globe is a contraindication to obtaining IOPs.

Ocular Ultrasound

Ocular US is performed with the linear or high-frequency transducer. Apply gel and the US probe to the exterior of the closed eye. Set the gain so that the structures in the posterior chamber are visible. Ask the patient to move the eye left to right and up and down. A retinal detachment

TABLE 3.3	Comparison of Anterior Chamber Pathology			
	Conjunctivitis[a]	**Iritis**	**Acute Glaucoma**	**Corneal Infection/Trauma**
Photophobia	None	Marked	Slight	Slight
Pain	None	Slight/marked	Marked	Marked
VA	Normal	Reduced	Reduced	Varies
Pupil	Normal	Smaller/normal	Large/fixed	Smaller/normal

VA, visual acuity.
[a]Not all red eyes are conjunctivitis.

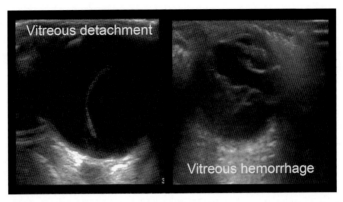

Figure 3.10: In a vitreous detachment the detached retina is tethered down at the optic nerve. Vitreous Hemorrhage on US appears as hyperechoic material in posterior chamber. Courtesy of Dr. Petra Duran, Jacksonville, FL.

(see **Figure 3.10**) will appear as a thick flap that is tethered to the posterior retina and is easily visualized on low gain. Increase the gain slowly while the patient moves their eye to check for posterior vitreous detachments (PVDs) and vitreous hemorrhage. PVDs are only loosely adherent and will float in the vitreous body, giving it the appearance of swaying seaweed. Vitreous hemorrhage will be seen as diffuse mobile opacities on high gain, taking on a "snow globe" appearance[3] (**Figure 3.10**).

The optic nerve sheath diameter (ONSD) can be used as a surrogate measure for intracranial pressure because the optic nerve sheath attaches to the posterior aspect of the globe and is contiguous with the subarachnoid space. To measure the ONSD, have the patient stare straight ahead without squinting and adjust the depth so that the eye fits within the entire screen. The gain should be adjusted to optimize optic nerve visualization in the posterior orbital fat. Measure the ONSD at a distance 3 mm posterior (deep) to the globe, where the US contrast is greatest. An ONSD greater than 5 mm in adults and 4 mm in infants suggests elevated intracranial pressure. In patients with increased intracranial pressure, the optic nerve sheath may also appear to have a crescent sign[4] (**Figure 3.11**).

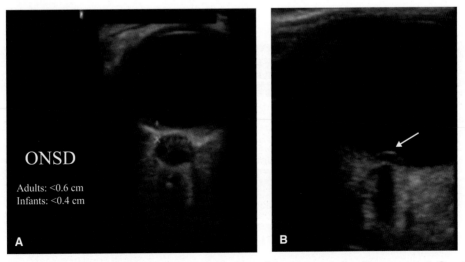

Figure 3.11: Optic nerve sheath diameter (ONSD; A) and the crescent sign (B, see arrow). Courtesy of Dr. Petra Duran, Jacksonville, FL.

CLINICAL DECISION-MAKING

Diagnosis of eye complaints can often be made with history and physical examination alone without the need for ancillary testing. Intraocular pathology usually presents with either a complaint of changes in vision or loss of vision with or without eye pain and can be divided into two categories: anterior chamber pathology, which most often presents with abnormal vision or sudden painful vision loss/changes, and posterior chamber pathology, which classically presents with complaints of floaters or sudden painless vision loss.

Extraocular pathology can present with complaints across the spectrum: visual changes with or without pain, unilateral or bilateral complaints, diplopia or visual field deficits, and other neurologic complaints. Pathologies causing a field cut interfere with the stimulus transmission between the retina and the visual cortex, whereas binocular diplopia usually occurs when ocular mobility is affected. Patients with retrobulbar or extraocular sign and symptoms will need further workup. Patients with a suspicion for systemic pathology such as hypertension, diabetes mellitus, myasthenia gravis, multiple sclerosis, thyroid disease, vascular disorders, or stroke should have appropriate ancillary testing. Patients presenting with eye complaints consistent with a stroke-equivalent CRAO or a neurologic finding consistent with brainstem pathology need emergent neuroimaging to determine whether possible interventional therapies are needed. The inflammatory markers erythrocyte sedimentation rate (ESR) and C-reactive protein (CRP) are nonspecific, but should be considered in older patients presenting with complaints of headache and abnormal vision or with a new-onset binocular diplopia to rule out vasculitis and other inflammatory conditions.

Patients with a suspicion for infectious or autoimmune pathology will need additional laboratory testing and imaging. Orbital infectious processes are readily visualized on contrast CT of the orbits; however, extraocular muscles are best imaged by MRI of the orbits with gadolinium and high-resolution cuts through the brainstem. If MRI of the orbits is not available, a contrast-enhanced cranial CT scan with fine cuts through the orbit can be used as a second-line option. Most patients presenting with binocular diplopia will need either CT or MRI imaging, with MRI being the study of choice in most cases. An MRI should be ordered when symptoms suggest a demyelinating process.

Lumbar puncture (LP) is diagnostic of CNS infections involving the eye and useful for inflammatory conditions that extend to the central nervous system. Neuroimaging is recommended before LP in patients with papilledema or focal neurologic findings.

Intraocular Pathology

Anterior Chamber Pathology

Anterior chamber pathology (**Table 3.4**) includes injury and disease of the cornea, hyphema, hypopyon, cataracts, lens dislocation, iritis/uveitis, endophthalmitis, and acute glaucoma. Eye pain associated

TABLE 3.4	Anterior Chamber Pathology	
	History and Physical Exam Finding	**Treatments**
Cornea Infection Abrasion/Ulcerations	• Pain • Redness • Tearing • Foreign body sensation • Fluorescein uptake	• Cycloplegic agent • Topical steroid—0.5% topical cyclosporine • Topical pain control • Broad-spectrum topical antibiotics—0.3% ciprofloxacin qid

Foreign body	• +/- Foreign body/rust ring	• Foreign body removal
		  • irrigation
		  • moistened cotton-tipped applicator
		  • sterile spud or a 25/27-gauge needle
		• +/- Ophthalmology consult

TABLE 3.4	Anterior Chamber Pathology (*continued*)	
	History and Physical Exam Finding	**Treatments**
Herpes Zoster Keratitis	• Dendritic lesion on fluorescein exam	• Topical: Trifluridine ophthalmic solution 1%—1 drop in affected eye 9 times/day for 7 days Ganciclovir ophthalmic gel 0.15%—1 drop in affected eye 5 times/day for 7 days • Oral: Acyclovir—400 mg 3-5 times/day for 7 days Valacyclovir—500 mg twice daily for 7 days Famciclovir—250 mg twice daily for 7 days
Hyphema	• Pain • Blurred vision • Blood in the anterior chamber	• Eye shield, limited activity, and head of bed elevation of at least 45 degrees • Topical corticosteroids • Topical cycloplegic agents (use in patients with significant ciliary spasm or photophobia) • TXA (for patients at higher risk for rebleeding)
Lens dislocation/subluxation	• Sudden vision change	• Urgent ophthalmology referral
Iritis/uveitis	• Decreased visual acuity • Photophobia • Ciliary flush • Cells and flares in the anterior chamber	• Traumatic: topical steroids, pain control and mydraitics/cycloplegic • Infectious: add antibiotics and/or antivirals with ocular penetrance in addition to above • Autoimmune: may need an immunosuppressive agent added • Elevated intraocular pressure: should be treated if present
Endophthalmitis	• Rapidly progressive blurred vision and eye pain • Decreased visual acuity • Lid swelling • Conjunctival and corneal edema • Cells and flares in the anterior chamber • +/− Hypopyon	• Emergent ophthamology consult • Intravenous antibiotics with ocular penetrance: ceftazidime, cefazoline, ciprofloxacin, gatifloxacin, or moxifloxacin • +/− Corticosteroids (avoided in suspected fungal infection)
Acute Glaucoma	• Sudden onset eye pain or headache • Nausea and vomiting • Decreased visual acuity • Red eye with a mid-dilated pupil • Steamy cornea • Elevated intraocular pressure (greater than 50 mm Hg)	Emergent Ophthalmology consult Decrease IOP (see Table 3.2). • Goal is to lower IOP to less than 40 mm Hg or by 25 % Surgery is the definitive treatment.

with cornea pathology will typically resolve with a topical anesthetic, whereas pain from more serious eye pathology, such as glaucoma, uveitis, and intraocular foreign body, will not. Most anterior chamber pathology will be diagnosed on physical examination without the need for further workup.

Posterior Chamber Pathology
See **Table 3.5**.

Central Retinal Venous Occlusion
CRVO presents with sudden, unilateral, painless vision loss, and findings that may include a blurred optic disc margin as well as areas of ischemia and hemorrhage ("blood and thunder") in the retina on physical examination (see Figure 3.8). Ophthalmology should be emergently consulted in patients with CRVO. The treatment is directed toward decreasing associated macular edema and inhibiting neovascular growth. Recent studies conclude that antivascular endothelial growth factor agents have superior efficacy and safety compared to other treatments.[5,6] Antithrombotic therapy, particularly low-molecular-weight heparins, has a role with improved visual acuity and fewer adverse outcomes.[7] Nonischemic etiologies are associated with an improved chance of a residual visual acuity better than 20/100, whereas ischemic cases fare much worse.

Central Retinal Artery Occlusion
Patients with a CRAO classically present with complete, sudden, painless, monocular vision loss. Patients may have a relative afferent pupillary defect regardless of their visual acuity, retinal edema, and a cherry red spot (the red background of the choroid in the central retina is sharply outlined by the edematous peripheral retina; see Figure 3.7). CRAO can be caused by an embolus, a thrombus, vasospasm, or a vasculitis that occludes the central retinal artery, leading to ischemia of the retina. Patients may also report waxing and waning symptoms of temporary monocular vision loss, that is, amaurosis fugax.

Amaurosis fugax may be a manifestation of proximal cerebrovascular disease or a TIA. Workup and disposition are the same as that for any TIA. In addition, amaurosis fugax may be the presenting symptom of other disease processes such as inflammation, arteritis, or a retinal migraine. Ancillary testing in younger patients without cardiovascular risk factors may be needed to rule out

TABLE 3.5 Posterior Chamber Pathology	Physical Exam Finding	Treatments
Retinal detachment	Floaters Photopsia Decreased vision Appearance of a fold or flap within the retina (Figure 7)	Emergent Ophthalmology consult Surgery is the definitive treatment.
Vitreous hemorrhage	Floaters Photopsia Decreased vision Blood posterior to the lens or in retina	Ophthalmology consult Stop any anticoagulation if possible
Central retinal vein occlusion (CRVO)	Sudden, unilateral, painless vision loss Blurred optic disk margin Areas of ischemia and hemorrhage ("blood and thunder") on exam	Emergent Ophthalmology consult Anti-vascular endothelial growth factor agents Antithrombotic therapy
Central retinal artery occlusion (CRAO)	Complete, sudden, painless, monocular vision loss Relative afferent pupillary defect Retinal edema Cherry red spot	Treat as a stroke equivalent emergent ophthalmology and neurology consults

other causes of transient vision loss. Retinal migraine, caused by reversible vasospasm, is a diagnosis of exclusion.

CRAO is a stroke and should be treated as such. Ancillary testing, including labs and imaging, should be tailored depending on individual findings, but may include complete blood count, metabolic panel, coagulation profile, CT head, computed tomography angiography (CTA) of the head and neck plus a CT diffusion scan, and/or MRI/magnetic resonance angiography (MRA) of the head and neck. Ophthalmology and neurology should be consulted in patients with recent onset of symptoms. Patients may need to be transferred to a stroke center for rapid diagnostics and treatment, although treatment is controversial and there is no accepted standard; see "Evidence" section. We recommend that stroke centers proactively establish a protocol for diagnosing and managing CRAO.

Optic Nerve Pathology

Optic Neuritis

Optic neuritis is a demyelinating inflammatory condition of the optic nerve that has many causes (**Table 3.6**), but is most often associated with multiple sclerosis. Half of the patients diagnosed with new-onset optic neuritis will ultimately be found to have multiple sclerosis. Optic neuritis typically presents as blurred vision or vision loss and pain on eye movement. It can be unilateral or bilateral, and may include field cuts, an afferent pupillary defect, and changes in color vision (dyschromatopsia). Adults more often present with unilateral optic neuritis, whereas children more commonly present with bilateral involvement. The diagnosis in the ED is largely clinical because the optic nerve most commonly appears normal on examination. Only 30% of patients will have an edematous optic disc of funduscopy.

The diagnosis is supported by the presence of an afferent pupillary defect and dyschromatopsia that is assessed by color plate testing and the red desaturation test. Testing of color vision complements the assessment of visual acuity in optic neuritis because the degree of dyschromatopsia may be proportionately greater than the degree of visual acuity loss. Persistent dyschromatopsia is common even after recovery of visual acuity in optic neuropathy. Optic neuritis, from causes other than multiple sclerosis, tends to have worse visual outcomes.

If the retina, in addition to the optic nerve, is involved, the diagnosis is neuroretinitis. In neuroretinitis, the disc is markedly swollen and a stellate figure composed of hard exudates is seen in the macula (in severe cases). Patients with neuroretinitis are not at increased risk for multiple sclerosis.

MRI of the orbit and brain, to look for inflammation of the optic nerve and demyelination in the brain, are the most important ancillary tests. Optic neuritis, with two or more non–contrast-enhancing lesions on MRI, is associated with a high risk of multiple sclerosis.

TABLE 3.6 Causes of Optic Neuritis

Multiple Sclerosis
Leber's disease (hereditary)
Infectious
- Tuberculosis
- Lyme disease
- Cryptococcal meningitis
- Herpes zoster
- Syphilis

Autoimmune
- Sarcoidosis
- Systemic lupus erythematosus
- Wegener's granulomatosis

Ischemia
Diabetes
Vitamin B12 deficiency
Methanol toxicity

Current guidelines for the treatment of optic neuritis are high-dose intravenous methylprednisolone at a dose of 500 to 1000 mg/day for 3 to 5 days.

Neuromyelitis Optica

Neuromyelitis optica (Devic syndrome), a rare demyelinating disease that presents with optic neuritis and transverse myelitis extending over at least two to three segments of the spinal cord, accounts for 1% to 3% of cases of optic neuritis. Patients more commonly present with bilateral optic neuritis plus weakness or numbness in the arms and legs and bowel or bladder incontinence, with sparing of the brain. Neuromyelitis optica can be seen in children, but is most common between ages 40 and 50. Optic neuritis is more often bilateral in neuromyelitis optica than in multiple sclerosis. Serum testing for antibodies to aquaporin-4, a water channel protein, is diagnostic, but may be absent in 20% of cases. Treatment for new-onset neuromyelitis optica is high-dose intravenous methylprednisolone and plasma exchange if there is no improvement.[8]

Anterior Ischemic Optic Neuropathy

Anterior ischemic optic neuropathy (AION) refers to ischemic damage to the optic disc. Patients will present with sudden, painless vision loss that can be unilateral or bilateral. Causes of AION include giant cell or temporal arthritis (arteritic or A-AION), diabetes, hypertension, systemic vascular disease, and other noninflammatory causes. A swollen optic disc should be seen on funduscopy and ED point-of-care ultrasound can aid in the diagnosis. Treatment is targeted at identifying and correcting the precipitant cause as well as discontinuing any contributing medications.

Giant cell or temporal arteritis (arteritic AION) is classically seen in patients older than age 50, with fever, malaise, headache or scalp tenderness, jaw claudication, and findings of polymyalgia rheumatica. The workup in these patients should comprise ancillary testing including an ESR. A significantly elevated ESR (>50) is common, but not always present.[9,10] Steroids are recommended for patients with a high clinical suspicion of giant cell arteritis, and patients should be admitted pending a temporal artery biopsy. The optimal dose of steroids remains undefined, but consensus statements recommend the equivalent of prednisone at 40 to 60 mg/day, with individualized tapering regimens based on response.[11] Methotrexate and other immunosuppressants are used as adjuncts to steroid therapy, but need not be started in the ED. If untreated, blindness frequently results, and symptoms may progress to involve both eyes.

Posterior Ischemic Optic Neuropathy

Posterior ischemic optic neuropathy (PION), which is also referred to as retrobulbar neuritis, is damage to the posterior or retrobulbar optic nerve. PION is less common than is AION, and is more difficult to diagnose, because the optic nerves appear normal initially. PION may be caused by giant cell arteritis, and is treated the same as in arteritic AION. Bilateral PION may also be seen in cases of watershed ischemia from significant acute blood loss, which may occur perioperatively. There is no treatment for nonarteritic PION disease and the process is irreversible.

Neuro-Ophthalmologic and Other Retrobulbar Etiologies (Extraocular Pathology)

Diplopia

Monocular diplopia, diplopia that does not resolve when one eye is closed, is an ophthalmologic problem related to distortions in the light path from dry eyes, a corneal irregularity, cataract, lens dislocation or, rarely, from retinal wrinkles involving the macula. In rare cases, monocular diplopia may be the presenting complaint in conversion disorder, but this is a diagnosis of exclusion.

The differential for binocular diplopia is extensive and requires the clinician to determine the cause of "ocular misalignment," which can be either gross or subtle. **Table 3.7** outlines some key causes of binocular diplopia. The most common cause of binocular diplopia is extraocular muscle dysfunction. Other causes of binocular diplopia are restrictive mechanical orbitopathies, neuraxial processes involving the brainstem and related CNs, systemic neuromuscular processes, or trauma. Observation of the eye movement velocity can help differentiate between categories. In neurogenic paresis, as the eyes move into the direction of the defect, the underacting eye moves smoothly but

TABLE 3.7	Differential for Binocular Diplopia
Orbital pathology	• Trauma • Infection/abscess • Craniofacial masses • Thyroid eye disease • Wegener granulomatosis • Giant cell arteritis • Systemic lupus erythematosus • Sarcoidosis • Rheumatoid arthritis

Cranial nerve palsies:
   Cranial nerve III
   Cranial nerve IV
   Cranial nerve VI
	• Multiple sclerosis
	• Hypertensive vasculopathy
	• Diabetic vasculopathy
	• Compression
	• Trauma
	• Cavernous sinus infection, mass, vasculitis or thrombosis
	• Orbital apex syndrome
	• Idiopathic intracranial hypertension

Neuroaxial process involving the brainstem and cranial nerves:	• Multiple sclerosis • Tumor • Stroke • Hemorrhage • Basilar artery thrombosis • Vertebral artery dissection • Ophthalmoplegic migraine • Basilar meningoencephalitis • Miller-Fisher or Guillain-Barré syndrome • Wernicke encephalopathy • Tick-borne diseases
Systemic disease	• Myasthenia gravis • Botulism

progressively slower than does the normal other eye. By contrast, in restrictive mechanical orbitopathies, eye movements will be smooth and symmetrical until the eye meets the point of obstruction, which causes abrupt slowing.

In general, diplopia secondary to brainstem lesions is accompanied by other neurologic symptoms including hemiparesis, abnormal movement, CN deficits, and cerebellar signs. However, a single ocular nerve palsy in the absence of other neurologic signs can be the presentation of more significant neurologic disease. Myasthenia gravis should be considered if the ocular motility restriction does not follow the distribution of any particular ocular motor nerve.

Cranial Nerve Palsies and Extraocular Muscle Dysfunction

Causes of an isolated oculomotor nerve palsy in CNs III (oculomotor nerve), IV (trochlear nerve), or VI (abducens nerve) include a demyelinating process (multiple sclerosis), trauma, or compression; however, the most common cause is hypertensive and diabetic vasculopathy. Diplopia that worsens on lateral gaze to one direction implies an issue with the abducens nerve (CN VI). Owing to its length, CN VI is the most common CN palsy, accounting for 50% of all CN palsies. Pain and speed of onset are differentiators. A sudden isolated CN III, IV, or VI palsy associated with orbital discomfort in a patient with chronic diabetes or hypertension strongly suggests microvascular ischemia as the cause. Owing to its length, CN VI is susceptible to increased intracranial pressure, and bilateral CN VI palsy may be the initial presentation of patients with elevated intracranial pressure.

A vertical or sometimes torsional diplopia that worsens on looking down and toward the nose implies a superior oblique (CN IV) palsy. A CN IV palsy makes descending stairs, reading, and watching television in bed difficult. CN IV is more susceptible to trauma because it sits against the tentorium.

The oculomotor nerve controls the inferior oblique and the medial, inferior, and superior recti muscles as well. It also innervates the levator palpebrae superior muscle and the ciliary and constrictor pupillae muscles, making it responsible for eyelid control and pupillary constriction. The patient with a complete CN III palsy typically reports diplopia in all directions of gaze, except on lateral gaze to the affected side, and an eye that is deviated down and out, with a dilated pupil and ptosis. Hypertensive and diabetic vasculopathy is the most common cause of CN III palsy, and classically presents with pupil sparing because the pupillomotor parasympathetic fibers run on the exterior of the nerve and are not affected by ischemia to the same degree as the deeper fibers. Patients presenting with a compressive lesion, such as an aneurysm, will often have pupillary mydriasis due to the compression of the fiber.

Most patients presenting with binocular diplopia will undergo CT or MRI in the ED, but imaging should be directed by the history and physical examination (**Figure 3.12**). Patients with a history of trauma and diplopia should undergo CT and/or MRI. For an isolated neuropathy of CN III, IV, or VI presenting without clinical suspicion of a ruptured aneurysm, the optimal study is MRI with fat-suppressed orbital imaging to assess for inflammation, neoplasm, or demyelination along the course of the nerves; see "Evidence" section.

In contrast to an isolated CN palsy, the combination of ipsilateral palsies of CN III, IV, and VI should raise concern for cavernous sinus or orbital apex pathology due to the nerves running in close proximity in those areas. The orbital apex is the posterior part of the orbit and houses the extraocular rectus muscles, CN III, CN IV, CN V, and CN VI, as well as the optic nerve. The cavernous sinus is a venous plexus located in the base of the skull. It occupies the space directly below the optic chiasm, directly medial to the sella turcica and above the sphenoid sinus and houses CN III, CN IV, CN V, and CN VI plus the internal carotid artery. Trauma, infection, tumor/mass, vasculitis, and thyroid disease can all cause pathology in the orbital apex or cavernous sinus. An orbital apex or cavernous sinus process will typically present with additional findings of exophthalmos, chemosis, and injection. Because the V1 and V2 branches of the trigeminal nerve travel through these structures, the patient may also have associated ipsilateral periorbital facial numbness or dysesthesia.

Cavernous sinus thrombosis occurs because of inflammation related to spread of infection from the surrounding structures, to include orbital cellulitis and abscess, sphenoid sinusitis, mastoiditis, and dental infections. Signs and symptoms include pain, diplopia, altered mental status, proptosis, orbital swelling, ophthalmoplegia, and headache. Cavernous sinus pathology may present initially with isolated CN VI involvement because it traverses through the cavernous sinus, as opposed to CNs III and IV that are located within its wall. In addition, bilateral eye findings may be present in cases of cavernous sinus thrombosis because the cavernous sinuses directly communicate.

For cavernous sinus pathology, a magnetic resonance venogram (MRV) or computed tomography venogram (CTV) of the brain and orbits should be ordered. An orbital apex syndrome is more commonly associated with decreased visual acuity because the optic nerve passes through the orbital apex. The extraocular muscles in an orbital apex syndrome are best imaged by MRI of the orbits with gadolinium and high-resolution cuts through the brainstem. If MRI of the orbits is not available, a contrast-enhanced cranial CT scan with fine cuts through the orbit can be used as a second-line option. An MRI should be ordered when symptoms suggest a demyelinating process.[11,12]

Cavernous sinus thrombosis should be treated with broad-spectrum antibiotics because septic thrombosis is the most common cause, with Streptococcal and Staphylococcal being the biggest culprits. Antifungal therapy may be added in patients who are at higher risk for fungal infections, for example, chronic sinusitis and diabetes. Anticoagulation is used unless contraindications are present; however, there are no prospective trials for this therapy, and evidence is from retrospective reviews and case reports only.[13] Corticosteroids are often given, but there is no evidence of benefit. Surgical decompression or drainage may be required for source control and definitive therapy.

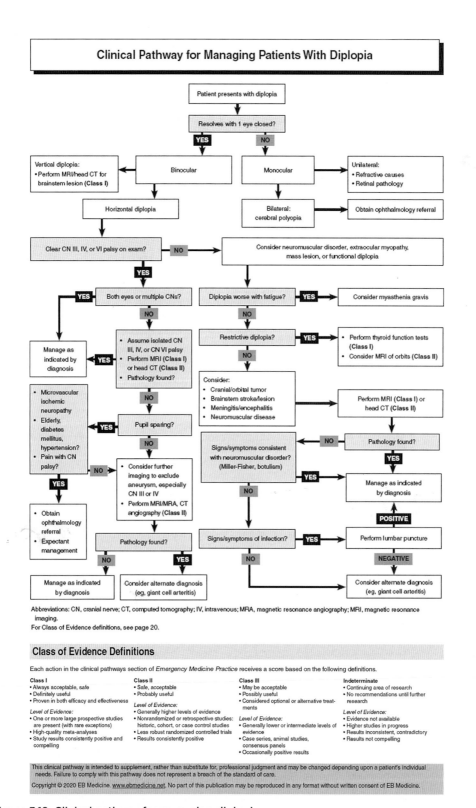

Abbreviations: CN, cranial nerve; CT, computed tomography; IV, intravenous; MRA, magnetic resonance angiography; MRI, magnetic resonance imaging.
For Class of Evidence definitions, see page 20.

Class of Evidence Definitions

Each action in the clinical pathways section of *Emergency Medicine Practice* receives a score based on the following definitions.

Class I	Class II	Class III	Indeterminate
• Always acceptable, safe • Definitely useful • Proven in both efficacy and effectiveness	• Safe, acceptable • Probably useful	• May be acceptable • Possibly useful • Considered optional or alternative treatments	• Continuing area of research • No recommendations until further research
Level of Evidence: • One or more large prospective studies are present (with rare exceptions) • High-quality meta-analyses • Study results consistently positive and compelling	*Level of Evidence:* • Generally higher levels of evidence • Nonrandomized or retrospective studies: historic, cohort, or case control studies • Less robust randomized controlled trials • Results consistently positive	*Level of Evidence:* • Generally lower or intermediate levels of evidence • Case series, animal studies, consensus panels • Occasionally positive results	*Level of Evidence:* • Evidence not available • Higher studies in progress • Results inconsistent, contradictory • Results not compelling

This clinical pathway is intended to supplement, rather than substitute for, professional judgment and may be changed depending upon a patient's individual needs. Failure to comply with this pathway does not represent a breach of the standard of care.

Figure 3.12: Clinical pathway for managing diplopia.
Used with permission of EB Medicine, publisher of *Emergency Medicine Practice. Kelly O'Keefe, Sarah Temple. An Evidence-Based Approach to Abnormal Vision in the Emergency Department. Emergency Medicine Practice.* 2020;22(4):1-28. © 2020 EB Medicine. www.ebmedicine.net

Mechanical Orbitopathy

A restrictive mechanical orbitopathy can be caused by orbital myositis, trauma, infection/abscess, or craniofacial masses, any of which can directly restrict movement of a single eye. A structural restriction of motion of a single eye, typically gradual in onset, may cause diplopia in a single or in multiple directions of gaze, depending on the type and extent of muscular involvement. A sensation of mass effect, discomfort, or pain in the culprit eye is a characteristic symptom. If the cause is infectious, the patient may have a history of fever. Signs of a structural orbitopathy or myositis include proptosis, periorbital swelling, edema, conjunctival or scleral hyperemia, and palpebral swelling involving a single eye.

Thyroid eye disease is a cause of restrictive orbitopathy caused by the enlargement or fibrosis of the extraocular muscles. It is most commonly seen in Graves disease; however, it can also be seen in other autoimmune thyroid conditions, and up to 10% of patients can be euthyroid or hypothyroid. Patients may present with isolated diplopia before the onset of systemic symptoms. Stigmata of thyroid eye disease include proptosis, eye lid retraction, diffuse conjunctival edema, and vascular injection.

PEDIATRIC ISSUES

- Optic neuritis is much less common in children than in adults, but is not rare and accounts for approximately a quarter of pediatric acute demyelinating syndromes. In addition, optic neuritis in children is most often postinfectious or postviral. Children younger than 10 years usually present with complaints of headache and with bilateral optic neuritis, whereas older children and adults usually present with unilateral optic neuritis. Children have a much lower probability of recurrent demyelinating events and a diagnosis of MS. The established treatment for children with optic neuritis is intravenous methylprednisolone 30 mg/kg/d (maximum 1 g daily) for 3 to 5 days.
- Children presenting with new-onset diplopia and a CN palsy should always undergo emergent MRI because compression is the most common cause of pathology in the pediatric population.

TIPS AND PEARLS

- Red flags for abnormal vision complaints: sudden change in vision, eye pain (with or without eye movement), visible abnormality of the retina or optic disk, diplopia or a visual field defect (by history or examination), presence of associated neurologic symptoms, and a history of HIV/acquired immunodeficiency disease syndrome (AIDS) or other immunosuppressive disorders.
- Sudden painless vision loss points to posterior chamber pathology and should be seen on ophthalmoscopy: retinal detachment or hemorrhage, CRVO, and CRAO.
- Sudden painful vision loss points to anterior chamber pathology: abrasion, ulceration, iritis/uveitis, acute glaucoma.
- Acute monocular vision loss with an afferent pupillary defect indicates a lesion of the eye or of the optic nerve (optic neuritis) anterior to the chiasm.
- The diagnosis of optic neuritis is largely clinical because the optic nerve most commonly appears normal, but is supported by the presence of an afferent pupillary defect and dyschromatopsia on examination.
- When assessing diplopia, look for isolated CN III, IV, and VI palsies first if no other associated symptoms are present.
- Hypertensive and diabetic retinopathies are the most common causes of diplopia.
- When evaluating a CN palsy, keep a high index of suspicion for systemic diseases such as multiple sclerosis, myasthenia gravis, and idiopathic intracranial hypertension.
- Bilateral, symmetric visual field defects suggest a lesion posterior to the chiasm.

SUMMARY

Abnormal vision complaints are common in the ED, and although most can be easily treated, they are alarming to the patient (**Table 3.8**). Likewise, eye complaints can be a challenge for the emergency clinician—the vague complaint of blurry or abnormal vision can be the presenting symptoms of a life-threatening neurologic or systemic disease. The history and physical examination generate the differential diagnosis and direct testing. Threats to sight or brain require rapid diagnosis, consultation, and treatment. It is essential that the emergency clinician have an understanding of evidence-based therapies to maximize the opportunity for full visual recovery.

EVIDENCE

Is there a role for thrombolytics in the treatment of CRAO?

The efficacy and safety of fibrinolysis, systemic thrombolytic therapy, or selective intra-arterial thrombolysis in CRAO remain unknown, and currently there is no generally accepted, evidence-based guideline for the treatment of non-arteritic CRAO.[14-18] One meta-analysis from 2015 found that patients with CRAO treated with fibrinolysis within 4.5 hours of symptom onset did better than the patients who were not treated (50% versus 17.7% improvement, with a number needed to treat of 4.0). However, there are no current prospective randomized controlled trials that support the meta-analysis.[19]

TABLE 3.8	Differential for Abnormal Vision
Painful vision abnormalities	• Trauma • Corneal infection/abrasion/ulceration/foreign body • Hyphema/hypopyon • Abscess • Craniofacial masses • Lens pathology • Iritis/uveitis/endophthalmitis • Acute glaucoma • Optic neuritis • Migraine • Idiopathic intracranial hypertension
Painless vision abnormalities	• Retinal detachment/hemorrhage • Central retinal artery occlusion • Central retinal vein occlusion • Anterior ischemic optic neuropathy/neuromyelitis optica
Diplopia	• Hypertensive/diabetic vasculopathy • Trauma • Aneurysm • Cavernous sinus infection, mass, vasculitis or thrombosis • Orbital apex syndrome • Thyroid eye disease • Giant cell arteritis • Systemic lupus erythematosus/sarcoidosis/rheumatoid arthritis • Multiple sclerosis • Tumor • Stroke/transient ischemic attack/hemorrhage • Basilar artery thrombosis • Vertebral artery dissection • Basilar meningoencephalitis • Miller-Fisher or Guillain-Barré syndrome • Wernicke encephalopathy • Myasthenia gravis • Botulism

Do patients with an isolated CN III, IV, or VI palsy and a history of diabetes and/or hypertension need an emergent neuroimaging study?

There is controversy as to whether patients presenting to the ED with an isolated CN III, IV, or VI palsy, a classic story, and vascular risk factors need emergent imaging. Consensus has been that patients older than 50 years, with vascular risk factors (hypertension, diabetes, smoking) and an isolated CN IV, VI, or a complete CN III palsy with pupil sparing (complete ptosis and no adduction, depression, or elevation; and a normal reactive isocoric pupil) due to microvascular ischemia, may not need neuroimaging because the yield regarding another pathology is low. Imaging may be deferred, absent other red flags, and only performed if symptoms persist past 3 months. However, some references state that with the availability of imaging in the ED and the small likelihood of more ominous pathology, all patients should undergo imaging.[20,21] If there is any equivocation or if there is ipsilateral involvement of more than one oculomotor nerve, imaging should be obtained in the ED because a small percentage of patients with risk factors may have a cause other than microvascular ischemia.[20,21]

Younger patients, or those without vascular risk factors, may require initial neuroimaging and should undergo evaluation for undiagnosed hypertension and diabetes because isolated CN palsy can be the initial clinical presentation of underlying disease. Children presenting with new-onset diplopia and CN IV or VI palsy should undergo emergent MRI because compression is the most common cause of pathology in the pediatric population.

In a patient with a third CN palsy, is an intact pupillary response sufficient to diagnose an ischemic optic neuropathy?

An intact pupillary response is not sufficient to diagnose an ischemic optic neuropathy. A 2017 study showed that 36% of compressive CN III palsies had pupil sparing. Other studies have reported lower percentages. Patients with a CN III palsy and an intact pupillary response can still have a compressive lesion, although the incidence varies depending on the study.[20,21]

Are ESR and/or CRP sensitive markers for temporal arteritis, and can clinical decision-making be based on the finding?

The inflammatory markers ESR and CRP are nonspecific, but should be considered in older patients presenting with complaints of headache and abnormal vision or with a new-onset binocular diplopia to rule out vasculitis and other inflammatory conditions. An elevated ESR greater than 50 is common, but not always present. A 2019 study showed ESR greater than 50 mm/hr and CRP greater than 20 mg/L to have similar sensitivity and specificity for temporal arteritis; however, other studies have shown that a small portion of patients will be diagnosed by biopsy despite normal ESR and CRP levels.[9,10]

Is an afferent nerve defect required to diagnose an optic neuritis?

Clinical practice suggests that an afferent nerve defect occurs in optic neuritis if the other eye is uninvolved and otherwise healthy. We have not been able to identify any studies that support or refute this finding. Also, of note, an afferent nerve defect can be present in other optic nerve pathology.

Is a color plate test required in the ED to assess optic neuritis?

Loss of color vision out of proportion to the loss of visual acuity is specific to optic nerve pathology. Abnormal color vision detection by color plates ranges from 88% to 94% depending on the color plates that are used. However, if color plates are not available in the ED, the red saturation test can be used to screen for color vision.

Are steroids beneficial in optic neuritis?

The Optic Neuritis Treatment Trial showed that treatment with methylprednisolone leads to more rapid recovery of vision in optic neuritis, but does not improve the final outcome with respect to visual acuity, fields, and perception of contrast and color when compared to oral prednisone and placebo. The trial also showed that patients who were treated with low-dose oral prednisolone only were twice as likely as the placebo group to have early recurrences (within 6 months) in their optic neuritis. Low-dose oral prednisolone alone is currently contraindicated for patients with typical optic neuritis.[8] The Optic Neuritis Treatment Trial showed that treatment with IV methylprednisolone (500-1000 mg/d for 3-5 days) leads to more rapid recovery of vision in optic neuritis, but does not improve the final outcome with respect to visual acuity, fields, and perception of contrast and color. Low-dose oral steroids lead to early recurrences in optic neuritis and are contraindicated for patients with typical optic neuritis.[8]

References

1. Vaziri K, Schwartz S, Flynn H, Kishor KS, Moshfeghi AA. Eye-related emergency department visits in the United States, 2010. *Ophthalmology*. 2015;123(4):917-919.

2. De Lott LB, Kerber KA, Lee PP, Brown DL, Burke JF. Diplopia-related ambulatory and emergency department visits in the United States, 2003-2012. *JAMA Ophthalmol*. 2017;135(12):1339-1344.

3. Gottlieb M, Holladay D, Peksa GD. Point-of-care ocular ultrasound for the diagnosis of retinal detachment: a systematic review and meta-analysis. *Acad Emerg Med*. 2019;26:931-939.

4. Hassen GW, Bruck I, Donahue J, et al. Accuracy of optic nerve sheath diameter measurement by emergency physicians using bedside ultrasound. *J Emerg Med*. 2015;48(4):450-457.

5. Brown DM, Campochiaro PA, Singh RP, et al. Ranibizumab for macular edema following central retinal vein occlusion: six-month primary end point results of a phase III study. *Ophthalmology*. 2010;117(6):1124-1133.e1121.

6. Gao L, Zhou L, Tian C, et al. Intravitreal dexamethasone implants versus intravitreal anti-VEGF treatment in treating patients with retinal vein occlusion: a meta-analysis. *BMC Ophthalmol*. 2019;19(1):8.

7. Lazo-Langner A, Hawel J, Ageno W, Kovacs MJ. Low molecular weight heparin for the treatment of retinal vein occlusion: a systematic review and meta-analysis of randomized trials. *Haematologica*. 2010;95(9):1587-1593.

8. Gal RL, Vedula SS, Beck R. Corticosteroids for treating optic neuritis. *Cochrane Database Syst Rev*. 2015(8):CD001430.

9. Li Ying CF, Lester S, Whittle SL, Hill CL. The utility of ESR, CRP and platelets in the diagnosis of GCA. *BMC Rheumatol*. 2019;3:14.

10. Buttgereit F, Dejaco C, Matteson EL, et al. Polymyalgia rheumatica and giant cell arteritis: a systematic review. *JAMA*. 2016;315(22):2442-2458.

11. Mahalingam H, Mani S, Patel B, et al. Imaging spectrum of cavernous sinus lesions with histopathologic correlation. *Radiographics*. 2019;39(3):795-819.

12. Badakere A, Patil-Chhablani P. Orbital apex syndrome: a review. *Eye Brain*. 2019;11:63-72.

13. Van der Poel NA, Mourits MP, de Win MML, et al. Prognosis of septic cavernous sinus thrombosis remarkably improved: a case series of 12 patients and literature review. *Eur Arch Otorhinolaryngol*. 2018;275(9):2387-2395.

14. Chronopoulos A, Schutz JS. Central retinal artery occlusion: a new, provisional treatment approach. *Surv Ophthalmol*. 2019;64(4):443-451.

15. Wolf A, Schumacher M, Neubauer AS, et al. [Comparison of superselective intraarterial fibrinolysis with conservative therapy. Use in patients with acute non-arteritic central retinal artery occlusion]. *Ophthalmologe*. 2010;107(9):799-805.

16. Schumacher M, Schmidt D, Jurklies B, et al. Central retinal artery occlusion: local intra-arterial fibrinolysis versus conservative treatment, a multicenter randomized trial. *Ophthalmology*. 2010;117(7):1367-1375.e1361.

17. Page PS, Khattar NK, White AC, et al. Intra-arterial thrombolysis for acute central retinal artery occlusion: a systematic review and meta-analysis. *Front Neurol*. 2018;9:76.

18. Mehta N, Marco RD, Goldhardt R, Modi Y. Central retinal artery occlusion: acute management and treatment. *Curr Ophthalmol Rep*. 2017;5(2):149-159.

19. Mac GB, Nackenoff A, Poli S, et al. Intravenous fibrinolysis for central retinal artery occlusion: a cohort study and updated patient-level meta-analysis. *Stroke*. 2020;51(7):2018-2025.

20. Tamhankar MA, Biousse V, Ying GS, et al. Isolated third, fourth and sixth cranial nerve palsies from presumed microvascular versus other causes: a prospective study. *Ophthalmology*. 2013;120:2264-2269.

21. Fang C, Leavitt JA, Hodge DO, Holmes JM, Mohney BG, Chen JJ. Incidence and etiologies of acquired third nerve palsy using a population-based method. *JAMA Ophthalmol*. 2017;135(1):23-28.

Weakness

Andy S. Jagoda

Melissa Villars

CLINICAL CHALLENGE

Neurologic weakness is a decrease in muscle strength or power; **weakness** is also a general term commonly used by patients to describe a state of low energy. Neurologic weakness may be a focal symptom, involving a single muscle group, or it may be generalized. A chief complaint of weakness requires a systematic history and physical to develop a working differential diagnosis and to direct testing. Clarification of what the patient means by "weakness" and a distinction between low energy versus diffuse motor weakness versus focal motor weakness is the starting point of the evaluation. The emergency department (ED) approach takes into account the possible, and at times rare, life-threatening causes including stroke, spinal cord lesions, toxic exposures, metabolic abnormalities, botulism, myasthenia gravis, and Guillain-Barré syndrome (GBS), among others. In evaluating weakness, the clinician must always consider disorders that can precipitously compromise the respiratory and functional status of the patient; see **Chapter 7: Myopathies and Neuromuscular Junction Disorders** for a more detailed evaluation of respiratory decompensation.

DIFFERENTIAL DIAGNOSIS

The differential diagnosis of the weak patient is divided into two broad categories: non-neurologic and neurologic causes, although there is overlap between the categories. Generally speaking, neurologic causes present with decreased neuromuscular power or focal abnormality on examination, whereas non-neurologic causes present as a feeling of global fatigue or asthenia and have a much broader list of possible differential diagnoses (**Figure 4.1**). The patient's age is an important consideration in developing the differential diagnosis of weakness. Elderly patients have a higher incidence of comorbid medical conditions than their younger counterparts and are at higher risk of acute central nervous system (CNS) and cardiovascular events. They are more likely to present with occult infections and metabolic disorders that are symptomatically manifested as weakness. In the pediatric age group, sepsis, dehydration, and electrolyte abnormalities are the leading causes of weakness. Infantile botulism and intussusception are two rare but important considerations. Infantile botulism may be seen in children days old to more than 1 year of age. This variant of botulism is much more common than food borne or wound botulism; it presents with weakness, poor tone, poor suck, and/or constipation.

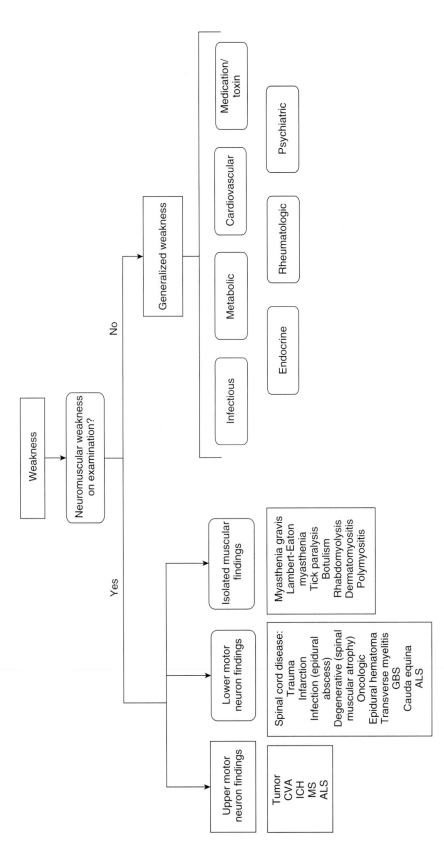

Figure 4.1: Weakness differential diagnoses. ALS, amyotrophic lateral sclerosis; CVA; GBS, Guillain-Barré syndrome; ICH, intracerebral hemorrhage; MS, multiple sclerosis.

Neurologic

Cerebral Lesions

Structural lesions in the CNS, such as tumors, strokes, and multiple sclerosis plaques, generally present with focal weakness though some lesions especially in the posterior circulation may present with nonfocal complaints, for example, difficulty swallowing, talking, or breathing, in addition to weakness. Strokes generally present with focal weakness in an anatomic distribution, see **Chapter 15: Stroke**. Intercranial hemorrhages may present with generalized weakness or have a focal finding on examination depending on the location and size of the hemorrhage.

Spinal Cord Lesions

Lesions in the spinal canal such as epidural hematoma and other vascular diseases, abscess, and metastatic disease can result in weakness that is either symmetric or asymmetric and distal to the site of compromise. Transverse myelitis is an infrequent yet debilitating demyelinating disease of the spinal cord presenting with an acute onset of back pain, lower extremity weakness or paralysis, and sensory deficit. This disease should be suspected in a patient with a recent viral illness presenting with both weakness and sensory deficit below a cord level; it should not be confused with GBS, which will typically demonstrate sparing of the anal sphincter and hyporeflexia with progressive weakness in an ascending pattern over days to a week. Clinical findings of transverse myelitis generally progress over 24 hours and include diminished or absence of strength and sensation below the level of involvement, sphincter dysfunction, hyperreflexia, and urinary incontinence or retention. Spinal epidural abscess also deserves special mention; early presentations can be nonspecific and thus the diagnosis initially missed may potentially lead to disastrous outcomes, see **Chapter XXX: CNS Infections**.

Neuromuscular Diseases

This group of diseases presents with weakness, the origin of which can be at the neuromuscular junction (eg, myasthenia gravis), the peripheral nerve (eg, GBS), or the muscle (eg, metabolic derangements, medications, and inflammatory states).

Non-neurologic

Infections

All infections can potentially cause weakness, either through general dehydration or through nonspecific mechanisms, such as those seen with mononucleosis or hepatitis. Specific toxins can also cause neurologic weakness, for example, poliomyelitis, botulism, or tick paralysis. The human immunodeficiency virus (HIV) can directly or indirectly cause the full spectrum of weaknesses, from nonspecific fatigue to neuropathies and myelopathies.

Metabolic

Metabolic derangements that can present with weakness include hypoxia, hyperthermia, and alterations in serum glucose and electrolytes. Frequently encountered metabolic causes of weakness include hypoglycemia, hypo- and hyperkalemia. Severe hypokalemia presents with generalized weakness and even paralysis. It can be medication induced as in the case of diuretic use, gastrointestinal loss, or rarely in association with genetic disorders such as familial periodic paralysis. Hyperkalemia not only can affect myocardial function but also may cause an ascending paralysis, ultimately leading to respiratory failure. During the summer, elderly patients with heat exhaustion will frequently present to the ED with generalized weakness because of dehydration and inability to regulate their temperature. A buildup of waste products like CO_2 in individuals with chronic obstructive pulmonary disease (COPD), urea in patients with renal failure, and bilirubin in liver failure can also lead to generalized weakness.

Cardiovascular

Acute myocardial infarction (AMI) may present with weakness as the only complaint, especially in the elderly. As the population ages, more patients will present with atypical complaints of myocardial infarction such as weakness or shortness of breath. Myocarditis is another serious but often missed cause of weakness in a patient with a recent viral infection, and these patients may present with a primary complaint of weakness without chest pain. Other cardiovascular causes of weakness associated with light-headedness or presyncope are due to transient decreased cerebral perfusion, for example, postural hypotension, cervical artery insufficiency, aortic stenosis, cardiac dysrhythmias, and states of decreased cardiac output.

Medications and Toxins

Prescription medications are a common cause of generalized weakness especially in the elderly (**Table 4.1**). Beta-blockers are particularly noteworthy. There are usually no focal findings on examination and individual muscle strength testing is normal. In one study of 106 patients with a chief complaint of weakness and dizziness, 9% of all patients and 20% of those older than age 60 had symptoms attributed to prescription medications.[1,2]

Certain toxins can present with the sudden onset of neurologic weakness: Organophosphates and carbamates act at the neuromuscular junction by inhibiting acetylcholinesterase. Patients present with a constellation of symptoms including lacrimation, defecation, salivation, and weakness, which can progress rapidly to paralysis and respiratory failure. In contrast, poisonings from heavy metals can be subtle and present with a slowly progressive course. Carbon monoxide may present with generalized weakness and headache as their only complaint. This diagnosis should be considered in patients presenting with weakness especially during the winter months when space heaters are often used.

Endocrine

Hypothyroidism is the most common endocrine cause of weakness and is frequently not diagnosed early in its presentation. Thyrotoxic periodic paralysis with alternations in potassium regulation can present with weakness as a primary complaint. Adrenal insufficiency, often induced by chronic

TABLE 4.1 Commonly Used Drugs and Other Substances Associated with Weakness
Myopathies
Steroids
Alcohol
Heroin
Clofibrate
Epsilon-aminocaproic acid
Diuretics
Laxatives
Amphotericin
D-Penicillamine
Cimetidine
Procainamide
Neuropathies
Carbon monoxide
Heavy metals
Polychlorinated biphenyls
Isoniazid
Nitrofurantoin
Gold
Neuromuscular Junction Disease
Organophosphates
Carbamates

steroid use, may present with weakness because of hypotension, hyperkalemia, and/or hyponatremia. The diabetic patient with hyperglycemia can present with generalized weakness from ketoacidosis, dehydration, or altered potassium. Cobalamin deficiency (vitamin B_{12}), which is most commonly seen with pernicious anemia, may present with lower extremity weakness, paresthesias, and tongue discomfort and has a macrocytic anemia on laboratory analysis.

Rheumatologic

Weakness is a prominent complaint of most rheumatologic diseases and occasionally is the primary presenting symptom. Diseases to consider include systemic lupus erythematosus, polymyositis, dermatomyositis, and polymyalgia rheumatica.

Psychogenic Weakness

A psychiatric diagnosis as a cause of weakness is one of exclusion and almost never made in the acute setting. Patients with conversion disorder may present with paralysis of a specific muscle group that is not anatomically consistent. The symptoms of these patients are subconscious, which is in contrast to the malingering patient, whose actions are purposeful and often have secondary gain. Patients with depression may also experience generalized weakness secondary to the profound fatigue common to the illness.

APPROACH

A key first step is differentiating loss of neuromuscular power from the sensation of generalized weakness. This may be complicated by the fact that presentations are not strictly binary; for example, hypothyroidism may present with general fatigue plus a myopathy. The history begins with elucidating the location of the complaint and whether it is symmetrical, focal, or generalized; other features include the acuity of onset and duration of symptoms, exacerbating and mitigating factors, and presence of associated symptoms.

Because neuromuscular weakness is the inability to perform a desired movement with normal force and power due to a reduction in muscle strength and function, these patients are likely to complain of an inability to perform specific tasks. Asking open-ended questions such as "what activities can you no longer do?" may be a good place to start with a patient having difficulty explaining their weakness in detail. Also, asking task-specific questions such as "are you having any difficulty brushing teeth, combing hair, rising from a chair, walking upstairs, opening a jar or door, etc." can be helpful primers to jump-start the dialogue for the patient. Patients who are unable to respond to questions about specific tasks and give more generalized histories of weakness are more likely to have a non-neuromuscular etiology.

Sudden onset of weakness suggests a vascular catastrophe, such as a spinal cord hemorrhage, and requires emergent evaluation. A slower progression of symptoms may suggest a metabolic disorder such as hyperkalemia, or disorders such as GBS or myasthenia gravis. A history of symmetric ascending weakness in a patient with a recent respiratory illness will aid in the diagnosis of GBS. The weakness of myasthenia gravis may fluctuate, and a careful history is needed to elicit a progression of symptoms throughout the day or an association with exercise, temperature extremes, such as hot showers, or repeated activity, such as chewing or combing one's hair.

Recent illness, other medical problems, occupational history, travel history, history of tick bites, use of medications, and use of recreational drugs are all important factors to assess in the patient complaining of weakness. A thorough review of systems includes inquiry about recent weight loss, fever or sweats, visual changes (including diplopia), difficulty swallowing, joint or muscle pain, palpitations, change in bowel habits, and skin rashes. Occupational or recreational exposures may indicate drug toxicity.

The physical examination begins with a full set of vital signs including oxygen saturation and a finger blood glucose. A blood glucose level should be obtained early during the evaluation, as hypoglycemia may present with an array of symptoms, including weakness. Capnometry may be useful in identifying and monitoring patients with weakness associated with compromised ventilation and is supplemented with obtaining a forced vital capacity or negative inspiratory force measurements. Tachycardia, with or without hypotension, suggests volume depletion including anemia, or toxic drug ingestion. Rectal temperature measurement is particularly important in that

TABLE 4.2	Motor Strength Grading System (Medical Research Council Scale)
Grade	**Definition**
5	Normal strength
4	Active movement against gravity and resistance
3	Active movement against gravity (no resistance from physician)
2	Active movement with gravity eliminated (no resistance from physician)
1	Flicker or trace contraction
0	No visible or palpable contraction

infections frequently present with nonspecific complaints, such as weakness. The ears, sinuses, thyroid, and cardiac status should be assessed, as well as a careful evaluation for signs of trauma, which may suggest physical abuse.

The neurologic examination begins early in the course of the patient's evaluation with an assessment of the mental status, for example, assessment of orientation and attention. Altered mental status, including confusion, slowness, or agitation, may represent underlying disease or toxic exposure. Suspicion of cognitive defects may prompt a formal mental status evaluation depending on the clinical setting. Cranial nerve testing in the patient with a complaint of weakness focuses on the motor examination. Ptosis can be an early sign of myasthenia gravis or hypothyroidism. When myasthenia is a consideration, having the patient hold an upward gaze for several minutes is helpful in assessing for fatigue. Difficulty with accommodation can be the earliest sign of weakness because of botulism and does not occur with myasthenia. Diplopia because of weak oculomotor muscles should be assessed, with an emphasis on the evaluation of the fourth and sixth cranial nerves that are the longest intracranial cranial nerves and sensitive to toxins such as botulism or to increased pressure from intracranial mass lesions.

The remainder of the neurologic examination in the patient complaining of weakness concentrates on motor strength, deep tendon reflexes, and assessment for muscle atrophy and fasciculations. **Table 4.2** lists the motor strength grading system (from 0 to 5) that permits standardization of documentation of the motor examination among examiners. Deep tendon reflexes are graded on a scale from 0, indicating areflexia, to 4, signifying hyperreflexia, with 2 being normal. ***Upper motor neuron*** diseases, such as multiple sclerosis, will typically present with hyperactive reflexes in comparison to the diminished or absent reflexes seen in diseases of the ***lower motor neuron***, as in GBS. Acute spinal cord lesions, such as in a conus medullaris lesion or transverse myelitis, can often initially present with areflexia early in its course. Cauda equina syndrome is due to impingement of the lumbar and sacral nerve roots, commonly from a ruptured vertebral disk. These patients will present with distal motor weakness, areflexia, urinary retention, and anesthesia in the saddle distribution.

Both upper and lower motor neuron diseases can initially present with the complaint of weakness. The important distinguishing characteristics are listed in **Table 4.3**. ***Upper motor neurons*** arise in the cerebral cortex, and their axons extend through the subcortical white matter, internal capsule, brainstem, and spinal cord, where they synapse directly with lower motor neurons or interneurons, fine-tuning motor activity. ***Lower motor neuron*** cell bodies lie in the brainstem motor nuclei and anterior horn of the spinal cord. Their axons extend to the skeletal muscles they innervate.

The weakness of ***upper motor neuron*** disease is generally unilateral, Babinski sign is present, muscle tone is increased, deep tendon reflexes are increased, and no fasciculations are visible or palpable. In general, distal muscle groups are more severely affected than are proximal groups. ***Lower motor neuron*** disease affects single muscle groups. Flexors and extensors are equally compromised in an extremity. Deep tendon reflexes and muscle tone are decreased with lower motor neuron disease. Muscle atrophy and fasciculation are long-term results of lower motor neuron lesions.

Amyotrophic lateral sclerosis (ALS) is a combined upper and lower motor neuron disease that can clinically present as a mixed picture. The etiology of ALS is unclear, but it is a disease involving

TABLE 4.3	Upper versus Lower Motor Neuron Weakness	
Clinical	Upper Motor Neuron	Lower Motor Neuron
Weakness	Weakness greater in the arm extensors and leg flexors; weakness often unilateral	Weakness often in one muscle group; extensor same as flexor
Deep tendon reflexes	Increased	Decreased
Muscle tone	Increased	Decreased
Fasciculation	None	Present
Muscle atrophy	None	Severe
Babinski sign	Present	Absent

the destruction of the anterior horn cells in the spinal column and the Betz cells in the motor cortex of the CNS. The clinical presentation is of asymmetric weakness in the distal motor groups with sensory sparing. Patients often exhibit both the muscle fasciculations of lower motor neuron disease and a positive Babinski sign with hyperreflexia as seen in upper motor neuron disorders.

Lower motor neuron diseases can arise from a muscle-based disorder, a neuropathic-based disorder, or a myoneural junction source. **Table 4.4** illustrates several symptoms, physical signs, and laboratory findings that distinguish the etiologies of lower motor neuron weakness. Weakness because of a myopathy tends to involve proximal muscle groups, whereas neuropathic disease (GBS) affects distal muscle groups. Neuromuscular junction diseases have a more distal distribution and are particularly inclined to affect respiratory and bulbar muscle groups (myasthenia gravis and botulism).

Spinal cord disorders from compressive or traumatic injury can also present with weakness involving motor function distal to the defect, as well as sensory and autonomic nerve dysfunction. In comparison to atraumatic cord disorders, such as in multiple sclerosis, traumatic cord lesions generally present acutely with distinct sensory and motor findings, as seen with the saddle anesthesia in patients with cauda equina syndrome. Autonomic dysfunction is also seen more commonly in spinal cord injuries manifesting with hypotension or priapism. Detailed history (including anticoagulation, recent fall or trauma, immune status, fever, intravenous drug abuse, spinal procedure, or surgery) is often necessary to make the diagnosis. An uncommon and occasionally overlooked diagnosis of spinal epidural abscess can be made in the setting of a patient with a history of intravenous drug abuse presenting with severe back pain, fever, and progressive lower extremity weakness.

TABLE 4.4	Clinical Findings in Neuromuscular Disease		
	Myopathy (eg, polymyositis)	Neuropathy (eg, Guillain-Barré syndrome)	Myoneural Junction (eg, Myasthenia gravis)
Distribution	Proximal > distal	Distal > proximal	Diffuse, especially bulbar and respiratory muscles
Reflexes	Decreased	Decreased	Normal
Sensory involvement	−	+	−
Atrophy	±	±	−
Fatigue	±	±	+
Serum CPK	Normal to elevated	Normal	Normal

CPK, creatine phosphokinase.

When psychogenic weakness is considered in the differential diagnosis, several maneuvers may be helpful. Weak muscles give way to pressure in a smooth fashion, but psychogenic weakness usually results in a jerking or sudden release. In a patient with upper extremity weakness from neuromuscular disease, making a fist should not result in wrist extension (unless there is an isolated lesion of the flexor tendons); in functional states, the wrist extends as the patient tries to make a fist. In patients with psychogenic bilateral lower extremity weakness, attempts to lift one leg against resistance result in the other leg firmly thrusting downward, whereas in patients with neuromuscular disease, the downward thrust is diminished or absent.

Diagnostic Testing

The history and physical should be able to distinguish motor weakness from more subjective complaints of weakness (fatigue, tiredness). If motor weakness is identified, it must be determined whether it is focal or generalized, proximal or distal and whether it is associated with a sensory deficit.

In general, a complete blood count, serum chemistry, and urinalysis should be obtained. A sedimentation rate and C-reactive protein may be helpful if rheumatologic disease is suspected. A monospot test, liver function tests, and thyroid function tests are sometimes indicated. Heavy metal screening, toxicologic screening, and red blood cell acetylcholinesterase level are indicated in selected cases. A serum creatine phosphokinase and aldolase are helpful in cases of suspected myopathy.

Pulse oximetry, capnometry, and arterial blood gas analysis are indicated in cases of suspected respiratory compromise. Pulmonary function testing, including vital capacity and maximum inspiratory force, is useful to assess respiratory function. An electrocardiogram and cardiac monitoring have a low diagnostic yield in patients with generalized weakness, though they may be helpful when dysrhythmias or electrolyte abnormalities are suspected; in patients at risk for cardiac disease, an electrocardiogram should be obtained to assess for a cardiac source. Rarely, more specialized laboratory testing including cerebrospinal fluid (CSF) analysis is indicated: Multiple sclerosis will typically have a pleocytosis on CSF examination, and electrophoresis may demonstrate oligoclonal bands of immunoglobulin G (IgG); GBS characteristically exhibits fewer than 50 lymphocytes per milliliter, a normal sugar, and an elevated protein.

Computed tomography (CT) and magnetic resonance imaging (MRI) with intravenous contrast are recommended when structural lesions in the brain or spinal canal are suspected. The CT angiography of the head and neck is indicated to evaluate brain lesions involving the posterior circulation. CT is not as sensitive in the evaluation of spinal cord lesions such as in spinal epidural hematomas and abscesses: If a patient presents with distinct weakness and sensory deficit below a cord level, an MRI with gadolinium is the test of choice. The MRI is also a useful imaging modality in the diagnosis of cauda equina syndrome as a cause of the lower extremity weakness in the setting of urinary dysfunction, saddle anesthesia, and impotence. An emergency MRI is indicated if an epidural abscess is suspected. If an MRI cannot be obtained, the patient should be stabilized, and consideration given to transfer to an appropriate facility.

DISPOSITION

Patients with progressive symptoms or those with a suspected or confirmed disease that has a progressive course or risk of respiratory compromise (eg, myasthenia gravis, GBS, or botulism) should be admitted to an intensive care setting regardless of their initial appearance. Acute, life-threatening causes of weakness are listed in **Table 4.5** and should be considered for every patient with rapid onset of symptoms. Early consultation with a neurologist or neurosurgeon is recommended, and a comprehensive management plan should be determined. Laboratory tests should not be ordered unless the results will be available before ED discharge or careful follow-up has been arranged.

TABLE 4.5	Acute Life-Threatening Causes of Weakness			
Cause	History	Physical	Laboratory	Treatment
Myasthenia gravis	Chronic weakness, improves with rest	Double vision, muscle fatigue, improves with rest	Positive ice bag test (or edrophonium if available)	Thymectomy, AChE inhibitors
Guillain-Barré	Recent infection, progressive weakness distal to proximal	Distal motor with/without sensory loss, absent reflexes, no visual deficits	CSF with elevated protein, <50 WBCs	Supportive care, plasma exchange, gamma globulin
Botulism	Acute onset; canned, pickled, smoked food	Blurred or double vision	None	Supportive care, equine antitoxin
Adrenal insufficiency	Acute weakness associated with stress	Hypotension, hyperpigmentation	Hyperkalemia, hyponatremia	Hydrocortisone
Organophosphate poisoning	Occupational exposure, progressive weakening	Miosis, fasciculations, muscarinic dysfunction	Decreased RBC AChE	Atropine, pralidoxime
Carbon monoxide poisoning	Occupational or social exposure	Nausea, vomiting, coma, headache, dizziness	Elevated carboxyhemoglobin	100% oxygen, hyperbaric oxygen
Hypokalemia	Familial, GI, or renal loss	Diffuse weakness	Low serum potassium	Potassium

AChE, acetylcholinesterase; CSF, cerebrospinal fluid; GI, gastrointestinal; RBC, red blood cell; WBCs, white blood cells.

TIPS AND PEARLS

- Patients with neurologic causes of weakness can generally identify specific tasks they can no longer do or tasks that they have difficulty performing.
- Determining if the loss of function involves proximal muscle or distal muscle groups is helpful in focusing the differential diagnosis: weakness of proximal muscles, that is, neck, shoulder, and/or hip girdle groups, suggests a problem at the level of the muscle (eg, myopathy), neuromuscular junction (eg, myasthenia gravis), or the peripheral nerves (eg, GBS).
- Distal upper extremity weakness can present as progressive difficulty with intrinsic muscles of the hand, and as such patients complaining of grip or finger extension difficulty, or a patient complaining of difficulty buttoning their shirt or drinking from a cup.
- In disorders involving only the muscle (myopathic disorders), patients often complain of positive symptoms such as stiffness, inability to relax the muscle (myotonia), pain (myalgias), cramping, or even contractures.
- A history revealing fluctuations in strength, particularly at the end of the day, suggests a neuromuscular junction disorder, for example, myasthenia gravis.
- Episodic periods of weakness or poorly localized weakness characterized by frequent relapses suggests multiple sclerosis, myasthenia gravis, or possibly periodic paralysis disorders.
- Insufficient airway protection (bulbar dysfunction) is secondary to weakness of the upper airway muscles: Patients may have difficulty swallowing, dysarthria, dysphagia, weak mastication, and clearing secretions and are at an increased risk of aspiration.

- Spinal epidural abscess should be suspected in patients complaining of lower extremity weakness with back pain, especially if the patient is immunocompromised or uses intravenous drugs.
- ALS should be suspected in patients complaining of weakness who have mixed upper and lower motor neuron findings.

SUMMARY

Neuromuscular weakness can present with variable histories and examinations. The most common presentations are with new-onset or worsening weakness. Sometimes patients can present with worsening respiratory symptoms, but these patients are often initially able to compensate for their weakness. Clinicians must recognize subtle historical and examination findings to assist with the diagnosis and proper workup as well as recognize when patients are at a state of impending respiratory failure, requiring mechanical ventilation.

EVIDENCE

How common is the chief complaint of weakness, and how frequently is it because of a serious underlying cause?

Weakness is a common presenting symptom in the ED and the frequency of this chief complaint increases as individuals age. A cross-sectional study examining all ED presentations over 6 months at a major university hospital in Switzerland found that weakness or "feeling unwell" comprised 14% of all chief complaints to the ED.[3] Of individuals older than 65 years, weakness is the fifth most common chief complaint based on a cross-sectional cohort study examining 575 million ambulance calls over 5 years.[4] Similarly, the likelihood of a serious underlying illness precipitating the weakness increases with age. In individuals older than 65 years presenting with weakness, an observational study of 273 patients found that 51% had a serious diagnosis.[5] The cross-sectional study of ambulance calls found 55% needed admission.[4] Among this elderly patient population, the most common diagnoses were non-neurologic (pneumonia [14%], urinary tract infection [13%], dehydration [13%], syncope [11%], and congestive heart failure [7%]).[4] These data give weight to the importance of a broad differential and thorough workup for the weak patient, especially the weak elderly patient.

How often do patients with acute myocardial disease present without chest pain but with a primary complaint of weakness?

In a retrospective cross-sectional study examining the symptoms of AMI, 4% of all patients presenting with an AMI did not experience chest pain and instead presented with a chief complaint of weakness.[6] The prevalence of atypical symptoms of AMI increases with age. In the elderly with autopsy-proven MI, 20% of the patients initially presented with weakness.[7] With regard to myocarditis, patients complain of weakness as part of a constellation of symptoms that include cough, dyspnea, myalgias, fever, vomiting, or diarrhea. In one study, up to 60% of patients with myocarditis did not have chest pain.[8]

How good is the neurologic examination in identifying neurologic weakness versus non-neurologic disease?

The sensitivity and specificity of the neurologic examination vary based on both the practitioner performing the examination and the underlying diagnosis. A small randomized study of medical student performance found a 78% sensitivity and 71% specificity for identifying focal neurologic deficits.[9] For patients with lower extremity weakness, one trial of examination reliability found 85% accuracy among both neurologists and other specialists in identifying an upper motor neuron deficit, whereas the Babinski sign only had 56% accuracy.[10] However, the neurologic examination is not a perfect diagnostic tool. In one study, six neurologists examined 46 patients with focal cerebral hemisphere lesions without obvious focal signs or symptoms, and 19 patients with no neurologic conditions. When examined by these blinded neurologists, the neurologic examination only identified 50% of the patients correctly. Pronator drift, finger and forearm rolling, and rapid alternating movements of the hands all helped to increase the sensitivity of the examination.[11] Although the neurologic examination is an important tool to use in evaluating patients with weakness, it is an imperfect one; thus, as always, it is important to keep the differential broad and supplement assessment with laboratory studies and imaging when appropriate.

How is impending respiratory failure from neuromuscular illnesses best assessed and what parameters are helpful in the decision to intubate?

Respiratory failure secondary to neuromuscular weakness is most commonly seen in GBS, myasthenia gravis, and ALS. Recognizing the indications for placing an advanced airway is key to management. The classic teaching is to monitor a patient's vital capacity and blood gas and consider intubation when vital capacity falls below 15 mL/kg or Po_2 is less than 70 mm Hg.[12] Early identification in patients with rapidly progressing disease, like GBS, is critically important for early intervention or appropriate level of monitoring. A retrospective survey of 114 patients admitted to the intensive care unit with GBS found that bulbar dysfunction, bilateral facial weakness, dysautonomia, and rapid disease progression were early indicators of subsequent progression to respiratory failure.[13] As vital capacity may be challenging to obtain in a busy ED, measuring single breath count (SBC) in conjunction with arterial blood gases (ABGs) can help to determine need for intubation. To do an SBC, the patient takes a maximal inspiration and then counts in a normal speaking volume; patients should be able to count above 40. Patients who are able to achieve an SBC above 7 are unlikely to need mechanical ventilation based on the results of a prospective cohort study of 96 patients.[14] Whereas early intubation is recommended for patients with GBS given their rapidly progressive course, other neuromuscular causes of respiratory failure can be initially trialed with noninvasive ventilation.[15,16] A small prospective cohort study of 17 patients found that noninvasive ventilation averted endotracheal intubation in 79% of patients with non-GBS causes of neuromuscular respiratory failure.[17]

References

1. Barin K, Dodson E. Dizziness in the elderly. *Otolaryngol Clin North Am*. 2011;44(2):437-454.

2. Chapman L, Miller S. Periodic paralysis: an unusual presentation of thyrotoxicosis. *Acute Med*. 2011;10(4):200-202.

3. Nemec M, Koller MT, Nickel CH, et al. Patients presenting to the emergency department with non-specific complaints: the Basel Non-specific Complaints (BANC) study. *Acad Emerg Med*. 2010;17(3):284-292.

4. Bhalla MC, Wilber ST, Stiffler KA, Ondrejka JE, Gerson LW. Weakness and fatigue in older ED patients in the United States. *Am J Emerg Med*. 2014;32(11):1395-1398.

5. Rutschmann OT, Chevalley T, Zumwald C, Luthy C, Vermeulen B, Sarasin F. Pitfalls in the emergency department triage of frail elderly patients without specific complaints. *Swiss Med Wkly*. 2005;135(9-10):145-150.

6. Gupta M, Tabas JA, Kohn MA. Presenting complaint among patients with myocardial infarction who present to an urban, public hospital emergency department. *Ann Emerg Med*. 2002;40(2):180-186.

7. Alexander KP, Newby L, Cannon CP, et al. Acute coronary care in the elderly, part I. *Circulation*. 2007;115(19):2549-2569.

8. Brady WJ, Ferguson JD, Ullman EA, Perron A. Myocarditis: emergency department recognition and management. *Emerg Med Clin North Am*. 2004;22(4):865-885.

9. Kamel H, Dhaliwal G, Navi BB, et al. A randomized trial of hypothesis-driven vs screening neurologic examination. *Neurology*. 2011;77(14):1395-1400.

10. Miller TM, Johnston SC. Should the Babinski sign be part of the routine neurologic examination? *Neurology*. 2005;65(8):1165-1168.

11. Anderson NE, Mason DF, Fink JN, Bergin PS, Charleston AJ, Gamble GD. Detection of focal cerebral hemisphere lesions using the neurological examination. *J Neurol Neurosurg Psychiatry*. 2005;76(4):545-549.

12. Ropper AH, Kehne SM. Guillain-Barré syndrome: management of respiratory failure. *Neurology*. 1985;35(11):1662-1665.

13. Lawn ND, Fletcher DD, Henderson RD, Wolter TD, Wijdicks EF. Anticipating mechanical ventilation in Guillain-Barré syndrome. *Arch Neurol*. 2001;58(6):893-898.

14. Kalita J, Kumar M, Misra UK. Serial single breath count is a reliable tool for monitoring respiratory functions in Guillain-Barré syndrome. *J Clin Neurosci*. 2020;72:50-56.

15. Bach JR. Noninvasive respiratory management of patients with neuromuscular disease. *Ann Rehabil Med*. 2007;41(4):519-538.

16. Wijdicks EF, Roy TK. BiPAP in early Guillain-Barré syndrome may fail. *Can J Neurol Sci*. 2006;33(1):105-106.

17. Servera E, Sancho J, Zafra MJ, Catalá A, Vergara P, Marín J. Alternatives to endotracheal intubation for patients with neuromuscular diseases. *Am J Phys Med Rehabil*. 2005;84(11):851-857.

Suggested Readings

1. Chew WM, Birnbaumer DM. Evaluation of the elderly patient with weakness: an evidence based approach. *Emerg Med Clin North Am*. 1999;17(1):265-278.

2. Ginde AA, Espinola JA, Camargo CA Jr. Trends and disparities in U.S. emergency department visits for hypoglycemia, 1993–2005. *Diabetes Care*. 2008;31(3):511-513.

3. Glick TH, Workman TP, Gaufberg SV. Suspected conversion disorder: foreseeable risks and avoidable errors. *Acad Emerg Med*. 2000;7(11):1272-1277.

4. Goldstein LB, Simel DL. Is this patient having a stroke? *JAMA*. 2005;293(19):2391-2402.

5. Hellman M, Mosberg-Galili R, Steiner I. Myasthenia gravis in the elderly. *J Neurol Sci*. 2013;325(1-2):1-5.

6. Koita J, Riggio S, Jagoda A. The mental status examination in emergency practice. *Emerg Med Clin North Am*. 2010;28(3):439-451.

7. Lin YF, Wu CC, Pei D, et al. Diagnosing thyrotoxic periodic paralysis in the ED. *Am J Emerg Med*. 2003;21(4):339-342.

8. Peppin J, Shields C. Advances in diagnosis and management of hypokalemic and hyperkalemic emergencies. *Emerg Med Pract*. 2012;14(2):1-17.

Fundamentals of Neuroimaging

Charles R. Wira III

Alex Janke

Over time in emergency medicine there has been greater accessibility to imaging modalities, such as non-contrast computed tomography (CT), computed tomography angiography (CTA), and computed tomography perfusion (CTP), as well as some systems having increased accessibility to magnetic resonance imaging (MRI). Emergency neuroimaging is generally focused on the detection of structural abnormalities (ie, intracerebral hemorrhage [ICH], cervical spine fracture). Recently, functional neuroimaging has also become available (ie, CTP) for some emergency conditions. Emergency medicine physicians need to be familiar with the increasing number of imaging modalities available so as to allow for the selection of the most appropriate imaging for neurologic emergencies, with them also having an approach to the interpretation of imaging sequences.

The imaging modalities routinely available in the hyperacute phase of care are predominantly CT and CTA. In some systems, CTP, and less likely MRI, may be available within the first 6 hours of care. This chapter reviews neuroimaging typically utilized in emergency situations and primarily focuses on brain rather than spinal cord imaging, with specific emphasis on the imaging sequences utilized for different stroke subtypes.

BASICS OF NEUROIMAGING

Computed Tomography (CT)

Over time, CT has evolved from a "slice-oriented" imaging modality to an "organ-oriented" modality. Helical CT, also known as spiral CT, has several advantages over older imaging techniques, such as eliminating interscan delay, its ability to produce overlapped images without overlapped scans, and having a more uniform sampling density.

CT scanners are differentiated by the number of tubes and detectors, classifying them as single- or dual-source scanners, and also by the number of slices that can be acquired per rotation. Currently, many centers utilize 64-slice scanners that generate 64 slices per rotation and acquire conventional axial and helical acquisitions with collimation ranges of 1 to 32 mm and 16 to 32 mm, respectively. In higher level applications, CTs may generate up to 320 slices per rotation, which could cover up to a 16-cm columnar length of a subject patient during a gantry rotation (ie, cardiac CT). Different gradations of tissue and substance density are acquired by CT imaging. This is represented by the Hounsfield unit (HU) CT density scale that ranges from −1000 for air to +1000 HU for bone, with 0 HU representing the density of water. The upper limit of the scale may be further differentiated (up to 4000 HU) for bone density and even different types of metals.

When an image is taken, the CT gantry, a circular rotating frame, rotates around the patient. Within the gantry, an x-ray tube is mounted on one side with a detector on the opposite side. The gantry rotates around a center point called the isocenter. This generates raw data representing the digitalized x-ray signal collected by the detector. Contrast resolution distinguishes between different densities and can generate sharp edges between small heterogeneously dense objects. Image processing utilizes pixels and voxels. Pixels are two-dimensional elements utilized to generate images on a display monitor. Voxels are three-dimensional volume representations derived from pixels. Pixels are the building blocks of an image matrix. Volume averaging describes when different objects are represented in the same voxel, thus only partially filling an individual voxel. Reformatted images are created from axial images and arrange axial data into other planes (ie, coronal, sagittal). Reconstruction algorithms are mathematical volumetric rendering techniques utilized to generate multidimensional views. Currently, there are a multitude of software packages available to generate three-dimensional reconstruction images for different pathologic conditions across the spectrum of clinical care (ie, diagnosis, surgical planning).

CTA utilizes intravenous (IV) iodinated contrast media to visualize the vasculature. Of note, because contrast media consist of small and highly diffusible molecules, they also give better interpretive resolution to certain organs with high perfusion. For example, in the non-neurologic realm, the liver, spleen, and kidneys may undergo contrast enhancement, thus improving the sensitivity of CT imaging to rule out traumatic injuries or pathologic conditions.

Angiography involves rapid contrast injection using mechanical injectors and standardized multiphase injection protocols. Contrast media travel from the right heart through the lungs to the left heart, and then distribute through the central arterial vasculature before entering different vascular beds and organs. The resultant attenuation in the vessels is influenced by the contrast injection rate, injection duration, cardiac output, tube voltage, and venous return. Thus, the timing of image acquisition relative to the contrast injection is critical and varies from patient to patient. One of the minimum prerequisites for more advanced CTA applications is a 64-slice scanner. Some applications, such as coronary CTA, are optimized further with higher slice scanners.

CTA has undergone recent evolution and may be categorized into different detection modes—single-phase and multiphase modes. Multiphase CTA provides angiographic images in three distinct phases after contrast injection: peak arterial phase, peak venous phase, and late venous phase. Traditional single-phase CTA only acquires images in the arterial phase and appears to give less accurate information about pial collateral arterial filling.

CTP provides a functional snapshot image of the ischemic penumbra, differentiating the region of the unsalvageable core from the salvageable region of the penumbra. Brain tissue flow may be described by several variables, including cerebral blood flow (CBF), cerebral blood volume (CBV), and mean transit time (MTT) (**Table 5.1**). Currently, a widespread version of CTP automatic processing using artificial intelligence (AI) is RAPID AI.[1] It provides a fast automated quantitative interpretation of the CTP, and was the software utilized in extended window thrombectomy trials.[2] RAPID AI is utilized following an initial CTA. A second, smaller volume contrast bolus (~40 mL) is administered as multiple sequential CT scans (from skull base to vertex) are obtained to capture the entire contrast passage (arterial inflow through venous outflow). Pixel data is interpreted by the RAPID software generating perfusion maps from CBV, MTT, time to peak concentration, and CBF. The final display generates an image (see **Figure 5.1**), with a nonsalvageable core (milliliter) and a penumbral volume of hypoperfusion (milliliter) amenable to reperfusion interventions. Target thresholds for core and mismatch volume are used to estimate benefit from thrombectomy in the extended window of stroke presentation (Table 5.1).

Magnetic Resonance Imaging (MRI)

MRI, and its many sequencing options, is an alternative to CT imaging, and free of ionizing radiation. It has several applications in the hyperacute phase of care. MRI can be utilized to confirm the onset of an acute ischemic stroke in the hyperacute phase. It gives information about stroke onset; enables arterial and venous imaging; identifies hemorrhages that may not be seen on CT; and it may also be utilized for assessing the etiology and severity of spinal cord injuries or syndromes in patients with fractures or new neurologic deficits.

TABLE 5.1	Key CT Perfusion Definitions and Penumbral Inclusion Criteria Definitions for the Extended Window DAWN and DEFUSE 3 Clinical Trials[2,17]

Key definitions:

- *Cerebral blood flow (CBF):* Volume of blood flowing through a selected volume region of the brain per unit time (mL blood per 100 g of brain tissue per minute).
- *Mean transit time (MTT):* The mean transit time of blood through a selected brain region (measured in seconds).
- *Time to maximum (Tmax):* Shows the severity in delays of contrast arrival time. Tmax >6 s is the threshold defining the penumbra volume. Tmax does include old strokes, so comparison to the non-contrast CT is compulsory.
- *Core:* unsalvageable infarct depicted by a CBF <30%.
- *Penumbra:* hypoperfused potentially salvageable tissue at risk for progression to irreversible infarct. Is the target area for reperfusion therapies. Is represented by the difference between the total volume of infarcted brain minus the core volume. Typically defined by the Tmax >6 s volume.
- *Penumbra-mismatch volume:* The total hypoperfusion volume minus the core volume. Is potentially salvageable brain tissue with reperfusion interventions.

Treatment criteria for extended window thrombectomy trials:

DEFUSE 3 Trial (6- to 16-h window)

- Ischemia core <70 mL
- Ratio of volume of ischemic tissue to initial infarct volume ≥1.8
- An absolute volume of potentially reversible ischemia ≥15 mL

DAWN Trial (6- to 24-h window)

- Group A: Age ≥ 80 y.o., NIHSS ≥ 10, infarct volume <21 mL
- Group B: Age < 80 y.o., NIHSS ≥ 10, infarct volume <31 mL
- Group C: Age < 80 y.o., NIHSS ≥ 20, infarct volume 31 to <51 mL

CT, computed tomography; NIHSS, National Institutes of Health Stroke Scale.

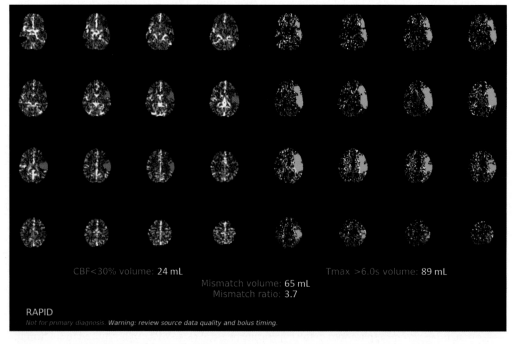

CBF<30% volume: **24 mL**   Tmax >6.0s volume: **89 mL**
Mismatch volume: **65 mL**
Mismatch ratio: **3.7**

RAPID
Not for primary diagnosis. **Warning: review source data quality and bolus timing.**

Figure 5.1: Sample Rapid Perfusion Map. Pink indicates the nonsalvageable core (24 mL) of the penumbra. Green indicates the ischemic tissue (89 mL). The mismatch volume (65 mL) is the potentially salvageable area: the penumbra.

The major components of an MRI include a superconducting magnet, gradient coils, and radiofrequency coils. The superconducting magnet ranges from the milli-Tesla range to 7 Tesla, with most conventional MRIs ranging between 1.5 and 3 Tesla. It defines the sequence time and imaging resolution. The superconducting magnet may, in some units, be cooled to almost absolute zero by liquid helium and mounted with a hollow bore to accommodate the patient. Gradient coils are used to provide intentionally measured variations in the magnetic field in the x, y, and z planes. Radiofrequency coils emit low-energy electromagnetic waves that emit a signal and receive a return signal.

Principles of quantum mechanics, namely, the atomic property of angular nuclear spin momentum, underlies the kinetics of magnetic resonance. Unlike some modalities of CT that focus on electrons, MRI focuses on protons. Essentially, the protons of hydrogen atoms, present in the total body water of a subject undergoing MRI, are influenced by the application of a strong external magnetic field. Without a magnet, there is a random alignment of protons. With the application of the magnetic field, alterations in angular spin cause an alignment to the magnetic field. In this magnetic-nuclear interaction, hydrogen nuclei may align either in parallel or perpendicular to the magnetic field depending on whether there is a low- or high-energy state. This is a reversible, modifiable, and measurable event. The term describing the change in orientation of the rotation axis of the spinning nucleus is *precession*.

The fraction of protons aligned with the magnetic field may be influenced by other modifiable forces, namely, radiofrequency energy pulse sequences. Application of a radiofrequency pulse can alter the net magnetic movement of protons. Upon cessation of the radiofrequency, relaxation phases occur; and echo waves are emitted by the protons, which can be measured. Time constant T1 refers to longitudinal relaxation time along the axis of the magnetic field, and is also known as spin-lattice relaxation time. It is the time constant by which anatomic spins align themselves to the magnetic field. Time constant T2 refers to the transverse relaxation time perpendicular to the magnetic field, and is also known as spin-spin relaxation time. It is the time constant for the loss of phase coherence among spins positioned at an angle to the magnetic field due to interactions between the spins. Thus, three distinct properties of materials can be determined by MRI: concentration of protons, T1, and T2. The utilization of radiofrequency pulse sequences allows the emphasis of one property over another, thus enabling contrast differentiation between different tissues dependent on the pulse sequence utilized.

Many different imaging sequences are derived from modulations of T1 and T2 relaxation times. T1-weighted images give the most anatomic representation of tissue planes. Fat rapidly aligns its longitudinal magnetization, appearing bright on image sequences. Water aligns at a slower rate, and thus has a dark appearance on sequences. This sequence can differentiate between central nervous system (CNS) gray and white matter. T2-weighted images alter with structural or metabolic changes in a tissue, making it able to identify pathologic changes in body tissue. The dominant signal intensities of different tissues are influenced by water and fat having a high signal intensity. Diffusion-weighted imaging (DWI) represents imaging sequences detecting the free diffusion of water and T2. In an acute ischemic stroke, signal abnormalities may be seen several minutes after onset due to swelling in the ischemic brain parenchyma that prevents water from diffusing freely from the extracellular to intracellular space. Fluid attenuation inversion recovery (FLAIR) sequences are fundamentally T2 sequences with subtraction of the cerebrospinal fluid (CSF). It is useful in evaluating many disorders of the CNS, including stroke and subarachnoid hemorrhage. It may also identify leptomeningeal diseases. Apparent diffusion coefficient (ADC) maps are images representing the actual diffusion values of water in tissue without T2 effects. Susceptibility-weighted imaging (SWI) is a sequence particularly adept at identifying compounds that distort the magnetic field (ie, deoxyhemoglobin, ferritin, hemosiderin), making it sensitive for identifying hemorrhage. Gadolinium contrast enhancement augments the T1 signal, and pathologic areas may have an increase in contrast accumulation. Fat suppression may be done for T1 and T2 sequences. Suppression can remove the high signal intensity from fat, enabling visualization of other underlying pathology (ie, the intramural thrombus of a craniocervical dissection). Finally, flow-sensitive sequences include magnetic resonance angiography (MRA), magnetic resonance venography (MRV), cine MRI utilized for CSF flow, and perfusion. Gadolinium contrast enhancement improves the diagnostic accuracy of MRA and MRV over non-contrast-enhanced "time-of-flight" (TOF) imaging sequences.

OBJECTIVES OF NEUROIMAGING

In the emergency phase of care, there is a broad spectrum of clinical presentations that merit consideration for neuroimaging. For some clinical symptom presentations, including, but not limited to, pediatric head trauma and adult trauma with potential cervical spine injuries, there are decision rules to guide the utilization of higher level neuroimaging (**Table 5.2**).

Non-contrast CT

Non-contrast CT of the head is the preliminary and most prevalent imaging modality utilized in the initial evaluation of ischemic and hemorrhagic stroke and traumatic brain injuries. Eligible patients with suspected acute ischemic stroke generally undergo a non-contrast CT of the head to exclude hemorrhage before treatment with IV tissue plasminogen activator (t-PA). However, the non-contrast CT may offer a wealth of other information in the acute phase for acute ischemic stroke presentations. It may differentiate acute (ie, loss of gray/white differentiation, sulcal effacement) from subacute changes (ie, well-defined hypodensity), may reveal a hyperdense vessel sign suggestive of a thrombus in a vessel causing a large-vessel occlusion (LVO), and may delineate the size of the infarct area (**Figure 5.2**). Of note, windowing, or gray-level mapping, is the process by which image brightness, image contrast, and the gray scale component of images can be manipulated to accentuate certain structures. Most viewing platforms have a "stroke" preset that will, for instance, highlight the differentiation between cerebral gray and white matter. There will also be a "brain" sequence preset that enables best identification of intracranial bleeding.

For acute ischemic stroke, a sample quantitative method validated to estimate the size of a penumbral core from the non-contrast CT is the ASPECTS score (Alberta Stroke Program Early CT Score).[3] ASPECTS is a 10-point non-contrast CT scoring system evaluating for early ischemic changes indicative of infarct and cytotoxic edema. In the middle cerebral artery territory, seven cortical and three subcortical territories are assessed for ischemic changes (**Figure 5.3**). A score of 10 reflects a normal scan without any early ischemic changes. Scores may be stratified into three groups: small-volume infarcts (ASPECTS 8-10), large-volume infarcts (ASPECTS $\leq$ 7), and very large-volume infarcts (ASPECTS $\leq$ 5). A score $\geq$8 correlates with better clinical outcomes after reperfusion therapies. A score $\geq$6 was a selection criterion for identifying patients with LVO stroke eligible for endovascular thrombectomy within 6 hours of stroke onset. Conversely, poor ASPECTS scores (low scores) correspond with a higher risk of developing a malignant middle cerebral artery syndrome

TABLE 5.2	Clinical Decision Rules Which May Be Utilized to Determine the Need for Advanced Imaging	
Clinical Decision Rule	**Purpose**	**Intended Population**
NEXUS	Clinically clears patients from cervical spine fractures or spinal cord injury without imaging	Adult patients
Canadian C-Spine Rule	Clinically clears patients from cervical spine fractures or spinal cord injury without imaging	Adult patients younger than 65 y
Canadian Head Injury Rule	Clinically clears patients with head trauma without imaging	Patients older than 15 y
PECARN Pediatric Head Injury/Trauma Algorithm	Predicts the need for brain imaging after pediatric head trauma	Pediatric patients
Ottawa Subarachnoid Hemorrhage Headache Evaluation Rule	Predicts the need for brain imaging and other diagnostic tests to rule out spontaneous subarachnoid hemorrhage	Patients older than 14 y

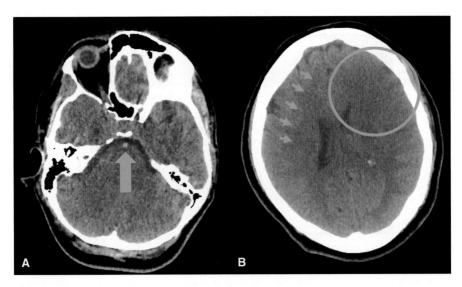

Figure 5.2: A, Hyperdense basilar artery sign. B, Loss of gray/white differentiation in the left frontal region, with preserved gray/white differentiation in the right hemisphere delineated by arrows.

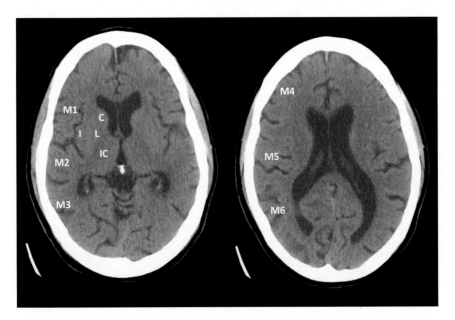

Figure 5.3: ASPECTS scoring regions. C, caudate; I, insular ribbon; IC, internal capsule; L, lentiform nucleus; M, middle cerebral artery territories at cortical (M1-M3) and supra-cortical levels (M4-M6).

from secondary edema, potentially necessitating a craniotomy. Non-contrast CT may also be utilized in the later phases of stroke syndromes to identify secondary complications of large territory strokes, including, but not limited to, hemorrhagic transformation, cerebral edema, mass effect, and herniation syndromes. Future investigation may identify and validate automated methods for calculating ASPECTS, as well as identifying other findings in the acute presentation (ie, hyperdense vessel signs).

Non-contrast CT of the head is also the principal imaging modality utilized to identify ICH, subarachnoid hemorrhage, and types of traumatic hemorrhages. It differentiates the type (subdural hematoma, epidural hematoma, traumatic subarachnoid hemorrhage) of hematoma, and can differentiate the age of some traumatic bleeds. Of note, blood has a different Hounsfield density depending

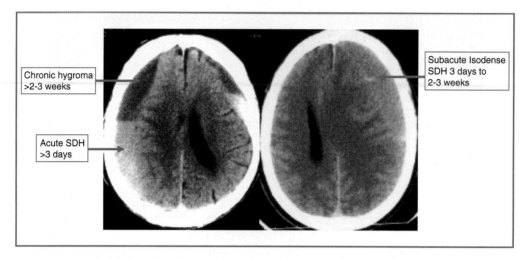

Figure 5.4: The different densities of blood in subdural hematomas.

on the age of the hematoma. For instance, for a subdural hematoma in the acute phase (<3 days), blood is hyperdense; in the subacute phase (3 days to 2-3 weeks), it is isodense; and for a chronic sub-dural (>2-3 weeks), it is hypodense from hemosiderin reabsorption resulting in a subdural hygroma (**Figure 5.4**).

For spontaneous ICH, non-contrast CT of the head can identify the size and location of an acute hematoma and can also identify secondary complications such as intraventricular extension, midline shift from mass effect, or herniation syndromes from the elevations in intracranial pres-sure. Non-contrast CT may be able to identify the etiology of the ICH, such as from a hemorrhagic cancer metastasis, or from a hypertensive bleed. The size of the intracerebral hematoma correlates with clinical outcomes and may be calculated by utilizing the ABC/2 formula[4]: A is the maximum length of the hematoma in centimeter, B is the length (cm) perpendicular to A in the same slice, and C can either be the number of slices with seen hematoma times the slice thickness. C could also be estimated by coronal reformats measuring the longest distance in centimeter from the top to bot-tom of the hematoma. Hematomas >30 mL (or cm^3) correlate with moderate disability, whereas hematomas >60 mL correspond to higher mortality rates.

Traumatic subarachnoid hemorrhages are typically identified with non-contrast CT of the head, with fairly good sensitivity in patients presenting within the golden hour of trauma time frame. Spontaneous subarachnoid hemorrhage, in 85% of cases due to rupture of cerebral aneu-rysms, also is initially evaluated for by non-contrast CT. On CT within the acute phase of presen-tation, high-density blood will be seen in the sulci, cisterns, and fissures. There may be associated intraventricular hemorrhage and a secondary hydrocephalus from the accumulation of blood in regions such as the aqueduct of Silvius. Reimaging is necessary if a patient undergoes clinical dete-rioration, because rebleeding may occur, which correlates with worse outcomes. In the later phases of aneurysmal subarachnoid hemorrhage presentation, ischemic stroke changes may be seen in the brain parenchyma from arterial vasospasm, causing secondary ischemic strokes.

The CT sensitivity to rule out a subarachnoid hemorrhage is improved with modern-day scanners, but diminishes over time as blood becomes more isodense. Sensitivity to rule out sub-arachnoid hemorrhage approaches 100% within the first 6 hours of onset of headache, whereas beyond 6 hours, sensitivity is 89%.[5]

CT Angiography

In this era of endovascular thrombectomy, CTA has a paramount role in identifying stroke sub-types with LVOs, and is also utilized to identify other entities such as cerebral dissections or cerebral aneurysms. It may also identify strokes resulting from aortic dissections and may identify patients with transient ischemic attack (TIA) at high risk for a stroke within 72 hours (ie, identification of a partial clot thrombosis or another critical lesion). For acute ischemic stroke, CTA is widely utilized at all levels of stroke centers to assess for clots potentially amenable to endovascular thrombectomy. To identify the most proximal parent vessel lesions serving as the etiology of a stroke, the most comprehensive imaging sequences include images from the aorta through the circle of Willis, giving visualization of the entire anterior (carotid) and posterior (vertebrobasilar) circulation. Smaller centers, or mobile stroke units (MSUs), may only have the capacity to perform brain CTA, which for thrombectomy treatment purposes is acceptable and will identify key culprit LVO lesions intervenable by thrombectomy. However, for some interventionalists, visualization of the entire aortic, carotid, and vertebral circulation can optimize preprocedural planning.

LVOs may be identified in the internal carotid arteries, anterior cerebral artery, territories of the middle cerebral artery (M1, M2, M3), vertebral arteries, basilar artery, and posterior cerebral arteries. Occlusions most amenable to stent retrieval device removal are those in the distal internal carotid artery, the proximal M1 segment of the middle cerebral artery, the middle M2 segments of the middle cerebral artery, or the basilar artery. Lesions in the proximal anterior cerebral artery may also be intervened upon. Some reports have attempted to treat lesions in the more distal middle cerebral artery territory (M3), but with current technology, these lesions are typically not accessible with stent retrieval devices. CTA may also elucidate clot characteristics, such as length and differentiating partial from complete vessel occlusions.

Recent evolution has occurred in CTA technology. Single-phase CTA evaluates contrast flow in the peak arterial phase, which can identify arterial occlusions, but may not be accurate in assessing collateral flow. Dual-phase CTA evaluates venous flow, but does not make a distinction between early and late venous flow, thus also having lesser accuracy. Multiphase CTA is an evolving technique utilized to assess collateral flow in the area of an LVO, and inform clinical decision-making and prognostication from interventional procedures. It can better differentiate early versus late collateral filling by providing angiographic images in three distinct phases: peak arterial, peak venous, and late venous.

CTA may also be utilized in the evaluation of ICH and aneurysmal subarachnoid hemorrhage. For ICH, up to 30% of patients may undergo hematoma expansion (by 30%) in the first 6 hours. There are clinical features placing patients at risk for hematoma expansion, including the use of anticoagulant medications and hypertension in the acute phase of presentation. Likewise, radiographic risk stratification may be performed with CTA. A "spot sign" from contrast extravasation into the hematoma corresponds with risk of hematoma growth and unfavorable outcomes.[6] Diagnostically, CTA may also identify the cause of an ICH, for example, by identifying arteriovenous malformations as the causative etiology.

For nontraumatic subarachnoid hemorrhage, up to 80% to 85% are caused by ruptured aneurysms. CTA is fairly sensitive and specific for identifying cerebral aneurysms larger than 3 mm and should be performed on all patients with a confirmed spontaneous subarachnoid hemorrhage on a non-contrast CT of the head. CTA may also identify specific features of individual aneurysms, or vessel wall characteristics suggesting a higher risk of rupture. In some realms, for patients presenting with acute-onset headaches with normal initial non-contrast CTs of the head, CTA is posed as being the next test to perform in lieu of performing a lumbar puncture.

In the setting of trauma, the most common utilization of CTA is evaluating for traumatic cerebrovascular dissections. This is routinely done for cervical spine fractures, where the vertebral arteries may have been secondarily injured by a cervical spine fracture adjacent to these vessels. In addition, cerebrovascular dissections may occur with direct blunt trauma to the neck, or in strangulation injuries overlying the common carotid arteries. They may also anatomically occur where the vessels penetrate the dura mater and are more susceptible to shearing forces.

CT Perfusion

CTP has become the most widely utilized imaging modality evaluating the ischemic penumbra. Modern platforms have the ability to quantify the core volume (destined to infarct), ischemic tissue (infarcted plus reversible ischemia). CTP penumbral imaging has become a criterion for endovascular thrombectomy patient selection in the extended window (see Table 5.2).

Magnetic Resonance Imaging

Many of the sequence modalities available in MRI may offer a wealth of information in the setting of acute ischemic stroke. The principal imaging sequences garnering the most interest include

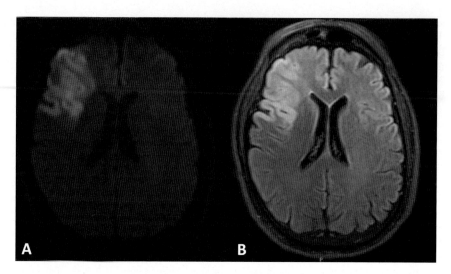

Figure 5.5: Stroke signal abnormalities on MRI. A, Restriction of diffusion in the right frontal region. B, Corresponding FLAIR signal abnormalities in the same region.

DWI, which may see a restriction of diffusion indicative of cerebral ischemia within minutes of stroke onset (**Figure 5.5**). This could be helpful in distinguishing a stroke mimic, such as a complicated migraine, Todd paralysis, or conversion reaction, from actual cerebral ischemia, which may influence treatment decisions in select cases where MRI is rapidly accessible. FLAIR image sequences also likewise see a signal abnormality in acute ischemic stroke, but findings are delayed up to 4.5 hours after stroke onset (Figure 5.5). Thus, MRI may serve as the "witness" as to when stroke onset occurred. Some investigators have reported using qualitative and quantitative diffusion/FLAIR mismatch ratios to identify patients eligible for thrombolysis when the onset of a stroke is unknown to the patient, patient surrogate, or providers (ie, wake-up strokes). Preliminary safety investigations have demonstrated positive results for thrombolytic therapy in the setting of wake-up strokes with regard to low symptomatic ICH rates related to reperfusion and t-PA.

Additional imaging sequences offering useful information in the evaluation of patients with acute ischemic stroke includes SWI, which is more accurate than is non-contrast CT in identifying small intracranial bleeds, including the very rare occurrence of small subdural hematomas and petechial hemorrhages. In addition, SWI may identify small punctate subacute to chronic microbleeds. Current guidelines do not recommend using SWI in lieu of non-contrast CT to determine t-PA eligibility, because these types of bleeds are profoundly rare occurrences. In addition, t-PA is typically not contraindicated in patients with parenchymal microbleeds on MRI.

Perfusion-weighted imaging (PWI) may be utilized on MRI, including qualitative perfusion maps and other quantitative imaging platforms, for select centers having hyperacute phase access to using MRI. MRA may be utilized in lieu of CTA in patients with contraindications to iodine contrast dye (ie, anaphylaxis). Of note, owing to the increased length of time to acquire images, often an MRA of the head, rather than of the head and neck, is performed looking for a culprit lesion amenable to treatment with a stent retrieval device. Very rarely, some patients, for example, those on dialysis with chronic kidney disease, may have an adverse reaction to gadolinium contrast resulting in a nephrogenic systemic fibrosis. This is a dermopathy resembling scleroderma, but it can also affect other internal organs such as the heart and lungs. In many institutions, the use of gadolinium is contraindicated in patients with severe renal disease. Imaging sequences may also differ depending on the age of a stroke (**Table 5.3**). ADC maps may emit a different signal dependent on how acute or chronic a stroke infarct core is. In the early to later phases of a stroke, ADC mapping will generate a low signal intensity. For chronic strokes, it will generate a high signal intensity. This may be useful in the evaluation of patients with prior strokes who present with new symptoms.

There are also additional MRI sequences that may be performed, including MRA, MRV, and cine MRI, to measure cerebral spinal flow. MRA is a longer examination, and, typically, only

TABLE 5.3	Key MRI Findings for Acute Ischemic Stroke across the Time Continuum		
	Hyperacute Phase (0-6 h)	Acute Phase (24 h to 1 wk)	Chronic Phase (>3 wk)
DWI	High signal intensity	High signal intensity	Variable signal intensity
FLAIR	Low signal intensity until 4.5 h after stroke onset	High signal intensity	Low signal intensity
ADC maps	Low signal intensity	Low signal intensity	High signal intensity

ADC, apparent diffusion coefficient; DWI, diffusion-weighted imaging; FLAIR, fluid attenuation inversion recovery; MRI, magnetic resonance imaging.

imaging sequences of the intracranial vasculature is performed rather than sequences going from the aortic arch to the circle of Willis. MRA has 87% to 99% sensitivity for ruling out carotid dissections.[7] However, sensitivity for smaller luminal diameter vessels (ie, vertebral artery dissections) is as low as 60%, in comparison to CTA that has sensitivities ranging from 74% to 100%. MRV may be utilized to identify cerebral sinus venous thrombosis not identified on conventional non-contrast MRI. Conventional MRI has 70% sensitivity because T1 and T2 sequences may see flow void or altered signal density in the venous system. Additional SWI sequences may reveal small parenchymal hemorrhages resulting from venous hypertension. MRV has greater accuracy and will reveal flow defects. CSF cine sequences are imaging sequences that may identify and localize impaired CSF flow in cases of hydrocephalus from intrinsic or structural causes.

In summary, advantages of having early access to MRI in the hyperacute phase of stroke care include being able to confirm the presence of a stroke with DWI, getting information regarding onset of stroke time by DWI/FLAIR mismatch, being able to confirm a stroke mimic presentation, in rare cases identifying small hemorrhages that may not be seen on CT, and viewing the arterial and venous vasculature when indicated. A major drawback is that MRI is currently not readily available in most emergency departments (EDs) for hyperacute phase imaging.

Outside of the stroke realm, MRI has many applications where it is superior to CT imaging. Some examples include providing a more sensitive and comprehensive evaluation of brain masses (**Figure 5.6**) or providing characteristic findings of increased signal on T2-weighted imaging for

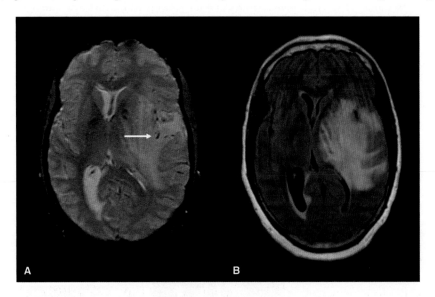

Figure 5.6: MRI of a left frontotemporal lobe glioblastoma. A, SWI sequence revealing mass effect and area of microhemorrhage (arrow). B, FLAIR sequence revealing edema contributing to mass effect midline shift.

posterior reversible encephalopathy syndrome (PRES). MRI can also yield information regarding CNS infections, with DWI enabling the identification of brain abscesses, abnormal meningeal enhancement occurring in meningitis, or temporal lobe signal abnormalities being seen in herpes simplex encephalitis. Outside of the emergency medicine realm, MRI is superior to CT for the identification of multiple sclerosis lesions, the workup for certain epilepsy syndromes, the initial dementia evaluation, working up cranial nerve palsies and abnormalities of the internal auditory canal, pituitary fossa lesions, metabolic disorders, and some congenital malformations.

Spine Imaging

For cervical spine imaging in the evaluation of adult patients with trauma, plain radiographs have traditionally been the most commonly utilized imaging modality for suspected fractures. The series includes an anterior posterior view, a cross-table lateral view, and an anterior posterior view of the odontoid. The lateral view must be able to visualize the top of the T1 vertebral body, and the odontoid view should show the lateral portions of the atlantoaxial articulation. If the T1 vertebral body is not well visualized, a lateral "swimmer's view" (with the patient's arm above the head) could traditionally be performed to better visualize the cervical thoracic junction. Limitations of plain radiographs include the need for multiple views, potentially missing fractures at any level, and incomplete views because of body habitus.

CT imaging with reconstruction techniques is more accurate in the identification of spine fractures than are traditional x-ray series, and is the standard of care at most trauma centers for evaluating the cervical spine. One series identified 100% sensitivity of CT to rule out cervical spine fracture, with a 3.2% false-negative rate of cervical spine x-rays.[8] Reconstruction views include the traditional axial views, but also coronal and sagittal views of vertebrae.

Although CT reconstruction imaging is better at identifying bony fractures, MRI enables an enhanced view of soft-tissue structures, most notably spinal cord injuries or ligamentous injuries (**Figure 5.7**). The protocol utilized in the assessment for spinal cord injury includes axial T2-weighted spin echo sequences and T2-weighted gradient-recalled echo sequences. It also includes sagittal T1- and T2-weighted spin echo sequences, T2-weighted gradient-recalled echo sequences, and sagittal short tau inversion recovery sequences. T2-weighted spin echo sequences can identify cord edema, and T2-weighted gradient-recalled echo sequences can identify hemorrhage. With these axial and sagittal sequences, the overarching objective of MRI in the setting of trauma is to determine the extent of injury to critical soft-tissue structures. Imaging is indicated for the majority of cervical spine fractures and for patients with neurologic findings suggestive

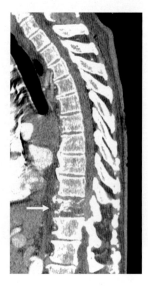

Figure 5.7: T11 fracture with retropulsion.

of spinal cord injury. MRI may identify pathologies such as traumatic disk herniation, anterior and posterior longitudinal ligament injury, cord contusions, epidural hematomas, and soft-tissue hematomas. In the non-trauma setting, MRI may be utilized in the evaluation of many pathologies, including, but not limited to, nontraumatic disk bulges, epidural abscesses, and transverse myelitis.

SPECIAL SITUATIONS

Neuroimaging in Pediatrics

Pediatric neurologic emergencies, although rare, do occur. Acute ischemic stroke may occur in patients with sickle cell disease, thrombotic disorders, or traumatic or spontaneous cerebrovascular dissections. Intracranial hemorrhages that typically result from traumatic mechanisms as spontaneous ICH or subarachnoid hemorrhage have profoundly low incidences. The threshold to perform neuroimaging in children is higher than in adults, stemming from the lower incidence of disease, the slightly higher lifelong risk of cancer from CT scan radiation exposure, and the higher incidence of needing conscious sedation for MRI. Clinical decision rules have been well established for pediatric head trauma, namely, the PECARN criteria, which provide decisional support for when to perform a CT, when to observe, or when to discharge.

Neuroimaging in Pregnancy

The overall incidence of acute ischemic stroke during pregnancy is low, but there are a variety of unique etiologies and sex-specific risk factors predisposing women in pregnancy and the postpartum phase. Likewise, ICH from eclampsia, arterial venous malformations, or aneurismal subarachnoid hemorrhage is also low, but more common in pregnancy rather than in the postpartum period. Early imaging of pregnant women presenting with symptoms is critical. Stroke system recommendations rely on consensus statements and extrapolation from existing practice guidelines.

An overarching principle for imaging selection in pregnancy is to optimize the risk/benefit balance (risk to the child, benefit to the mother). Practice guidelines and consensus recommendations have been established by radiology and obstetric associations and advocacy organizations. In occasions where there is a moderate to high suspicion of a life-threatening or significantly debilitating neurologic emergency, imaging selection might be extrapolated from guidelines for nonpregnant persons and may also influenced by immediate accessibility to imaging.

In pregnancy, radiation dosages <5 rads are typically safe in all trimesters, whereas dosages from 5 to 10 rads have uncertain effects, and dosages >10 rads may induce spontaneous abortions or cause malformations in the first trimester (weeks 3-10), and cause neurocognitive deficits in later phases of pregnancy (weeks 11-27).[9] In general, the radiation exposure from cranial neuroimaging results from radiation scatter (ie, from deflecting off the skull) as opposed to being in the direct line of radiation (ie, a CT of the abdomen/pelvis). Neuroimaging with CT in pregnancy has a radiation dose from a non-contrast CT of the head of <0.01 rads, contrasted to lumbar spine CT imaging estimated at 0.28 to 2.4 rads.[10] For cervical spine imaging, CT delivers 2.6 rads to the neck contrasted to 0.18 rads by radiographs. The utilization of IV iodine contrast has not been demonstrated in animal models to have teratogenic side effects, but may have a theoretical risk of causing neonatal hypothyroidism. Thus, contrast is reserved for exceptional circumstances, and when utilized, neonatal thyroid testing is recommended.

The principal benefit of MRI is the absence of radiation exposure. When stroke systems can support the utilization of MRI, it should be utilized in favor of CT imaging. Although there is the theoretical risk of harm from a minimal increase in body temperature from the magnets, there is no definitive data suggesting harm. Conversely, gadolinium utilization in pregnancy should be limited to situations where it will significantly enhance the diagnostic yield, because it has been demonstrated in animal models to have teratogenic effects or result in spontaneous abortion.[10]

TIPS AND PEARLS

- Non-contrast CT of the head may have early abnormal findings in acute ischemic stroke, is sensitive for ruling out intracranial bleeding from trauma or intraparenchymal hemorrhage, and has good sensitivity for ruling out subarachnoid hemorrhage in patients presenting within an early time frame.
- CTA is a critical test for patients with acute ischemic stroke for identifying LVOs that may be amenable to mechanical thrombectomy.
- CTP software can identify a favorable penumbral profile for selecting patients for thrombectomy in the extended time window of presentation.
- MRI may detect strokes in the hyperacute phase of presentation (restriction of diffusion) and may serve to indicate when stroke onset occurred (diffusion/FLAIR mismatch).
- MRI has many applications where it is superior to CT.
- CT imaging of the spine is more accurate than are plain radiographs. MRI can detect soft-tissue spinal cord injuries.

SUMMARY

Acute neuroimaging is a critical pillar of stroke and trauma systems of care. Great evolution has occurred over the past decade in advanced neuroimaging, which has improved accuracy, giving clinicians a greater ability to understand the individual patient's pathophysiology of disease, and has enabled a better and more widespread evaluation of patients with neurologic emergencies.

EVIDENCE

Can neuroimaging be used to extend the time from onset to reperfusion?

Both the time from last normal and imaging are useful in the decision to thrombolyse, and each may complement and enhance medical decision-making. With regard to IV t-PA utilization, time will always be a critical piece of information determining whether a patient is eligible for this therapy because many smaller health care systems may not have access to higher level imaging (ie, MRI, CTP). In other systems, time delays may occur if higher level imaging is always required before determining t-PA eligibility. In the future, advanced imaging may select treatment candidates presenting with an unknown time of onset (ie, wake-up strokes) given that MRI may serve as the "witness" to when stroke onset occurred if a diffusion/FLAIR mismatch is identified. Likewise, CTP may identify patients with stroke in the extended window of presentation who might safely receive IV t-PA when there is a demonstrated penumbral mismatch.[11] For mechanical thrombectomy, several trials demonstrated benefit for patients presenting within 6 hours of stroke onset, so findings on imaging may not overturn the decision to treat in the early time window. Likewise, in this early time period, CTP may falsely overestimate the initial size of the infarct core (also known as "ghost core").[12] In the extended time window, advanced penumbral imaging is typically incorporated into treatment decisions.

In ruling out aneurysmal subarachnoid hemorrhage, is there a benefit to obtaining a CTA, and can CTA finding negate the need for a lumbar puncture?

This is a complex topic that generates a lot of discussion. In some cases, it may be reasonable to perform a CTA; but if done on all patients, there may be drawbacks. For background, 85% of spontaneous subarachnoid hemorrhages are caused by aneurysms. For patients presenting with acute headaches, the history and physical examination are integral prerequisites before selecting any type of imaging. Historical features, such as thunderclap headache or a family history of cerebral aneurysms, enable the clinician to generate a rough pretest probability for aneurysmal subarachnoid hemorrhage. In addition, new focal neurologic deficits found on examination typically mandate a more thorough evaluation with vessel imaging. Currently, there are no validated scoring systems to quantify risk estimates for patients with normal neurologic examinations. Another key piece of information is the duration of symptoms. As mentioned in the chapter, a non-contrast CT of the head has excellent sensitivity in ruling out subarachnoid hemorrhage within 6 to 12 hours of symptom onset. Beyond that time, blood may be isodense, limiting interpretive accuracy. Although CTA is fairly sensitive to rule out aneurysms, the decision to perform vessel imaging on all patients with headache may also have drawbacks and overburden a system. If the initial non-contrast CT of the head is normal within the high-sensitivity 6-hour window, no further testing is typically necessary. If patients present in the extended window, traditional teaching recommends a lumbar puncture afterward to rule out subarachnoid hemorrhage, with older literature suggesting this is a safe approach. Drawbacks include the invasiveness of the procedure, and that xanthochromia takes roughly 12 hours to develop. In select cases, if lumbar puncture is not feasible, CTA or MRI/MRA may be considered.[13] However, further prospective investigation, including the validation of clinical decision rules, is necessary before this approach can be widely instituted.[14]

What imaging is necessary for patients with transient neurologic deficits who may be discharged from the ED?

TIA is considered to be a tissue-based, rather than a time-based, diagnosis, with up to 34% of patients with transient neurologic symptoms having signs of a cerebral infarction on MRI.[15] It is recommended that patients with suspected TIA symptoms have CTA performed to determine whether they have a high-risk parent vessel lesion placing them at risk for a stroke within 48 to 72 hours. Examples include a cerebrovascular dissection, critical stenosis, large-vessel thrombus causing a partial occlusion, or other lesions creating a critical stenosis or posing risk for artery to artery embolization. Regarding MRI, the specificity for infarct is 95% within 24 hours of symptom onset. Thus, it is most optimal to perform an MRI to differentiate a TIA (no infarct) from a nondisabling acute ischemic stroke, given the variance in recurrent stroke risk. In addition, MRI may also suggest a cardioembolic etiology of stroke if there are focal infarcts seen in multiple vessel territories.

Is the accuracy of an MSU CT sufficient for t-PA and thrombectomy decision-making?

In many systems utilizing MSUs, there is a great reduction in door-to-needle times for the administration of IV t-PA to eligible patients with acute ischemic stroke, and outcomes appear to be significantly improved. In addition, MSUs can rapidly identify hemorrhagic strokes or acute ischemic strokes with LVOs that would need to be transported directly to a comprehensive stroke center with neurosurgical, neurocritical care, or neurointerventional capabilities rather than a non-thrombectomy center only equipped for administering IV t-PA. MSUs typically utilize a 16-slice CT/CTA. Although there are no direct data per our knowledge reporting the sensitivity/specificity of MSU CT/CTAs, they are regarded as having adequate sensitivity to rule out ICH before the field administration of IV t-PA, and are thus regarded as being adequate for t-PA decision-making. They also are regarded as having suitable sensitivity/specificity for ruling in or out LVO strokes, with many MSU systems having routing eligible plans dependent on the results of imaging.

Are there portable neuroimaging devices?

Authors evaluating portable CTs report that the quality of images is reduced compared to standard conventional scanners. However, they contend that the diagnostic accuracy and reliability is unchanged.[16] In the real world, portable CTs are typically utilized in neuroscience intensive care units to get serial CTs on patients who may not be able to be transported to neuroradiology for serial imaging. Such CTs are most commonly 32-slice units with a cost starting range of $100,000. Although the utilization of a portable CT in the ED may decrease the door-to-imaging benchmark, at this time, there is limited, if any, utilization of portable CTs in the ED setting on a regular basis for initial point-of-care neuroimaging. Low-dose magnet portable MRI units have recently been generated and are available at select sites. Investigation is ongoing to establish the sensitivity and specificity thresholds of different imaging sequences for a spectrum of neurologic emergencies.

What is the optimal study to identify spinal epidural abscess?

For spinal epidural abscess, gadolinium-enhanced MRI is the test of choice, with a >90% sensitivity and specificity. Repeat interval testing may be required in cases of a negative or an equivocal result when there remains a moderate to high clinical suspicion. Imaging the entire spine merits consideration to evaluate for noncontiguous collections. Contrast-enhanced CT may reveal signs suggestive of epidural abscess (ie, findings of osteomyelitis or diskitis), but is neither sensitive nor specific to adequately inform clinical decision-making.

References

1. Lansberg MG, Lee J, Christensen S, et al. RAPID automated patient selection for reperfusion therapy: a pooled analysis of the echo planar imaging thrombolytic evaluation trial (EPITHET) and the diffusion and perfusion imaging evaluation for understanding stroke evolution (DEFUSE) study. *Stroke*. 2011;42(6):1608-1614.

2. Nogueira RG, Jadhav AP, Haussen DC, et al. Thrombectomy 6 to 24 hours after stroke with a mismatch between deficit and infarct. *N Engl J Med*. 2018;378(1):11-21. doi:10.1056/NEJMoa1706442

3. Barber PA, Demchuk AM, Zhang J, Buchan AM. Validity and reliability of a quantitative computed tomography score in predicting outcome of hyperacute stroke before thrombolytic therapy. ASPECTS Study Group. Alberta Stroke Programme Early CT Score [published correction appears in *Lancet* 2000 Jun 17;355(9221):2170]. *Lancet*. 2000;355(9216):1670-1674. doi:10.1016/s0140-6736(00)02237-6

4. Kleinman JT, Hillis AE, Jordan LC. ABC/2: estimating intracerebral haemorrhage volume and total brain volume, and predicting outcome in children. *Dev Med Child Neurol*. 2011;53(3):281-284. doi:10.1111/j.1469-8749.2010.03798.x

5. Dubosh NM, Bellolio MF, Rabinstein AA, Edlow JA. Sensitivity of early brain computed tomography to exclude aneurysmal subarachnoid hemorrhage: a systematic review and meta-analysis. *Stroke*. 2016;47(3):750-755. doi:10.1161/STROKEAHA.115.011386

6. Hotta K, Sorimachi T, Osada T, et al. Risks and benefits of CT angiography in spontaneous intracerebral hemorrhage. *Acta Neurochir (Wien)*. 2014;156(5):911-917. doi:10.1007/s00701-014-2019-7

7. Mehdi E, Aralasmak A, Toprak H, et al. Craniocervical dissections: radiologic findings, pitfalls, mimicking diseases: a pictorial review. *Curr Med Imaging Rev*. 2018;14(2):207-222.

8. Griffen MM, Frykberg ER, Kerwin AJ, et al. Radiographic clearance of blunt cervical spine injury: plain radiograph or computed tomography scan? *J Trauma*. 2003;55(2):222-227.

9. ACR–SPR practice parameter for imaging pregnant or potentially pregnant adolescents and women with ionizing radiation. Accessed April 2, 2020. https://www.acr.org/-/media/ACR/Files/Practice-Parameters/Pregnant-Pts.pdf

10. Klein JP, Hsu L. Neuroimaging during pregnancy. *Semin Neurol*. 2011;31(4):361-373.

11. Ma H, Campbell BCV, Parsons MW, et al. Thrombolysis guided by perfusion imaging up to 9 hours after onset of stroke. *N Engl J Med*. 2019;380(19):1795-1803.

12. Boned S, Padroni M, Rubiera M, et al. Admission CT perfusion may overestimate initial infarct core: the ghost infarct core concept. *J Neurointerv Surg*. 2017;9(1):66-69. doi:10.1136/neurintsurg 2016-012494

13. Maher M, Schweizer TA, Macdonald RL. Treatment of spontaneous subarachnoid hemorrhage: guidelines and gaps. *Stroke*. 2020;51(4):1326-1332. doi:10.1161/STROKEAHA.119.025997

14. Carpenter CR, Hussain AM, Ward MJ, et al. Spontaneous subarachnoid hemorrhage: a systematic review and meta-analysis describing the diagnostic accuracy of history, physical examination, imaging, and lumbar puncture with an exploration of test thresholds. *Acad Emerg Med*. 2016;23(9):963-1003.

15. Brazzelli M, Chappell FM, Miranda H, et al. Diffusion-weighted imaging and diagnosis of transient ischemic attack. *Ann Neurol*. 2014;75(1):67-76.

16. Rumboldt Z, Huda W, All JW. Review of portable CT with assessment of a dedicated head CT scanner. *Am J Neuroradiol*. 2009;30(9):1630-1636.

17. Albers GW, Marks MP, Kemp S, et al. Thrombectomy for stroke at 6 to 16 hours with selection by perfusion imaging. *N Engl J Med*. 2018;378(8):708-718. doi:10.1056/NEJMoa1713973

Section II

Clinical Presentations

Altered Consciousness and Behavior

Andrew Bissonette and Joseph B. Miller

THE CLINICAL CHALLENGE

Patients presenting with altered mental status (AMS) to the emergency department (ED) are common and challenging. Although etiologies for AMS include benign diagnoses, such as alcohol intoxication, many are associated with the potential for negative outcomes and require immediate stabilizing or life-saving interventions. Once rapidly reversible life threats are addressed, there often remains a broad differential diagnosis to consider requiring a systematic approach, including a careful history and neurologic examination, and judicious use of diagnostic tools.

PATHOPHYSIOLOGY

Consciousness has two components: arousal and content.[1] Deficits in either result in altered consciousness. Arousal refers to the level of alertness or wakefulness. This is maintained by multiple cerebral foci, including the brainstem, hypothalamus, thalamus, and basal forebrain—all with broad cortical connections through the reticular activating system. Deficits in arousal cause AMS. Delirium represents a subset of AMS that is characterized by acute changes in arousal that follow a fluctuating course.

Content refers to the awareness of self and the environment and allows for interaction with the environment. This process is carried out in the cortical regions via widespread neural networks. Loss of consciousness refers to loss of both content and arousal, and requires bilateral cortical impairment or brainstem impairment.

PREHOSPITAL CONSIDERATIONS

AMS in the prehospital setting is often associated with life-threatening conditions that require emergent interventions, such as hypoglycemia, hypoxemia, seizures, or opiate overdose. A brief history and examination focused on life threats is indicated. History should focus on pertinent information from witnesses and environmental observations. Time course and prodromal symptoms are tremendously useful, as is information about the patient's medical history, medications, and any substance abuse or recent illness.[2]

Physical examination should focus on vital signs, oxygen saturation, signs of trauma, and a standardized assessment of alertness, such as the Glasgow Coma Scale (GCS). Although the GCS

- Airway, breathing, circulation
- Glasgow Coma Scale, pupils, vital sings
- Assess for signs of trauma
- Assess and treat for hypoglycemia
- Intravenous or intraosseous access
- Treat seizure
- Treat suspected opiate overdose
- Key history: time last seen normal, prodromal symptoms, bystander report, context and environment

Figure 6.1: Prehospital checklist. Derived from Cadena RS, Sarwal A. Emergency neurological life support: approach to the patient with coma. *Neurocrit Care*. 2017;27:74-81.

was derived for assessment of head injury, it is a reasonable means of documenting changes in mentation due to any etiology. Critical tests in the field include glucose level and stroke screen if clinical suspicion warrants. All patients with AMS should be placed on a cardiac monitor with pulse oximetry. Treatment should be administered in the prehospital setting, according to local protocols for the suspected etiology. **Figure 6.1** shows a checklist of prehospital considerations most relevant to the management of patients with AMS.

APPROACH/THE FOCUSED EXAMINATION

Approach

The approach to AMS is to rapidly identify and manage critical life-threatening or disabling conditions. This requires a consistent approach to managing conditions as they are identified and an active differential diagnosis so that less common or evident conditions are not overlooked. A common mnemonic for the differential diagnosis of most AMS cases is "AEIOU-TIPS" (see **Table 6.1**). One

TABLE 6.1	Mnemonic "AEIOU-TIPS" for Altered Mental Status
Mnemonic	**Things to Consider**
Alcohol	Alcohol levels, serum osmoles
Epilepsy/endocrine/electrolytes/ encephalopathy	EEG, referral to neurology, TFTs, cortisol, chemistry panel, LFTs/NH_3
Insulin	Glucose
Oxygen/opiates	Spo_2, ABG, hypoxia presents with agitation, hypercarbia presents with somnolence; Look for needle marks
Uremia	BUN/Cr Things changing serum osmolarity affect mental status. Uremia, sodium, glucose, and alcohol are common etiologies
Trauma/temperature	CT head, C-collar, CT C-spine
Infection	CBC, BCx, UA, UCx, CXR, LP/CSF Sepsis and CNS infections are more important. However, even simple fever may cause AMS in elderly and kids
Poisoning/psychosis	Drug levels (eg, lithium, digoxin)
Shock/stroke/SAH/space-occupying lesion	ECG, troponin, CT head, LP

ABG, arterial blood gas; AMS, altered mental status; BCx, blood cultures; BUN, blood urea nitrogen; CBC, complete blood count; CNS, central nervous system; Cr, creatinine; C-collar, cervical collar; C-spine, cervical spine; CSF, cerebrospinal fluid; CT, computed tomography; CXR, chest x-ray; ECG, electrocardiogram; EEG, electroencephalogram; LFTs, liver function tests; LP, lumbar puncture; NH_3, ammonia; SAH, subarachnoid hemorrhage; Spo_2, oxygen saturation; TFTs, thyroid function tests; UA, urinalysis; UCx, urine culture.

can also classify AMS into the following categories: primary central nervous system (CNS)/structural, metabolic/autoregulatory, toxic/pharmacologic, and infectious. The ED needs to assess and treat readily reversible causes of altered mentation, including hypoglycemia, opioid intoxication, and Wernicke encephalopathy. Rapid treatment prevents clinical deterioration and may prove diagnostic.

Focused History

History obtained from witnesses and emergency medical services may suggest a cause of the patient's altered consciousness. Establishing the time course of altered consciousness should be a priority. A sudden onset suggests ischemic stroke, hemorrhage, seizure, or cardiac event with decreased cerebral perfusion.[3] Subacute onset points more toward infectious or toxic-metabolic causes of altered consciousness. The history should include infectious symptoms, recent trauma, illicit drug use, or alcohol use in addition to current medications, recent medication changes, and medication compliance.

Determining baseline cognitive function and similar previous episodes aids in assessing etiologies. Known medical problems that can guide initial evaluation include cirrhosis (hyperammonemia), chronic kidney disease (uremia), obstructive or restrictive lung disease (hypercapnia), epilepsy, immunocompromise, and psychiatric disease.

Abcs and Cervical Spine Precautions

As in the prehospital setting, the ED approach begins with an assessment of the patient's airway, breathing, circulation (ABC), disability, and exposure to trauma (**Figure 6.2**). Maintaining a patent airway and adequate respirations is critical for preventing secondary neural injury from hypercapnia and/or hypoxia. If head or neck trauma cannot be ruled out, immobilize the cervical spine.

Maintaining an appropriate mean arterial pressure (MAP) sustains cerebral perfusion pressure (CPP) to the potentially injured brain. The goal MAP varies according to the underlying etiology of altered consciousness, and goal MAP may additionally be guided by intracranial pressure (ICP) monitoring in some cases. Nevertheless, during the initial resuscitation and before a clear etiology of AMS is determined, treatment to maintain a MAP >65 mm Hg is suggested.

In the setting of trauma, the GCS is a critical indicator of disability. Patients with traumatic brain injury (TBI) are categorized as severe TBI (GCS $\leq$ 8), moderate TBI (GCS 9-12), and mild TBI (GCS 13-15); see **Chapter 12: Head Trauma: Severe**.

Assessing pain response and movement in all four extremities provides a vital neurologic baseline in those with decreased arousal, especially if the patient will require intubation and administration of a long-acting paralytic agent, or require heavy sedation with agents that are not quickly reversible. Lastly, rapid exposure and initial assessment for notable examination findings of the head, neck, chest, back, abdomen, and extremities can provide key diagnostic information.

Neurologic Assessment

Level of Consciousness

The GCS is useful to quantitatively and serially measure level of consciousness. Limitations of the GCS include its limited capacity for monitoring changes in hemiparesis, aphasia, or brainstem abnormalities. When assessing level of consciousness, serially increase stimulation from a normal tone command to a loud command and then to physical stimulation followed by noxious peripheral (eg, nail bed pressure) and central stimuli (eg, sternal rub, trapezius muscle squeeze, and supraorbital pressure) as needed to elicit a response. Qualitative level of consciousness is best documented and communicated by directly describing what responses were seen with a particular level of stimulation.

Motor Response

Assess the motor responses looking for spontaneous movement, then responses to verbal or tactile stimulation. Purposeful movements must be distinguished from reflex movements. Examples of purposeful movement include localizing to noxious stimuli, including reaching for an endotracheal tube. Instances of reflexive activity include flexion, flexion-withdrawal, and extensor posturing to noxious stimuli, which are findings associated with midbrain compression or injury. Notably, grasp can be a

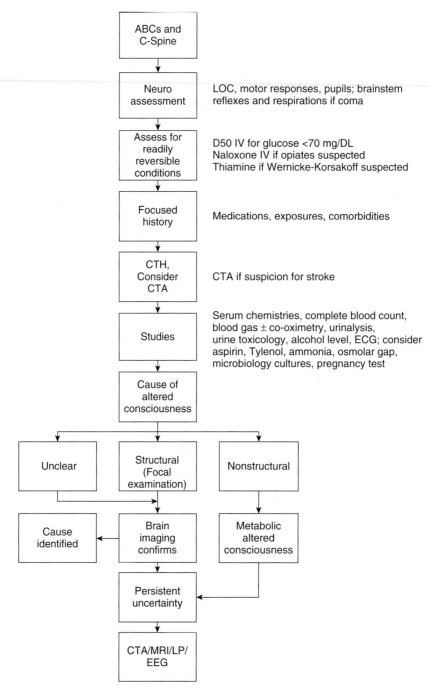

Figure 6.2: Approach to altered mental status. ABCs, airway, breathing, circulation; C-spine, cervical spine; CTA, computed tomography angiography; CTH, computed tomography of the head; ECG, electrocardiogram; EEG, electroencephalogram; IV, intravenous; LOC, level of consciousness; LP, lumbar puncture; MRI, magnetic resonance imaging. Derived from Cadena RS, Sarwal A. Emergency neurological life support: approach to the patient with coma. *Neurocrit Care.* 2017;27:74-81.

reflex, and does not indicate purposeful movement unless the patient is reliably able to let go of the grasp as well. In addition to motor responses, muscle tone and extremity reflexes should be tested and compared bilaterally. Symmetric findings do not rule out structural causes of altered consciousness, but symmetry does increase the likelihood of a nonstructural source of altered consciousness.

Pupil Assessment

Pupil assessment includes size, reactivity, and symmetry. Especially in those with depressed arousal or abnormal motor responses, pupil assessment can rapidly alert the physician to potentially reversible life-threatening conditions, such as cerebral herniation; see **Table 6.2** and **Chapter 3: Abnormal Vision, Pupils, and Eye Movements**.

TABLE 6.2	Pupillary Abnormalities and Associated Diseases	
Miotic	**Mydriatic, Reactive**	**Anisocoric**
Structural	Structural	Structural
Medial or bilateral pontine damage	Midbrain damage (pretectal area)	Unilateral CN III compression (eg, uncal herniation, PCOM aneurysm)
Bilateral Horner syndrome		
Toxic	Toxic	Unilateral pontine damage
Opioids	Stimulants (eg, cocaine, methamphetamine)	Unilateral Horner syndrome
Clonidine		Edinger-Westphal nucleus damage
Barbiturates	Hallucinogens (eg, PCP, LSD)	Traumatic
GHB		Subarachnoid hemorrhage
Typical and atypical antipsychotics		Carotid dissection (via unilateral Horner syndrome)
Cholinergic agents	**Mydriatic, Unreactive**	
β-Blocker eye drops	Structural	Post-traumatic iridocylitis
Infectious	Midbrain damage	Iatrogenic
Argyll Robertson pupils	Bilateral CN III compression	Ophthalmologic mydriatics (ie, red bottle cap)
Pseudo-Argyll Robertson pupils (more likely mid-sized)	Metabolic	
	Global cerebral anoxia, brain death	Local drug effect (eg, ipratropium nebulizer)
	Hypothermia	
	Toxic	Ocular prosthesis
	Barbiturates	Other
	Anticholinergics	Acute angle closure glaucoma
		Holmes-Adie pupil
		Physiologic anisocoria

CN, cranial nerve; GHB, γ-hydroxybutyrate; LSD, lysergic acid diethylamide; PCOM, posterior communicating artery; PCP, phencyclidine.

Brainstem Assessment

In the comatose patient, additional cranial nerve (CN) brainstem reflexes include corneal (afferent CN V1, efferent CN VII), response to visual threat (afferent CN II, efferent CN VII), oculocephalic reflex or doll's eyes (afferent CN VIII, efferent CNs III, IV, VI), gag (afferent CN IX, efferent CN IX, X), and cough (afferent CN X, efferent CN X). Of note, the oculocephalic reflex should not be tested if there is concern for cervical spine injury.

Hypothermia (including induced hypothermia) and neuromuscular blockade both reversibly impair CN reflexes. Locked-in syndrome, fulminant Guillain-Barré syndrome, and unrecognized intoxication (eg, tricyclics, lidocaine, baclofen, barbiturates, anticholinergics, and organophosphates) can also impair CN reflexes and mimic brain death. Barbiturates represent one of the most notorious iatrogenic brain death mimics.

Breathing Pattern

Breathing pattern can help localize CNS injury. Hyperventilation can result from primary pontine or midbrain insults as well as metabolic encephalopathy, especially metabolic acidosis. In addition to CHF and metabolic encephalopathy, insults to the diencephalon (ie, thalamus, hypothalamus, epithalamus, and subthalamus) can produce Cheyne-Stokes breathing. Primary pontomedullary insults can lead to cluster (Biot) breathing. Bilateral pontine lesions can result in apneusis (deep, gasping inspiration with a pause at full inspiration followed by a brief, insufficient release). Ventrolateral medulla damage bilaterally can produce primary neurologic apnea. Intracerebral hemorrhage can induce yawning.

Additional High-Yield Examination Findings

Depending on the patient's clinical status, a comprehensive physical examination may be completed before or after imaging. On lung auscultation, evidence of pneumonia or chronic obstructive pulmonary disease can point to an infectious etiology or hypercarbia, respectively. Heart and extremity examination can raise suspicion for heart failure or endocarditis. Skin examination may show track marks suggesting intravenous drug abuse or may reveal jaundice suggesting liver disease. The skin examination might also reveal a petechial rash, such as that seen in meningococcemia.

Perhaps most importantly, a thorough neurologic examination should be performed, looking for motor, sensory, reflex, and cerebellar abnormalities with particular focus on detecting focal deficits. In addition, all patients should be checked for meningeal signs. Asterixis can point toward cirrhosis or uremia. Otherwise, unexplained nystagmus should raise the possibility of nonconvulsive status epilepticus (NCSE), posterior circulation stroke, or drug overdose. Funduscopy (retinal hemorrhages, papilledema) or ultrasound measurement of optic nerve sheath diameter ($\geq$5 mm when measured 3 mm behind the globe) may raise suspicion for increased ICP.[4] Once time-critical management has concluded, a comprehensive head-to-toe examination is necessary, searching for findings such as unexposed trauma (especially posterior), medication patches, and septic joints as well as infected dialysis lines, implanted pacemakers, and sacral decubitus ulcers.

Diagnostic Studies

Computed Tomography

If no clear diagnosis is found after assessing for readily reversible causes and performing a focused history and neurologic assessment, we recommend obtaining noncontrast computed tomography (CT) of the head, especially in the presence of anticoagulation or focal neurologic deficits. Imaging should not be delayed until initial laboratory evaluation is completed. If stroke is suspected, a CT angiography of the head and neck should be strongly considered in addition to a noncontrast CT of the head.

CT head with and without contrast is indicated when a CNS infection is suspected to evaluate for abscess, hydrocephalus, or hemorrhagic changes. As shown in Figure 6.2, we recommend that a CT head should be obtained before lumbar puncture (LP) in any patient with an altered level of consciousness. Although there is controversy regarding this recommendation when there is strong suspicion for acute bacterial meningitis, current guidelines recommend CT before LP in adults if patients have a history of immunocompromise, CNS disease, new seizure, papilledema, or focal neurologic deficits on examination.[5,6] In children and adolescents, guidelines recommend against

LP, even if a CT finding is negative, when clinical signs of increased ICP are present, including GCS <9 or a drop in GCS of 3 or more, relative bradycardia and hypertension, focal neurologic signs, papilledema, abnormal posturing, or unequal, dilated or poorly responsive pupils.[7]

If initial finding of CT head does not confirm suspected structural pathology, further imaging with CT angiogram of the head/neck, a CT perfusion scan, or magnetic resonance imaging (MRI) may be indicated.

Laboratory Testing

In the absence of a clear diagnosis, diagnostic studies should include a complete blood count with differential, coagulation studies, and serum chemistries (basic metabolic panel, ionized calcium levels, and liver function tests) to look for a metabolic etiology. In addition to acid-base information, a blood gas can reveal hypercapnia that might not otherwise have been appreciated. Additional blood gas co-oximetry should be considered in those at risk for carbon monoxide, cyanide, or methemoglobinemia. Urinalysis is indicated in most patients with AMS, especially the elderly. We do recommend that both urine toxicology and serum alcohol be analyzed.

Salicylate, acetaminophen, and ammonia levels are indicated in the correct clinical scenario. Ammonia levels should be strongly considered in those taking valproic acid (VA); VA toxicity causes hyperammonemia, which may be missed if one ascribes the patient's altered consciousness to underlying seizure or bipolar disorder rather than to VA's inhibition of the acyl-carnitine pathway.[8] For patients on antiepileptic agents, drug levels are indicated when feasible. In the correct clinical setting, thyroid function tests, cortisol, vitamin B_{12} levels, and human immunodeficiency virus (HIV) testing can be revealing. When concerned for rheumatologic etiologies such as lupus cerebritis, erythrocyte sedimentation rate, complement levels, antinuclear antibodies, and appropriate autoimmune serologies based on suspected diagnosis can be helpful in establishing a diagnosis.

Finally, urine pregnancy testing should be obtained in all females of child-bearing potential for multiple reasons, including ruling out eclampsia.

Chest X-ray

A chest x-ray is indicated for concern for thoracic pathology or in the setting of sepsis of unclear etiology. In these cases, blood, urine, and/or cerebrospinal fluid (CSF) cultures should also be considered.

Electrocardiogram

The electrocardiogram (ECG) can provide evidence for multiple cardiac sources of altered consciousness (eg, arrhythmia, ischemia) but also can clue physicians into possible ingestions, such as a prolonged QTc from antipsychotics or QRS prolongation and an elevated R wave (>0.3 mm) in aVR from tricyclic antidepressants or other sodium channel blockers.

Lumbar Puncture

An LP is indicated when there is concern for CNS infection, autoimmune disorders, or suspected CNS involvement of hematologic cancer or solid organ cancers.[9,10] Typically, CSF analysis should include cell count and differential, protein, glucose, gram stain, and bacterial culture as well as additional studies that may be considered depending on the clinical scenario; see **Table 6.3**. Given the broad differential diagnosis, it is wise to freeze spin and store a vial of CSF for any future additional testing that may become necessary.

Electroencephalography

In patients with persistent and unexplained altered consciousness, a high suspicion for NCSE is warranted, and an electroencephalography (EEG) should be obtained. Special consideration should be given to NCSE in those with seizure history, with seizure activity noted during their clinical course, or with twitches, abnormal eye movements, or fine tremors while persistently altered. However, the absence of these findings does not rule out NCSE. In addition, NCSE must be on the differential diagnosis of any patient suspected to have a prolonged postictal phase. Critically ill patients with unexplained altered consciousness are at particular risk for NCSE.

Data suggest that prompt EEG in patients with seizure or AMS improves diagnostic capability and may change treatment course. A recent review of five studies including 478 patients showed

TABLE 6.3	CSF Studies to Consider in Altered Mental Status[a]
All Patients	**Encephalitis Suspected**
Cell count and differential	Viral PCR
Protein	Enterovirus
Glucose	WNV
Gram stain and bacterial culture	EBV[a]
PCR for HSV-1, HSV-2, and VZV	IgG and IgM
Known History of Malignancy	WNV[b]
Cytology and flow cytometry	Saint Louis encephalitis[b]
Immunocompromised	EBV
PCR	Additional serologies depending on season and geography
CMV	Bacterial PCR
HHV6	Rickettsia[b]
JC virus	*Mycobacterium tuberculosis*
Bacterial culture notifying laboratory of suspicion for *Nocardia*	ELISA and Western blot
Galactomannan if aspergillosis suspected	VDRL
India Ink if cryptococcus suspected	*Borrelia burgdorferi*[b]
	Acid-fast bacilli smear and culture
	Fungal culture
	Fungal Species
	Cryptococcus antigen
	Histoplasma antigen[b]
	Coccidiodes immunodiffusion or complement fixation[b]
	IgG index and oligoclonal bands
	Paraneoplastic and limbic encephalitis antibody panel

CMV, cytomegalovirus; CSF, cerebrospinal fluid; EBV, Epstein-Barr virus; ELISA, enzyme-linked immunosorbent assay; HHV6, human herpesvirus 6; HSV-1, herpes simplex virus 1; HSV-2 herpes simplex virus 2; IgG, immunoglobulin G; IgM, immunoglobulin M; JC, John Cunningham; PCR, polymerase chain reaction; VDRL, Venereal Disease Research Laboratory; VZV, varicella zoster virus; WNV, West Nile virus.
[a]*Can be falsely positive with blood contamination (perform with EBV IgG and IgM).*
[b]*Depends on season, geography, and travel history.*
Derived from Douglas VC, Josephson SA. Altered mental status. Continuum (Minneap Minn). 2011;17:967-983.

the prevalence of NCSE in patients with AMS ranged from 8% to 30% (overall prevalence of 21.5%, 95% CI: 18%-25%), suggesting that the prevalence of NCSE is sufficiently high to consider routine use of urgent EEG in select patients.[11] A recent portable device that syncs with cloud monitoring and can be applied by any emergency clinician shows promise in providing early diagnostic information.[12] In addition, portable, quantitative EEG-based brain function monitoring may provide important diagnostic and functional information on brain injury.[13]

At the conclusion of the initial evaluation, clinicians can usually classify patients into a structural or a nonstructural cause of their altered consciousness. If brain imaging confirms a structural etiology, emergent medical or surgical intervention and advanced neuromonitoring, such as ICP monitoring, may be needed.

MANGEMENT

General Principles

Although sometimes overlapping, the management of structural pathology is often quite distinct from the management of nonstructural pathology.

There remains an ongoing need to determine strategies to effectively manage delirium in the ED that can hasten its resolution and reduce long-term sequelae. Sedative treatment of agitated delirium has been well studied,[14] but pharmacologic or nonpharmacologic treatments that improve patient-centered outcomes for delirium in the ED are generally lacking and present a fertile area for future innovation.

Given the potential for medications to worsen altered consciousness, we recommend that pharmacologic treatment of altered arousal only occur where treatment is required for patient or staff safety. Low-dose typical or atypical antipsychotics are frequently used, but come with the potential to prolong the QTc, extrapyramidal side effects (especially in Lewy body dementia), anticholinergic side effects, and anti-alpha side effects. Both antipsychotics and benzodiazepines may potentially prolong the overall length of the episode of altered arousal despite temporarily relieving symptoms. Moreover, given the lack of evidence for efficacy in undifferentiated altered consciousness, benzodiazepines are not clearly recommended and are known to have deleterious effects on critically ill and elderly inpatients.[15] Although further research is pending, the clinician must currently weigh the pros and cons of various delirium management options in light of each patient's particular clinical circumstances. That said, alcohol withdrawal, seizure/status epilepticus, and a number of toxidromes (eg, sympathomimetic, anticholinergic, serotonin syndrome, and neuroleptic malignant syndrome) are known to benefit from treatment with benzodiazepines.

Distinguishing Delirium from Dementia and Depression

Dementia syndromes include Alzheimer, vascular, Lewy body, and frontotemporal dementia. Emergency management of dementia is largely supportive; however, the clinician should actively guard against anchoring on a dementia diagnosis when evaluating a patient with dementia who is presenting with an acute change in behavior. It is important to distinguish between dementia and delirium, because the latter is commonly associated with treatable medical illness. Advanced age and baseline cognitive dysfunction are the most consistently identified risk factors for delirium. In addition, depression in the elderly is a common mimic of dementia, which is a very treatable condition. See **Table 6.4** for a comparison of these three disorders.

For recognizing the gap in delirium detection, particularly among older adults, research has demonstrated the high sensitivity of the Delirium Triage Screen (DTS) and the high specificity of the Confusion Assessment Method for the Intensive Care Unit (CAM-ICU) or the brief CAM for recognizing delirium in the ED.[16,17] Whether routine use of these or related tools can lead to long-term improvements in ED patient care remains unknown.

When patients without a known predisposing condition experience delirium with a relatively minor insult, such as a urinary tract infection (UTI), consideration for outpatient screening for a neurodegenerative disease should be considered. If the patient does not steadily improve after removal of the precipitant, workup for alternative sources of altered consciousness should be considered.

Structural Diagnoses

Structural pathology should be suspected in any patient who has a focal neurologic deficit. However, some structural pathology can present without focal findings, such as nondominant parietal strokes. For those in whom elevated ICP is a concern, prevention of hypoxia and hypotension is paramount. Other standard measures include head positioning (ie, head of bed elevated to 30° and face midline), minimizing noxious stimuli, analgesia and sedation as necessary, maintenance of normothermia, avoidance of hyponatremia, and steroids in select conditions (ie, brain tumors, abscess, and noninfectious neuroinflammatory disorders). Neurosurgery consult for further medical management recommendations and possible definitive treatment should be swift. See **Chapter 12: Head Trauma: Severe** for further discussion of ICP management.

TABLE 6.4	Differentiating Depression, Delirium, and Dementia		
	Depression	Delirium	Dementia
Onset	Weeks to months	Hours to days	Months to years
Mood	Low/apathetic	Fluctuates	Fluctuates
Course	Chronic; responds to treatment	Acute; responds to treatment	Chronic, with deterioration over time
Self-awareness	Likely to be concerned about memory impairment	May be aware of changes in cognition; fluctuates	Likely to hide or be unaware of cognitive deficits
Activities of daily living (ADLs)	May neglect basic self-care	May be intact or impaired	May be intact early, impaired as disease progresses

Ischemic Stroke

Acute ischemic stroke typically presents with focal neurologic deficits rather than alterations in arousal. However, infarcts involving the reticular activating system in the brainstem (eg, basilar artery thrombosis) can lead to decreased arousal and coma, whereas posterior cerebral artery (affecting the paramedian territory) and nondominant parietal lobe infarcts can result in increased arousal (often agitated delirium) and other behavior changes. Subacute ischemic stroke can lead to decreased arousal via edema resulting in elevated ICP.

Ischemic stroke results in numerous deficits in content with many well-defined clinical syndromes (please see **Chapter 15: Acute Stroke** for further detail). Two notable ischemic causes of altered content that can easily be mistaken for psychiatric pathology include abulia (ie, lack of will, drive, or initiative for action, speech, or thought) in thalamic or orbital frontal infarcts and the more common Wernicke/receptive aphasia (difficulty understanding written and spoken language with preserved speech fluency that tends to lack content or meaning) resulting from infarcts in the Wernicke area of the posterior temporal lobe.[3] Locked-in syndrome from basilar artery thrombosis affecting the pons can cause quadriplegia and aphasia, where the patient is aware but cannot move or speak except for vertical eye movements and blinking. It is often initially mistaken for coma, vegetative state, or even brain death. Subtle movements may be the only sign of locked-in syndrome, basilar ischemia, or NCSE.

Intracranial Hemorrhage

Noncontrast CT imaging of the head is the best imaging modality for intracranial hemorrhage (ICH). ICH is a common cause of altered consciousness. Each affected area is associated with particular alterations in arousal and content. Although focal deficits are common, patients may present with only altered arousal. ICH can result from both traumatic and nontraumatic insults, such as aneurysmal subarachnoid hemorrhage. Moreover, even in the absence of intracranial hemorrhage, TBI can lead to alterations in content and arousal, such as in diffuse axonal injury.

Posterior Reversible Encephalopathy Syndrome

Posterior reversible encephalopathy syndrome (PRES) occurs classically in the setting of severely elevated blood pressure, eclampsia, or calcineurin inhibitors. Most patients present with altered arousal (28%-92%), seizures (74%-87%), and headaches (26%-53%).[18] Focal alterations are less common, with hemiparesis and visual field deficits seen in < 50% of patients.[18] Imaging can show reversible vasogenic subcortical edema without infarction in the parieto-occipital white matter, although atypical imaging findings are frequent. Magnetic resonance imaging or CT-perfusion scan may be useful in making the diagnosis. Treatment centers on the reversing the precipitating cause, including control of hypertension and withdrawal of offending agents, such as calcineurin inhibitors. Antiepileptic therapy can be discontinued when the acute phase of PRES has resolved.

Hydrocephalus

Hydrocephalus is typically detected by CT brain imaging, and can be noncommunicating, communicating, normal pressure, or *ex vacuo*. Neurology or neurosurgery consultation is usually indicated for the management of symptomatic hydrocephalus. Noncommunicating hydrocephalus is caused by a focal obstruction in CSF flow, most commonly at the cerebral aqueduct. It can occur anywhere in the ventricular system, with imaging findings and symptoms dependent on the location of CSF flow obstruction. Causes include tumor, edema, cysts, hemorrhage, thrombosis, and malformations, such as Chiari and Dandy-Walker malformations. Communicating hydrocephalus is the result of impaired CSF reabsorption in the absence of CSF flow obstruction between the ventricles and subarachnoid space. It presents with diffuse ventricular dilation on imaging. It can result from subarachnoid or intraventricular hemorrhage, meningitis, or congenital absence of arachnoid villi.

Normal pressure hydrocephalus is an important consideration in elderly patients with delirium. It is a chronic form of communicating hydrocephalus with dilated ventricles but typically normal CSF pressure. It presents with a classic triad of urinary incontinence, altered mentation, and gait apraxia (which may mimic a Parkinsonian gait).

Hydrocephalus *ex vacuo* occurs when brain matter shrinks with a reactionary increase in CSF to fill the newly open space. Examples include loss of brain matter because of aging, Alzheimer disease, stroke, or alcohol abuse.

Tumor

Depending on type, location, and associated complications, tumor presentation and management can vary widely. In addition to compressing adjacent cerebral tissue, tumors can lead to pathology via surrounding vasogenic edema, hemorrhagic conversion, and noncommunicating hydrocephalus. Treatment should occur in concert with an oncologist and neurosurgeon as appropriate. Vasogenic edema is a common reason for acute alterations in consciousness in patients with intracranial malignancy, and may be accompanied by headache, seizure, or motor/sensory deficits. Initial medical management typically includes dexamethasone.

Dural Vein Sinus Thrombosis and Cavernous Sinus Thrombosis

Dural vein sinus thrombosis (DVST) is an important structural pathology to consider; the diagnosis requires that the clinician order venous phase imaging (CT or MRI) of the head in addition to noncontrast and/or arterial-phase imaging. The clinical presentation of DVST is highly variable, and can be acute, subacute, or chronic. It can present structurally with focal weakness, aphasia, papilledema, and multiple CN palsies. However, because it can cause an isolated intracranial hypertension syndrome, DVST can also mimic nonstructural pathology and present with headache, visual disturbances, altered arousal, or seizure without focal findings.

Cavernous sinus thrombosis (CST) is a sub-type of DVST that most commonly results from contiguous spread of infection from the nares, sinuses, or dental tissue. It commonly presents with CN palsies. CN VI palsy is the most common CN abnormality in CST given its medial position within the cavernous sinus. In addition, CNs III, IV, V_1, and V_2 are frequently affected as they course through the lateral portion of the cavernous sinus. Owing to impaired venous drainage from the eye, CST can also present with chemosis, decreased vision, and exophthalmos.

Nonstructural Diagnoses

Metabolic Alterations

Hypoglycemia is one of the most common and readily reversible etiologies of AMS. It usually presents with global deficits, although focal motor and sensory findings may occur. Rapid treatment usually produces immediate return to baseline mental status; prolonged and severe episodes of hypoglycemia can precipitate hypoglycemic encephalopathy or lead to irreversible injury. Although concomitant treatment with thiamine is reasonable, the evidence that dextrose administration can precipitate Wernicke encephalopathy is poor.[19,20] Hyperglycemia is also a common etiology of altered consciousness, particularly when it leads to diabetic ketoacidosis and hyperosmolar hyperglycemic nonketotic coma.

In adults, outside of hyper/hyponatremia, most mild-moderate electrolyte abnormalities are not the etiology of a patient's altered mentation. Severe hyponatremia and hypernatremia with rapid correction have been associated with central pontine myelinolysis and cerebral edema, respectively, along with AMS.

Hypercalcemia can cause fatigue, headache, impaired memory, drowsiness, depressed arousal including coma; hypocalcemia can cause irritability and anxiety, paresthesia, seizure, and Chvostek and Trousseau signs. Hypermagnesemia results in loss of deep tendon reflexes (8.5-12 mg/dL), respiratory paralysis (12-16 mg/dL), impaired cardiac conduction (>18 mg/dL), and cardiac arrest (>30 mg/dL). Hypophosphatemia is associated with altered consciousness, muscle weakness, numbness, weak reflexes, and seizures. Note, ionized calcium levels avoid the potential shortcomings of total calcium measurements and corrected calcium calculations, especially in the critically ill.[21]

Uremia can present with progressive weakness, muscle atrophy, peripheral neuropathy, tremors, disruption of the sleep-wake cycle, memory and concentration deficits, headache, seizure, and altered consciousness including coma. It often co-occurs with a metabolic acidosis in the setting of renal failure. Treatment requires reversal of the underlying renal disorder or dialysis. Dialysis disequilibrium syndrome (DDS) is an important complication of treatment, thought to be caused by reverse osmotic shift because of the rapid clearance of urea or other osmoles in the serum. It is typically seen during the first hemodialysis session of a patient with a markedly elevated blood urea nitrogen (BUN; ie, >150 mg/dL) and is more prevalent in the elderly and those with preexisting neurologic disease. DDS can present with headache, blurred vision, or restlessness, and can progress to somnolence, seizure, coma, or even death. Treatment with mannitol or hypertonic saline may be indicated in coordination with a nephrologist.

Although common among patients with cirrhosis, care must be taken not to anchor on the diagnosis of hepatic encephalopathy. Such patients are at risk for concomitant infection (including spontaneous bacterial peritonitis) or intracranial bleeding (coagulopathy of liver failure, thrombocytopenia), and the presence of hyperammonemia is not specific for hepatic encephalopathy.[22] Both hyperammonemia and co-occurring sodium dyscrasias can also produce structural pathology in the form of cerebral edema with or without herniation. Clinical suspicion for structural pathology and consideration of neuroimaging should remain high in patients with liver disease. Physical examination should focus on brisk deep tendon reflexes, asterixis, and abnormal Babinski. Guidelines note that altered mentation in a patient with cirrhosis is an indication for paracentesis to rule out spontaneous bacterial peritonitis.[23] Treatment for hepatic encephalopathy aims to reverse any underlying causes in addition to enhancing ammonia elimination via administration of lactulose. The addition of rifaximin should be considered in patients with severe, acute hepatic encephalopathy.

Hypercapnia

Given the high prevalence of advanced chronic obstructive pulmonary disease (COPD), obesity hypoventilation syndrome, and obstructive and central sleep apnea, hypercapnia is a common cause of altered consciousness that can be easily missed without blood gas analysis. In addition, many disorders leading to altered consciousness can secondarily produce hypoventilation and hypercapnia. Thus, we recommend the liberal use of blood gases (venous or arterial) in patients with altered consciousness; venous blood gas (VBG) has been shown to be a reliable alternative to arterial blood gas (ABG) analysis; see **Table 6.5.** The literature supports that Pco_2, pH, and bicarbonate levels from peripheral or central VBGs are similar to those from ABGs with minor adjustments, with the exception of extreme values.[24-31] For the purpose of ruling out acute or chronic hypercapnia significant enough to lead to altered consciousness, clinically reliable conclusions can be reached with VBG analysis alone. In the absence of a blood gas, elevated bicarbonate can be a clue to hypercapnic conditions.

Thiamine Deficiency (Wernicke-Korsakoff Syndrome)

Thiamine deficiency is typified by the classic triad of deficits in mentation, oculomotor function, and gait ataxia, although all components of this classic triad are rarely present. Metabolic stress, often due to infection, is a common precipitant of Wernicke encephalopathy. At-risk patients include those with alcohol dependence, diabetes, gastric bypass, and chronic intestinal disorders.[32]

TABLE 6.5	Estimated Corrections for Converting VBG Values to ABG Values	
	Central	**Peripheral**
pH	Add 0.03-0.05 pH units	Add 0.02-0.04 pH units
Pco_2	Subtract 4-5 mm Hg	Subtract 3-8 mm Hg
HCO_3	No correction	Subtract 1-2 meq/L

ABG, arterial blood gas; HCO_3, bicarbonate; meq/L, milliequivalents per liter; mm Hg, millimeters of mercury; Pco_2, partial pressure of carbon dioxide; VBG, venous blood gas.

Korsakoff syndrome is a *chronic* cerebral pathology resulting from damage to the medial temporal lobes; it is typically seen as a late neuropsychiatric manifestation of Wernicke encephalopathy. It classically presents with anterograde and short-term retrograde memory deficits with relative preservation of long-term memory. Confabulation is classically described, but not always present.

Treatment with intravenous thiamine is broadly indicated for patients with altered consciousness and any potential for alcohol use disorder or nutritional deficiencies that could put them at risk for Wernicke encephalopathy. In cases of high clinical suspicion, high-dose thiamine (500 mg IV 3 times daily) administration is indicated. Wernicke encephalopathy is reversible if treated promptly. Prognosis for recovery is slightly better in Wernicke encephalopathy than in Korsakoff syndrome, although both disorders have low rates of recovery when treatment is delayed. Owing to poor bioavailability, oral thiamine is not recommended in the ED treatment of suspected Wernicke encephalopathy, but can be considered at high doses (ie, 2,000 mg) if intravenous thiamine is unavailable.[33]

Vitamin B12 Deficiency

Vitamin B_{12} (cobalamin) deficiency is well known to be associated with subacute cognitive decline and delirium as well as visual impairment and subacute combined degeneration (SCD) of the spinal cord. SCD results from degeneration of the posterior and lateral spinal columns, and is classically associated with pernicious anemia. It can also be seen with deficiencies in vitamin E and copper. Degeneration of the posterior spinal column results in decreased sensation of vibration and proprioception, resulting in a positive Romberg test result. Degeneration of the lateral corticospinal column results in upper motor neuron findings, including bilateral spastic paresis and a positive Babinski sign. Treatment is vitamin replacement, which can reverse symptoms if not too long-standing. Intramuscular or intravenous routes of vitamin replacement should be utilized in those whose vitamin B_{12} deficiency is the result of altered gastrointestinal absorption.

Seizure

Seizure can alter consciousness in a broad array of patterns. Depending on type, seizure can have structural or nonstructural etiologies. For example, previous stroke represents a structural source of seizure, whereas medications that lower the seizure threshold represent a nonstructural source. Moreover, physical examination findings can suggest a nonstructural source when there is a structural focus (eg, a seizure that secondarily generalizes from focal source) or suggest a structural source when there is no anatomic defect (eg, Todd paralysis in a patient with epilepsy).

Convulsive seizures are typically apparent, although atypical seizure manifestations are notoriously difficult to classify and often require extended EEG monitoring to confirm epileptiform activity. In addition, there are atypical seizure manifestations so unusual that history and physical examination findings may not suggest a seizure etiology at all, potentially leading to a missed diagnosis. As mentioned earlier, a high suspicion for nonconvulsive seizure is warranted in patients with a prolonged postictal phase after a seizure or in those patients with persistent and unexplained altered consciousness.

A rare but important consideration is the possibility of limbic seizures in patients with out-of-character aggression or brief periods of psychosis, especially in the presence of previous head trauma and in the absence of a known psychiatric disorder. Toxicologic etiologies of seizure are also important considerations and include anticholinergic drugs, tricyclics, cocaine, carbamates, carbon monoxide, glycols, ethanol, lead, lithium, and salicylates.

Endocrinopathy

Hyperthyroidism is notorious for presenting with psychiatric symptoms, such as mania and anxiety, and severe thyrotoxicosis can present with delirium. Apathetic hyperthyroidism, more commonly affecting the elderly, can conversely present with depression and apathy. Similarly, hypothyroidism can lead to symptoms of depression or decreased arousal, including frank coma when severe. Measurement of thyroid stimulating hormone and free thyroxine levels is often rapidly available in the ED to diagnose thyroid disorders. Endogenous and iatrogenic cortisol excess as well as adrenal insufficiency (typically Addisonian crisis) can lead to psychosis or agitated delirium. Characteristics of excess cortisol include muscle weakness, moon faces, weight gain, hyperglycemia, hypernatremia, and hypokalemia. Characteristics of adrenal insufficiency include fatigue, muscle weakness, postural hypotension, skin hyperpigmentation, hyponatremia, hyperkalemia, and eosinophilia. Although formal diagnosis should be determined in consultation with an endocrinologist, a midnight cortisol level should be measured if cortisol excess is suspected, and an 8:00 a.m. cortisol level should be checked if cortisol deficiency is suspected.

Treatment of adrenal insufficiency in the ED typically combines both glucocorticoids (eg, prednisone or hydrocortisone) and mineralocorticoids (eg, fludrocortisone). Stress doses of glucocorticoids should be considered during illness, surgical procedures, and hospitalization.

Infection

CNS infection, including meningitis, encephalitis, and HIV-associated neurocognitive disorders (HANDs), can cause AMS. UTIs have classically been associated with new neuropsychiatric symptoms or exacerbation of existing neuropsychiatric disorders in the elderly. We recommend a screening urinalysis in all patients presenting with altered consciousness, especially because the urinalysis can yield important findings, such as the presence of ketones, in addition to findings consistent with infection.

In sepsis, a combination of neurodegenerative pathways and neurovascular injury commonly result in septic encephalopathy and long-term neurologic sequelae among sepsis survivors. Manifestations range from mild confusion to convulsions or even coma. Diagnosis is clinical and often difficult, given that there is no clear criteria for the disorder as well the common presence of multiple potential alternate etiologies (eg, pharmacologic sedation, metabolic derangements). There is no targeted therapy for septic encephalopathy, so treatment centers on management of the underlying infection and supportive care.

Toxic Causes and Illicit Drug Use

Illicit substance abuse and withdrawal syndromes as well as toxicologic exposures are critical considerations in the ED evaluation of altered consciousness. Clinical features that should prompt consideration of toxicologic pathology include history of substance abuse, history of overdose, suicidal ideation or prior suicide attempt, psychiatric illness, agitation, stupor or coma, seizures, hyperthermia or hypothermia, muscle rigidity, rhabdomyolysis, bronchospasm, and unexplained cardiac arrythmia.[34] General laboratory prompts for potential toxicologic ingestion include an osmolar gap >10 mOsm, an arterial saturation gap (the measured SaO_2 on ABG minus Spo_2 on pulse oximetry) >5%, an elevated anion gap, and specific drug levels as well as acute renal or liver failure. Vigilance for toxic syndromes should be maintained to increase the chance of detecting an otherwise occult toxic exposure; see **Table 6.6**.

Owing to limited history or lack of patient candor, withdrawal syndromes leading to altered consciousness may not be readily apparent. Especially in those who present with a concurrent medical illness that precluded the ingestion of a typical medication or illicit substance, it can be easy to miss a superimposed withdrawal syndrome.

Hematologic/Oncologic

Altered consciousness due to thrombotic thrombocytopenic purpura (TTP) is commonly misdiagnosed as sepsis, transient ischemic attack (TIA), malignant hypertension, lupus flare, preeclampsia, eclampsia, or HELLP (hemolysis, elevated liver enzymes, and low platelets) syndrome of pregnancy. The full pentad of fever, thrombocytopenia, microangiopathic hemolytic anemia, renal impairment, and neurologic abnormalities is not typically present. A high index of suspicion should be maintained, with current guidelines stating that a combination of microangiopathic hemolytic anemia and thrombocytopenia without alternate explanation is sufficient to diagnose and treat TTP.

TABLE 6.6 Toxidromes

	Onset	Medications	Mental Status	Diaphoresis	Pupils	Bowel Sounds	Neurologic Findings
Opioid	Variable	Natural and synthetic opioids	Depressed	↓	Pinpoint	↓	Nonfocal
Sedative-hypnotic	Variable	Multiple	Depressed	↓	Normal	Normal	Nonfocal
Cholinergic	Variable	Prescription, carbamates, organophosphates	Variable	↑	Pinpoint	↑	Nonfocal
Sympathomimetic[a]	Variable	Multiple	Agitated delirium	↑	Dilated	↑	Nonfocal
Anticholinergic	<12 hr	Multiple	Agitated delirium	↓	Dilated	↓	Nonfocal, ataxia, bladder retention
NMS	1-3 days	Dopamine antagonist, recently discontinued dopamine agonist	Agitated delirium → Depressed	↑	Normal	Normal	Lead pipe rigidity in all muscle groups, bradyreflexia
Serotonin syndrome	<12 hr	Serotonergic agent (including recently discontinued SSRIs with long half-lives)	Agitated delirium → Depressed	↑	Dilated, ocular clonus	↑	Clonus, hyperreflexia (lower > upper)
Malignant hyperthermia	30 min-24 hr, typically with 10 min of succinyl choline	Succinyl choline, inhalational anesthetics	Agitated delirium	↑	Normal	↓	Rigor mortis-like rigidity, hyporeflexia

Toxidromes below the line have significant clinical overlap and require care to differentiate. Red elements are helpful discriminators.
Attention should be paid to axilla (moisture), leg tone, reflexes, bowel sounds, timing of symptoms, and both current and recently withdrawn medications to work through the differential diagnosis.
[a]Includes GABAergic withdrawal (eg, alcohol, benzodiazepines, barbiturates).
GABA, γ-aminobutyric acid; NMS, neuroleptic malignant syndrome; min, minutes.

Similarly, paraneoplastic neurologic syndromes and carcinomatous meningitis are easily misdiagnosed in altered oncologic patients given wide differential diagnoses.

Rheumatologic Pathology and Vasculitis

Connective tissue diseases may directly affect the brain via vasculitis or thrombosis. They can also produce altered consciousness because of their end-organ damage and resultant metabolic abnormalities. More common etiologies include lupus, Sjögren syndrome, neurosarcoidosis, and limbic encephalitis.

PEDIATRIC CONSIDERATIONS

The evaluation of pediatric patients with altered consciousness is similar to that of adults and should follow the abovementioned algorithm with pediatric-appropriate modifications. One important alteration includes the use of the pediatric GCS scale to grade level of consciousness in children younger than five years old. An additional high-yield physical examination maneuver is palpation of the fontanel in an infant, which may raise suspicion of elevated ICP.

In the setting of infantile altered consciousness and, especially, seizure, a careful feeding history with detail on formula preparation is crucial given the prevalence of infantile hyponatremia. Capillary blood gas electrolytes can quickly confirm or refute potential causative electrolyte dyscrasias.

Pediatric patients can present with a myriad inborn errors of metabolism, resulting in various metabolic derangements that can cause altered mentation. If suspected, we would recommend pediatric consultation and screening with the following studies: glucose, ketones, basic metabolic panel (BMP), blood gas with lactate, and ammonia.[35] Similarly, pediatric patients can present with new onset of endocrine disorders, such as congenital adrenal hyperplasia.

It is critical to recall that pyridoxine (vitamin B_6) deficiency is a well-described etiology for refractory pediatric seizure, and prompt replacement can be lifesaving in the setting of pediatric status epilepticus.

Childhood absence epilepsy (CAE) deserves special mention because it is a common pediatric epilepsy syndrome (accounting for 10% of all pediatric epilepsies), and is easily misdiagnosed as "staring spells" or even attention deficit hyperactivity disorder, which unfortunately is concomitantly seen in about one-third of patients with CAE.

History of home birth in the setting of neonatal altered consciousness should raise suspicion for possible vitamin K deficiency and associated intracranial hemorrhage. In addition, lack of prenatal care in combination with home birth likely increases the risk of group-B streptococcal, *Neisseria*, chlamydial, and herpes infections.

Altered mentation in a neonate almost invariably leads to consideration of meningitis and/or encephalitis in the absence of a clear, alternative diagnosis, especially in the setting of fever.

In all pediatric patients with altered consciousness, providers must remain vigilant for occult and nonaccidental trauma.

TIPS AND PEARLS

- Acutely altered consciousness often suggests stroke, hemorrhage, seizure, or cardiac event with decreased cerebral perfusion.
- Subacute altered consciousness more commonly is the result of infectious or toxic-metabolic causes of altered consciousness.
- Common nonstructural causes of altered consciousness include medication side effects or overdose, illicit drug use, toxic ingestion, metabolic alterations, systemic or primary CNS infections, seizure, and endocrinopathy.
- Key initial steps managing patients with altered consciousness include the evaluation of the ABCs, and assessing for hypoglycemia, opiate overdose, seizure, and trauma.
- Altered patients should be assessed for level of consciousness and their motor responses. A rapid brainstem assessment and appraisal of breathing pattern is advised for those patients who are comatose.

- Key findings on neurologic examination of altered patients can identify changes to suggest toxic syndromes that can lead to rapid treatment of coma.
- Subtle movements may be the only sign of basilar ischemia, locked-in syndrome, and NCSE.
- CT head should be obtained before LP in any patient with an altered level of consciousness.
- Patients on valproic acid with an AMS should be assessed for hyperammonemia.

EVIDENCE

Is it necessary to provide thiamine before giving glucose in patients with AMS from hypoglycemia?

Although a commonly repeated myth, there is no data that demonstrates that glucose administration to correct AMS due to hypoglycemia precipitates Wernicke encephalopathy.[19,20] Glucose administration need not be delayed to administer thiamine, and thiamine treatment can be determined on the basis of alcohol use and risk for nutritional deficiencies.

Is the GCS score helpful in the prognosis of nontraumatic coma?

Relatively little research exists regarding the use of the Glasgow Coma Score in nontraumatic coma, and noted limitations include poor brainstem evaluation, lack of pupillary assessment, and confounders produced by intubation. An early sentinel study showed that GCS was a strong, independent predictor of 2-week outcomes in patients presenting with nontraumatic coma; patients with a GCS score of 6 to 8 were 7 times more likely to waken at 2 weeks than were those with a score of 3 to 5.[36] More recently, a study of 286 patients older than age 16 who were hospitalized for nontraumatic coma demonstrated that prehospital GCS performed similarly to prehospital Mainz Emergency Evaluation System (MEES) and to day-of-admission Acute Physiology and Chronic Health Evaluation (APACHE) II scores in terms of predicting mortality. There were no statistically significant differences among the performance of the three scales (using optimized cutoffs of 5 for GCS, 18 for MEES, and 19 for APACHE), with GCS (81.9%) demonstrating a higher raw correct prediction rate for mortality than MEES (78.3%) and APACHE II (79.9%).[37] Citing its accuracy, simplicity, and rapidity of completion, the authors concluded that the GCS was the best prediction score for patients in an emergency situation. More specifically, GCS has proved a strong prognostic indicator in patients with posterior circulation stroke and following cardiac arrest.[38,39] Despite low quality of evidence, the GCS is still recommended as a component of monitoring of comatose adult patients with acute brain injury by the Neurocritical Care Society and the European Society of Intensive Care Medicine.[40]

Does a normal CT rule out a CNS lesion as a cause of coma?

CT alone cannot rule out a CNS lesion as a cause of coma. MRI provides superior imaging of the soft tissue and of the posterior fossa, detecting lesions that can be missed by CT.[41] In trauma, specifically, MRI has been demonstrated to detect diffuse axonal injury in patients with discrepancy between their neurologic status and their otherwise unremarkable CT head.[42] In one study, patients remaining in coma at least 24 hours after initial trauma despite minimal sedation had a 64% chance of a brainstem lesion detected by MRI that was missed by CT.[43]

Do all strokes with AMS have focal finding on neurologic examination?

Not all strokes or TIAs present with focal findings on neurologic examination. Posterior circulation strokes, specifically, often present with nonfocal findings.[44] A study of 1265 patients with TIA or minor stroke revealed that one in five patients had nonfocal symptoms, especially when ischemia was located in the posterior circulation.[45]

Does a normal urine drug screen rule out a toxicologic etiology of AMS? Does a positive drug screen change management?

Urine drug screens using automated chemistry analyzers for limited screening of drugs of abuse have several limitations compared to analysis by gas chromatography/mass spectrometry, limiting their ability to reliably rule out a toxicologic etiology of AMS.[46] That said, automated screens can be useful when the finding is positive. A recent prospective observational study showed that toxicology screening tests are helpful in undifferentiated patients with decreased arousal, psychiatric symptoms, or neurologic symptoms, which fits the demographic of this chapter.[47] Notably, this same study showed that screening tests were mostly unhelpful in patients who, upon admission, were already known to be intoxicated.

References

1. Posner JB PF. *Plum and Posner's Diagnosis and Treatment of Stupor and Coma.* 5th ed. New York: Oxford University Press; 2019.

2. Cadena RS, Sarwal A. Emergency neurological life support: approach to the patient with coma. *Neurocrit Care.* 2017;27:74-81.

3. Douglas VC, Josephson SA. Altered mental status. *Continuum (Minneap Minn).* 2011;17:967-983.

4. Robba C, Santori G, Czosnyka M, et al. Optic nerve sheath diameter measured sonographically as non-invasive estimator of intracranial pressure: a systematic review and meta-analysis. *Intensive Care Med.* 2018;44:1284-1294.

5. Tunkel AR, Hartman BJ, Kaplan SL, et al. Practice guidelines for the management of bacterial meningitis. *Clin Infect Dis.* 2004;39:1267-1284.

6. April MD, Long B, Koyfman A. Emergency medicine myths: computed tomography of the head prior to lumbar puncture in adults with suspected bacterial meningitis—due diligence or antiquated practice? *J Emerg Med.* 2017;53:313-321.

7. National Institute for Health and Care Excellence. Meningitis (bacterial) and meningococcal septicaemia in under 16s: recognition, diagnosis and management. 2010. Updated February 1, 2015. Accessed March 24, 2021. https://www.nice.org.uk/guidance/cg102/chapter/Key-priorities-for-implementation

8. Baddour E, Tewksbury A, Stauner N. Valproic acid-induced hyperammonemia: incidence, clinical significance, and treatment management. *Ment Health Clin.* 2018;8:73-77.

9. Sarwal A, Stern-Nezer S, Tran DS. Emergency neurological life support: approach to the patient with coma. *Neurocrit Care.* 2019.

10. Tunkel AR, Glaser CA, Bloch KC, et al. The management of encephalitis: clinical practice guidelines by the Infectious Diseases Society of America. *Clin Infect Dis.* 2008;47:303-327.

11. Zehtabchi S, Abdel Baki SG, Malhotra S, Grant AC. Nonconvulsive seizures in patients presenting with altered mental status: an evidence-based review. *Epilepsy Behav.* 2011;22:139-143.

12. Hobbs K, Krishnamohan P, Legault C, et al. Rapid bedside evaluation of seizures in the ICU by listening to the sound of brainwaves: a prospective observational clinical trial of ceribell's brain stethoscope function. *Neurocrit Care.* 2018;29:302-312.

13. Hanley D, Prichep LS, Badjatia N, et al. A brain electrical activity electroencephalographic-based biomarker of functional impairment in traumatic brain injury: a multi-site validation trial. *J Neurotrauma.* 2018;35:41-47.

14. Lee S, Gottlieb M, Mulhausen P, et al. Recognition, prevention, and treatment of delirium in emergency department: an evidence-based narrative review. *Am J Emerg Med.* 2020;38:349-357.

15. Lonergan E, Luxenberg J, Areosa Sastre A, Wyller TB. Benzodiazepines for delirium. *Cochrane Database Syst Rev.* 2009;(4):Cd006379.

16. Han JH, Wilson A, Vasilevskis EE, et al. Diagnosing delirium in older emergency department patients: validity and reliability of the delirium triage screen and the brief confusion assessment method. *Ann Emerg Med.* 2013;62:457-465.

17. Han JH, Wilson A, Graves AJ, et al. Validation of the confusion assessment method for the intensive care unit in older emergency department patients. *Acad Emerg Med.* 2014;21:180-187.

18. Lee VH, Wijdicks EF, Manno EM, Rabinstein AA. Clinical spectrum of reversible posterior leukoencephalopathy syndrome. *Arch Neurol.* 2008;65:205-210.

19. Hack JB, Hoffman RS. Thiamine before glucose to prevent Wernicke encephalopathy: examining the conventional wisdom. *JAMA*. 1998;279:583-584.

20. Schabelman E, Kuo D. Glucose before thiamine for Wernicke encephalopathy: a literature review. *J Emerg Med*. 2012;42:488-494.

21. Hu ZD, Huang YL, Wang MY, Hu GJ, Han YQ. Predictive accuracy of serum total calcium for both critically high and critically low ionized calcium in critical illness. *J Clin Lab Anal*. 2018;32:e22589.

22. Ge PS, Runyon BA. Serum ammonia level for the evaluation of hepatic encephalopathy. *JAMA*. 2014;312:643-644.

23. Runyon B; American Association for the Study of Liver Diseases. Management of adult patients with ascites due to cirrhosis: update 2012. *Hepatology*. 2009;49:2087-2107.

24. Malinoski DJ, Todd SR, Slone S, Mullins RJ, Schreiber MA. Correlation of central venous and arterial blood gas measurements in mechanically ventilated trauma patients. *Arch Surg*. 2005;140:1122-1125.

25. Walkey AJ, Farber HW, O'Donnell C, Cabral H, Eagan JS, Philippides GJ. The accuracy of the central venous blood gas for acid-base monitoring. *J Intensive Care Med*. 2010;25:104-110.

26. Gokel Y, Paydas S, Koseoglu Z, Alparslan N, Seydaoglu G. Comparison of blood gas and acid-base measurements in arterial and venous blood samples in patients with uremic acidosis and diabetic ketoacidosis in the emergency room. *Am J Nephrol*. 2000;20:319-323.

27. Brandenburg MA, Dire DJ. Comparison of arterial and venous blood gas values in the initial emergency department evaluation of patients with diabetic ketoacidosis. *Ann Emerg Med*. 1998;31:459-465.

28. Malatesha G, Singh NK, Bharija A, Rehani B, Goel A. Comparison of arterial and venous pH, bicarbonate, Pco_2 and PO_2 in initial emergency department assessment. *Emerg Med J*. 2007;24:569-571.

29. Chu YC, Chen CZ, Lee CH, Chen CW, Chang HY, Hsiue TR. Prediction of arterial blood gas values from venous blood gas values in patients with acute respiratory failure receiving mechanical ventilation. *J Formos Med Assoc*. 2003;102:539-543.

30. Kelly AM, Kyle E, McAlpine R. Venous pCO(2) and pH can be used to screen for significant hypercarbia in emergency patients with acute respiratory disease. *J Emerg Med*. 2002;22:15-19.

31. McKeever TM, Hearson G, Housley G, et al. Using venous blood gas analysis in the assessment of COPD exacerbations: a prospective cohort study. *Thorax*. 2016;71:210-215.

32. Sinha S, Kataria A, Kolla BP, Thusius N, Loukianova LL. Wernicke encephalopathy-clinical pearls. *Mayo Clin Proc*. 2019;94:1065-1072.

33. Smithline HA, Donnino M, Greenblatt DJ. Pharmacokinetics of high-dose oral thiamine hydrochloride in healthy subjects. *BMC Clin Pharmacol*. 2012;12:4.

34. Hall J, Schmidt GA, Kress J. *Principles of Critical Care*. 4th ed. New York: McGraw-Hill; 2015.

35. Guerrero RB, Salazar D, Tanpaiboon P. Laboratory diagnostic approaches in metabolic disorders. *Ann Transl Med*. 2018;6:470.

36. Sacco RL, VanGool R, Mohr JP, Hauser WA. Nontraumatic coma. Glasgow coma score and coma etiology as predictors of 2-week outcome. *Arch Neurol*. 1990;47:1181-1184.

37. Grmec Š, Gašparovic V. Comparison of APACHE II, MEES and Glasgow coma scale in patients with nontraumatic coma for prediction of mortality. *Crit Care*. 2000;5:19.

38. Tsao JW, Hemphill JC, 3rd, Johnston SC, Smith WS, Bonovich DC. Initial Glasgow Coma Scale score predicts outcome following thrombolysis for posterior circulation stroke. *Arch Neurol*. 2005;62:1126-1129.

39. Schefold JC, Storm C, Krüger A, Ploner CJ, Hasper D. The Glasgow coma score is a predictor of good outcome in cardiac arrest patients treated with therapeutic hypothermia. *Resuscitation*. 2009;80:658-661.

40. Le Roux P, Menon DK, Citerio G, et al. Consensus summary statement of the International Multidisciplinary Consensus Conference on Multimodality Monitoring in Neurocritical Care: a statement for healthcare professionals from the Neurocritical Care Society and the European Society of Intensive Care Medicine. *Neurocrit Care*. 2014;21(Suppl 2):S1-S26.

41. Haupt WF, Hansen HC, Janzen RWC, Firsching R, Galldiks N. Coma and cerebral imaging. *SpringerPlus*. 2015;4:180.

42. Paterakis K, Karantanas AH, Komnos A, Volikas Z. Outcome of patients with diffuse axonal injury: the significance and prognostic value of MRI in the acute phase. *J Trauma Acute Care Surg*. 2000;49:1071-1075.

43. Firsching R, Woischneck D, Diedrich M, et al. Early magnetic resonance imaging of brainstem lesions after severe head injury. *J Neurosurg*. 1998;89:707.

44. Sparaco M, Ciolli L, Zini A. Posterior circulation ischaemic stroke-a review part I: anatomy, aetiology and clinical presentations. *Neurol Sci*. 2019;40:1995-2006.

45. Plas GJJ, Booij HA, Brouwers PJAM, et al. Nonfocal symptoms in patients with transient ischemic attack or ischemic stroke: occurrence, clinical determinants, and association with cardiac history. *Cerebrovasc Dis*. 2016;42:439-445.

46. Reisfield GM, Goldberger BA, Bertholf RL. "'False-positive" and "false-negative" test results in clinical urine drug testing. *Bioanalysis*. 2009;1:937-952.

47. Lager PS, Attema-de Jonge ME, Gorzeman MP, Kerkvliet LF, Franssen EJF. Clinical value of drugs of abuse point of care testing in an emergency department setting. *Toxicol Rep*. 2018;5:12-17.

Myopathies and Neuromuscular Junction Disorders

Rebecca Elizabeth Traub

Neuromuscular disorders include all diseases of the peripheral nervous system that extends from the anterior horn of the spinal cord to the muscles and small peripheral nerves in the extremities. There are acute or emergency presentations of diseases at every level of the peripheral nervous system, including myopathies, neuromuscular junction disorders, peripheral neuropathies, disorders of the brachial and lumbosacral plexus, and spinal nerve root and motor neuron disease. This chapter focuses on primary diseases of muscle (myopathies) and the neuromuscular junction.

MYOPATHIES

Myopathies include a broad range of diseases primarily affecting muscle itself. Most, but not all, cause elevation in the serum creatine kinase (CK); however, there are nonmyopathic disease processes that can also cause the CK to be elevated (**Table 7.1**).

There are three broad categories of primary muscle disease: genetic or inherited, inflammatory, and toxic-metabolic. Inflammatory or toxic-metabolic myopathies are more likely to be seen in the emergency setting, but even patients with preexisting genetic myopathies may present with acute worsening of weakness affecting cardiac or respiratory function.

INFLAMMATORY MYOPATHIES

Inflammatory myopathies include the group of immune-mediated muscle diseases that cause inflammation and damage in skeletal muscle, and, in severe cases, may also affect cardiac or respiratory muscle. Types of myositis include polymyositis (PM), dermatomyositis (DM), necrotizing autoimmune myopathy (NAM), and inclusion body myositis (IBM).

The Clinical Challenge

The incidence of DM and PM combined has been estimated at 2 per 100,000 annually. NAM is probably less common. DM, PM, and NAM share similar clinical features, with proximal muscle weakness being a hallmark feature, that are difficult to distinguish on initial presentation. Any patient presenting with subacute proximal muscle weakness without sensory symptoms and an

TABLE 7.1	**Causes of Weakness with Elevations in the Serum Creatine Kinase (CK)**
Myopathies	
Inflammatory	• Dermatomyositis—*accompanying rash* • Polymyositis—*history of connective tissue disease* • Necrotizing autoimmune myopathy—*history of statin exposure or underlying malignancy* • Inclusion body myositis—*indolent onset and progression*
Genetic	• Muscular dystrophy • Congenital myopathy • Metabolic myopathy—*recurrent episodes of rhabdomyolysis*
Toxic	• Alcohol • Cocaine • Corticosteroids—*CK is usually normal* • Statin medications
Non-Myopathic Processes That Can Increase CK (usually <1000 IU/L)	
• Neurogenic processes that can increase CK (usually <1000 IU/L)	• Motor neuron disease (including amyotrophic lateral sclerosis) • Rapidly progressive peripheral neuropathies, including chronic inflammatory demyelinating polyneuropathy
Neuroleptic malignant syndrome—*in association with altered mental status, fever, rigidity*	

elevated CK on laboratory testing is suspicious for an inflammatory myopathy. The presence of typical rash suggests the specific diagnosis of DM.

Uncommonly, inflammatory myopathies affect cardiac muscle and can cause cardiomyopathy or cardiac conduction abnormalities. Any patient in whom inflammatory myopathy is suspected should undergo cardiac testing to assess for myocardial involvement. It is also rare for respiratory function to be affected in inflammatory myopathies, but in severe cases, respiratory failure requiring mechanical ventilation can occur.

Interstitial lung disease (ILD) can occur in association with PM or DM in 10% of cases, most often with antisynthetase antibodies. In patients with a history of DM or PM and respiratory symptoms, ILD should be strongly considered.

Patients with known diagnosis of inflammatory myopathies are often on corticosteroid or other immune-suppressing medications. Such patients are at increased risk for infectious complications. Any patient with inflammatory myopathy on immune-suppressing therapy who presents in the emergency setting should be considered for infectious complications of treatment.

Pathophysiology

DM, PM, and NAM are autoimmune conditions causing inflammation in and destruction of muscle. DM is a vasculopathy of muscle and skin, typically presenting with rash, proximal muscle weakness, and high CK. Muscle pathology shows perimysial and perivascular inflammation involving the sheath of connective tissue that groups muscle fibers into bundles.

PM presents with clinical features similar to that of DM, without the associated rash. Pathology, however, shows primarily endomysial inflammation and muscle fiber necrosis involving the connective tissue that ensheathes each muscle fiber, or myocyte. DM, more than PM, can occur as a paraneoplastic syndrome, and thus patients should be screened for underlying cancer. NAM is a distinct autoimmune myopathy presenting with symptoms similar to that of PM, but often with more severe and treatment-refractory weakness. The pathology of NAM is distinct, with myofiber necrosis with little or no inflammatory response. It is often seen in association with anti–signal recognition particle (SRP) antibodies or 3-hydroxy-3-methylglutaryl coenzyme A reductase (HMG CoA reductase or HMGCR) antibodies, sometimes associated with statin medication exposure.

IBM is a distinct subset of acquired muscle disease that has both inflammatory and neuro-degenerative features. The exact pathophysiology underlying IBM is not well understood. The clinical progression is much more indolent, often over many years. The typical pathology on muscle biopsy includes endomysial inflammation with congophilic rimmed vacuoles.

Prehospital Concerns

Prehospital concerns in inflammatory myopathies relate primarily to rare patients with cardiac or respiratory muscle involvement of the muscle disease. In these cases, supportive measures include mechanical ventilation, in rare cases, and close cardiac monitoring.

Approach/The Focused Examination

Inflammatory myopathies share clinical features of proximal muscle weakness, affecting the arms and legs. The history will often reveal difficulty getting up from a chair or toilet, or with reaching overhead, combing hair, or brushing teeth. Neurologic examination should include confrontation testing of both proximal and distal muscle groups, including ability to stand from a seated position and gait assessment. Muscle pain, or myalgias, may be present. Sensory symptoms and examination findings are absent unless there is a coexisting reason for the patient to have neuropathy (eg, diabetes). In more severe cases, there may be facial or bulbar weakness. Ocular muscles are typically spared. Respiratory weakness can be present in severe cases. In severe or more longstanding cases, muscle atrophy may be present. Deep tendon reflexes are typically normal.

IBM has distinct clinical features, with more indolent progression of weakness—often over many months to years. The distribution of weakness in IBM is also different from that of the other inflammatory myopathies, with the greatest weakness and atrophy in the forearm flexors, quadriceps, and peroneal compartment of the lower leg. In advanced cases, facial and bulbar weakness occurs.

The diagnosis of DM should be specifically considered in the patient presenting with proximal muscle weakness and rash. The typical skin findings of DM can include Gottron papules (erythematous papules or scaling over the dorsum of the hands and fingers), heliotrope eruption over the eyelids, facial erythema, and rash over sun-exposed sites—most typically over the chest and upper back ("shawl sign").

PM should be more strongly considered as a diagnosis in patients with a previous history of connective tissue disorders. In these patients, the myositis "overlap syndrome" occurs in association with their other preexisting rheumatologic disorder.

Serum CK is nearly always elevated in inflammatory myopathies. Inflammatory markers, such as erythrocyte sedimentation rate (ESR) and C-reactive protein (CRP), may be variably elevated. In any patient with subacute proximal weakness and elevated serum CK, inflammatory myopathy should be highly considered. Additional tests used to confirm diagnosis include myositis-specific antibodies, electrodiagnostic testing, skin biopsy, and muscle biopsy.

Management

Treatment strategies for DM, PM, and NAM are similar. IBM is clinically distinct, does not typically respond well or at all to immunotherapy, and is addressed separately. The initial treatment for most inflammatory myopathies is glucocorticoids, either intravenous (IV) methylprednisolone or high-dose oral corticosteroids (usually prednisone); see **Table 7.2**. Pending clinical and laboratory response to corticosteroids, the doses are slowly tapered over many months, along with the addition of steroid-sparing therapy. Typical steroid-sparing medications used for inflammatory myopathies include methotrexate, mycophenolate, azathioprine, intravenous immunoglobulin (IVIG), and rituximab.

In the emergency setting, additional management is supportive, assessing for cardiac or respiratory muscle involvement, and treating associated muscle pain. In the acute setting, nonsteroidal anti-inflammatory medications and short-term opiate pain medications may be used. Long-term agents for neuropathic pain, such as gabapentin, pregabalin, duloxetine, and others are used for management of muscle pain. Patients on immunosuppressing treatment should be carefully monitored for infectious complications. Patients on IVIG treatment are at increased risk for venous and arterial thrombotic events.

TABLE 7.2	Treatments for Inflammatory Myopathies
Drug Name	**Typical Dosing**
Corticosteroids	
IV methylprednisolone (acute therapy)	1 g daily ×3-5 days
Prednisone	60-80 mg daily starting dose, tapered over months
Intravenous immunoglobulin (IVIG)	1-2 g/kg q2-4 wk
Methotrexate	10-25 mg PO or IM once weekly
Mycophenolate	500-1500 mg PO BID
Azathioprine	100-250 mg PO daily
Rituximab	1 g IV q2 weeks ×2 doses every 6 mo

BID, twice daily; IM, intramuscular; IV, intravenous; PO, orally.

IBM has pathologic features shared with the inflammatory myopathies, but typically does not respond, or responds minimally to the immune-suppressing treatments used for the other autoimmune myopathies. Some patients with IBM do improve partially with immunotherapy and thus may be treated with corticosteroids, IVIG, or oral steroid–sparing treatments, but most patients ultimately will not be maintained on these medications and the management is primarily supportive. In late-stage disease, IBM often causes dysphagia and occasionally causes respiratory muscle weakness. Some patients elect to have a percutaneous gastrostomy tube placed and use noninvasive ventilation for respiratory support.

Pediatric Issues

Juvenile dermatomyositis (JDM) and juvenile polymyositis (JPM) are inflammatory myopathies occurring in the pediatric population. NAM is rarely seen in the pediatric population. Clinical features are similar to the adult population, and diagnostic testing is similar, including laboratory antibody testing, electromyography (EMG), and muscle biopsy. The differential diagnosis emphasizes the genetic myopathies. Treatments for inflammatory myopathies in childhood are similar to those used in adults, including corticosteroids and steroid-sparing medications.

Viral myositis is also more common in childhood, most often associated with influenza and coxsackie infections. Typical viral syndrome symptoms accompanied or followed by myalgias and elevated serum CK levels are characteristic of viral myositis. The syndrome is transient and resolves within a week without intervention. Supportive measures, including IV fluids if there is associated rhabdomyolysis, and pain control as needed, are appropriate.

GENETIC MYOPATHIES

Genetic myopathies include a broad range of inherited muscle diseases, including muscular dystrophies, congenital myopathies, metabolic myopathies, and periodic paralysis disorders. Onset is usually in childhood, but some milder phenotypes can present in adulthood. They can demonstrate a range of phenotypes, with either proximal or distal weakness, typically without sensory symptoms. Depending on the genetic mutation, there may be involvement of cranial muscles. Cardiac involvement is present in some genetic subtypes. Most genetic myopathies will present for outpatient evaluation with slowly progressive weakness, but emergency presentations may occur with infectious or metabolic stressors or cardiopulmonary complications of disease. A list of genetic myopathies associated with cardiac involvement is shown in **Table 7.3**.

Of the muscular dystrophies, the most common relate to mutations in the *dystrophin* gene, with an X-linked inheritance pattern. Duchenne muscular dystrophy (DMD) presents in early childhood and causes proximal weakness, pseudohypertrophy of the calf muscles, and prominent cardiac and respiratory muscle involvement. Becker muscular dystrophy (BMD) also results from mutations in the *dystrophin* gene, but those resulting in a still partially functioning protein and thus a milder phenotype, often presenting later in childhood or adulthood. Treatment with corticosteroid

TABLE 7.3	Genetic Myopathies with Increased Risk of Cardiac Involvement
Myopathy	
Dystrophinopathies	• Duchenne muscular dystrophy (*DMD*) • Becker muscular dystrophy (*BMD*)
Myotonic dystrophy	• Type 1 myotonic dystrophy (*DMPK*) • Type 2 myotonic dystrophy (*CNBP*)
Emery-Dreifuss muscular dystrophy	• *EMD, LMNA, SYNE1, SYNE2, FHL1, TMEM43, TOR1AIP1, SUN1, SUN2*
Some limb girdle muscular dystrophies	• *MYOT, LMNA, DNAJB6, SGCG, SGCA, SGCB, SGCD, TCAP, TRIM32, FKRP, TTN, POMT1, FKTN, POMT2, POMGnT1, DAG1*
Myofibrillar myopathies	• *DES, CRYAB, MYOT, LDB3, FLNC, BAG3, KY, PYROXD1, TTN*
Specific congenital myopathies	• Nemaline myopathy • Central core disease • Minimulticore disease • Centronuclear myopathies
Mitochondrial myopathies	

medications has been shown to slow decline in strength in DMD, and thus these patients can incur complications of long-term steroid treatment.

Other muscular dystrophies and inherited myopathies include Emery-Dreifuss muscular dystrophy (EDMD); myotonic dystrophy, including types 1 and 2; limb girdle muscular dystrophy (LGMD); facioscapulohumeral muscular dystrophy (FSHD); myofibrillar myopathies; and genetically diverse congenital myopathies. Inherited myopathies associated with *RYR1* mutations, or central core disease, is associated with an increased risk of malignant hyperthermia, for which anesthesia precautions must be taken.

Metabolic myopathies include the group of muscle diseases associated with genetic defects in energy storage and metabolism. Subgroups of metabolic myopathies include disorders of glycogen metabolism, disorders of lipid metabolism, and mitochondrial disorders. Disorders of glycogen metabolism can lead to episodes of acute rhabdomyolysis, often precipitated by physical activity, illness, or other metabolic stress, and must be treated supportively.

The common management strategies for all of the genetic myopathies include close monitoring for cardiac arrhythmia or associated cardiomyopathy, supportive measures for respiratory muscle weakness, high index of suspicion for pneumonia or aspiration in patients with respiratory muscle weakness, and avoidance of myotoxic medications.

PERIODIC PARALYSIS

Periodic paralysis syndromes are a rare group of neuromuscular disorders related to muscle channel ion defects that result in episodes of muscle weakness, often triggered by exercise, fasting, or high carbohydrate intake.

Hypokalemic periodic paralysis, related to either calcium channel or sodium channel mutations, presents with episodes of weakness associated with low serum potassium levels. Attacks can be precipitated by exercise, high-carbohydrate meals, and other metabolic stressors. Episodes of paralysis typically last hours to days at a time. Weakness is generalized, but typically spares ocular, bulbar, and respiratory muscles. During episodes of hypokalemia, cardiac arrhythmia can occur; thus, electrocardiogram and cardiac monitoring are indicated. Diagnosis is made on the basis of typical history and laboratory findings, family history, electrodiagnostic testing, and genetic testing.

Acute treatment of hypokalemic periodic paralysis involves potassium repletion and management of any underlying metabolic stressor. The recommended dosing regimen for acute hypokalemic periodic paralysis is 60 to 120 mEq of oral potassium chloride, given in 30 mEq doses every 30 minutes, with frequent laboratory checks to avoid rebound hyperkalemia. IV fluids containing dextrose should be avoided because they can worsen the hypokalemia. Long-term prophylactic treatment may include acetazolamide (250 mg twice daily) or dichlorphenamide (50 mg twice daily), and sometimes potassium-sparing diuretics, such as spironolactone.

More common than the rare genetic hypokalemic periodic paralysis is generalized weakness seen in the setting of hypokalemia due to other medical causes, such as renal or gastrointestinal (GI) wasting. Hyperthyroidism can also cause a clinical picture mimicking hypokalemic periodic paralysis. In these cases of weakness due to hypokalemia of other causes, correction of the metabolic derangement will result in rapid improvement in strength.

Hyperkalemic periodic paralysis, a disease related to sodium channel mutations, presents with episodes of muscle weakness associated with high serum potassium levels. Attacks can be precipitated by cold exposure, fasting, following exercise, or potassium intake. Weakness during attacks is generalized, but usually spares cranial and respiratory muscles. Between attacks, physical examination may demonstrate clinical myotonia. Laboratory testing will usually demonstrate normal or mildly elevated serum potassium levels. Diagnosis is established on the basis of typical history, electrodiagnostic testing, and genetic testing.

Treatment of acute attacks in hyperkalemic periodic paralysis, when mild, can include oral sugar or brief exercise. More severe attacks can be treated with thiazide diuretics, inhaled albuterol, and IV calcium. Arrhythmia associated with episodes of hyperkalemia has been reported, so electrocardiogram and cardiac monitoring are indicated. Prophylactic treatment to avoid attacks includes dietary strategies and treatment with oral acetazolamide or dichlorphenamide.

TOXIC MYOPATHIES

Myopathies may occur as a result of direct toxicity of prescribed, illicit, or recreational medications and drugs. Glucocorticoids commonly cause a proximal myopathy, without elevation of CK, that improves with reduction in dose or cessation of the medications. Statin medications, prescribed for hyperlipidemia, commonly cause myalgias, but less often cause myopathy and elevated serum CK levels. Other commonly prescribed medications that can cause myopathy include hydroxychloroquine, chloroquine, colchicine, and some antiviral medications used for human immunodeficiency virus (HIV).

In addition to direct toxicity, some medications can induce an inflammatory myopathy. Rarely, statin medications can trigger a NAM associated with HMGCR antibodies. Tumor necrosis factor (TNF)-α inhibitor medications and penicillamine have also been reported to trigger inflammatory myopathies. More recently, checkpoint inhibitor chemotherapy agents have been associated with a broad range of autoimmune complications, including myositis.

Alcohol can cause either a chronic myopathy, with or without peripheral neuropathy, due to long-term use, or acute myopathy from binge drinking, sometimes causing rhabdomyolysis. Cocaine can also precipitate an acute episode of rhabdomyolysis.

In any patient presenting with weakness and elevated CK, the clinician must evaluate all prescribed medications and consider alcohol and illicit substances as possible contributors.

RHABDOMYOLYSIS

Rhabdomyolysis is the syndrome of acute muscle pain, weakness, elevated serum CK, and myoglobinuria causing dark or brown urine. Muscle swelling may also be present. CK can be very elevated, usually over 1000 IU/L and as high as 100,000 IU/L. When the degree of muscle breakdown is severe, secondary electrolyte abnormalities can occur, including life-threatening hyperkalemia. Acute kidney injury can occur because of the effects of myoglobin on the kidneys. Rarely, rhabdomyolysis can trigger disseminated intravascular coagulation (DIC) due to the release of prothrombotic materials from damaged muscle. There are a number of potential causes or triggers for rhabdomyolysis, listed in **Table 7.4**.

In patients presenting with acute myalgias, weakness, and color changes in urine, testing with serum CK and urinalysis for myoglobinuria are indicated to evaluate for rhabdomyolysis. Additional testing should be directed at underlying triggers or causes. Further testing directed at an underlying myopathy, including EMG, muscle magnetic resonance imaging (MRI) and muscle

TABLE 7.4	Causes of Rhabdomyolysis
Cause	
Trauma	• Compression • Prolonged immobilization • Compartment syndrome • Electrical injury
Extreme exertion	
Hyperthermia	
Genetic metabolic myopathies	
Infection	• Influenza • Coxsackie
Toxic	• Alcohol • Cocaine • Amphetamines • Statins • Herbal weight loss supplements

biopsy are not typically indicated unless there are recurrent episodes of rhabdomyolysis or an inflammatory myopathy is considered in the differential diagnosis.

Treatment of rhabdomyolysis in the emergency setting involves assessment for and management of electrolyte derangements, treatment of any underlying or triggering conditions, and aggressive IV fluids for prevention of acute kidney injury. Isotonic IV fluids should be started as soon as muscle injury is suspected or detected and continued until the serum CK level is clearly stabilized or improving. The exact amount and rate of fluid resuscitation must be guided by the severity of muscle injury and risk for volume overload–associated complications. Typical recommendation for initial treatment is isotonic saline given at 200 to 1000 mL/h. Some recommend bicarbonate therapy in more severe cases of rhabdomyolysis; typical dosing is to alternate each liter of normal saline with 1 L of 5% dextrose plus 100 mmol of bicarbonate, adjusting the dose to achieve a urine pH greater than 6.5. Arterial pH and serum calcium need to be monitored during bicarbonate therapy. Very severe cases or life-threatening hyperkalemia may require hemodialysis.

TIPS AND PEARLS

- Myopathy should be considered in patients presenting with symmetric proximal muscle weakness without sensory loss.
- Checking the serum CK is a good screening test for myopathic disease process.
- Myopathy with subacute presentation, rapid progression, or associated rash should raise suspicion for an autoimmune or inflammatory myopathy.
- More long-standing, slowly progressive myopathy may indicate an underlying genetic cause.
- Patients with myopathic disorders may be at risk for involvement of cardiomyopathy, cardiac conduction abnormalities, or neuromuscular respiratory weakness.
- Consider toxic or infectious myopathies in patients with acute presentations of weakness and muscle pain, including a careful review of prescribed medications.
- Periodic paralysis disorders associated with hypo- and hyperkalemia require careful management and close monitoring of potassium levels.

EVIDENCE

Is there evidence that supports the treatment of autoimmune myopathies?

There are no large randomized controlled studies for use of corticosteroids in inflammatory myopathies, but consensus guidelines recommend this treatment as first line for PM and DM.[1] There have been small randomized and retrospective studies demonstrating benefit of azathioprine and methotrexate as steroid-sparing therapy.[2] There are case series reporting benefit of IVIG in refractory cases of myositis.[3]

Do IV fluids prevent acute kidney injury in rhabdomyolysis?

The evidence for fluid resuscitation in rhabdomyolysis is extrapolated from studies of rhabdomyolysis related to trauma or crush injuries. A number of studies of patients injured from trauma or during a natural disaster reported reduced risk of acute kidney injury with aggressive fluid administration.[4] There is not clear evidence supporting the use of bicarbonate therapy in patients with rhabdomyolysis, but some studies have shown benefit it more severe cases.[5]

Are there guidelines for the management of genetic myopathies?

With the exception of a few genetic myopathies for which there is available enzyme replacement or interfering RNA therapies, the management of inherited muscle diseases is supportive and symptomatic. Involvement of a multidisciplinary team, including rehabilitation services, respiratory therapy, speech therapy, and other medical specialists (cardiology, pulmonary medicine) are important for extending life expectancy and improving quality of life.[6]

NEUROMUSCULAR JUNCTION DISORDERS

Neuromuscular junction disorders include diseases that affect both the postsynaptic process of neuromuscular transmission (primarily myasthenia gravis [MG]), and those that affect the presynaptic processes (botulism and Lambert-Eaton myasthenic syndrome [LEMS]). All neuromuscular junction disorders can present with acute initial presentations, or acute worsening of weakness, including dysphagia and respiratory muscle weakness, making their appropriate identification and prompt management critical.

MYASTHENIA GRAVIS

The Clinical Challenge

MG is an autoimmune disease affecting the postsynaptic neuromuscular junction, preventing the transmission of motor neuron action potentials to muscle fibers. Patients present with fatigable weakness, often affecting the cranial muscles, causing diplopia, ptosis, facial weakness, dysphagia, and dysarthria. Limb weakness is often present, and weakness of the respiratory muscles can be life-threatening.

The prevalence of MG is approximately 1 per 10,000, making it a relatively rare disease. The relapsing-remitting nature of the disease and the many factors that can trigger an exacerbation or weakness or respiratory crisis means that the disorder will be seen in the emergency department (ED) setting.

There is the initial challenge of identifying the possible diagnosis of MG in any patient presenting with generalized weakness, particularly when associated with diplopia, ptosis, or bulbar symptoms. Many other neurologic disorders may mimic these symptoms, but MG should be highly considered, particularly in the presence of these ocular and bulbar symptoms.

In patients with a known diagnosis of MG, one challenge is identifying those patients with disease exacerbation requiring treatment with immunotherapy and close respiratory monitoring from patients taking high doses of pyridostigmine (> 120 mg every 4 hours). Pyridostigmine can cause a cholinergic crisis that must be considered in the differential of MG exacerbation. This entity produces muscle weakness, but is typically associated with other signs of cholinergic toxicity, including bronchospasm, increased salivation, diarrhea, and abdominal cramping. Involvement of the consultant neurologist is usually recommended for these patients, but in the emergency setting, the clinician should err on the side of close monitoring because these patients can quickly decompensate from a respiratory perspective and may require mechanical ventilation.

The additional challenge in patients with known MG is avoiding medications that can worsen or exacerbate weakness because of their pharmacologic effects on the neuromuscular junction. Medications often administered in the ED for other clinical conditions, including IV magnesium, β-blocker and calcium channel medications, and a number of antibiotic medications can precipitate myasthenic worsening or even crisis. When encountering a patient with an MG diagnosis, it is critical to review a medication's potential effect on this condition before prescribing. A list of high-risk medications in MG is listed in **Table 7.5**.

Pathophysiology

MG is an autoimmune disorder of the postsynaptic neuromuscular junction. Neuromuscular transmission occurs by release of the neurotransmitter acetylcholine from the presynaptic motor nerve terminal. 80% to 90% of MG patients have antibodies present to the acetylcholine receptor (AChR), blocking the ability of the neurotransmitter to bind to the postsynaptic receptors and reducing the number of these receptors. The loss of AChRs on the postsynaptic muscle membrane reduces the "safety factor" in neuromuscular transmission and resulting in the fatigable weakness of clinical disease. Five percent to 10% of patients lacking AChR antibodies instead have antibodies to the muscle-specific kinase (MuSK), a transmembrane protein component of the postsynaptic neuromuscular junction, affecting the clustering of AChRs. These patients are phenotypically similar to patients with AChR antibody–positive MG, but often have more bulbar weakness. Treatments for MuSK MG are overlapping, but somewhat different from AChR MG, because of its immunoglobulin (IgG)4-mediated pathophysiology. The remaining 5% to 10% of patients with MG are "seronegative," meaning they lack antibodies to AChR and MuSK. Novel antibodies, including to LRP4 and agrin, are being identified in some of these patients.

Diagnostic testing used to confirm the diagnosis of MG includes the antibody tests as noted earlier, and electrodiagnostic testing as well. Nerve conduction studies, with repetitive stimulation, and single-fiber electromyography (SFEMG) are used to confirm the diagnosis of MG.

TABLE 7.5	Cautionary Drugs for Patients with Myasthenia Gravis
Type	**Drugs**
Anesthetics	• Neuromuscular blocking agents
Antibiotics	• Aminoglycosides • Fluoroquinolones • Ketolides • Macrolides
Botulinum toxin	

Cardiac medications	• Antiarrhythmics
	  • Quinine
	  • Procainamide
	  • Other sodium channel antiarrhythmics
	
	• β-Blockers
	• Calcium channel blockers

Corticosteroids[a]	
D-Penicillamine	
Chemotherapy	• Immune-checkpoint inhibitor chemotherapy
Magnesium[b]	
Other medications[c]	• Iodinated contrast[c] • Statin medications[c]

IV, intravenous; MG, myasthenia gravis.
[a]Often used for the treatment of MG but can cause worsening when first started.
[b]Particularly IV.
[c]Possible risk, monitor for worsening.

Ten percent to 12% of patients diagnosed with MG have an associated thymic tumor (thymoma) underling the disease. For this reason, all patients newly diagnosed with MG must undergo CT or MRI of the chest to evaluate for thymic neoplasm.

Prehospital Concerns

Prehospital management of patients with MG primarily focuses on monitoring and management of respiratory weakness associated with the disease. Patients with MG can have rapid deterioration of respiratory status due to weakness of the diaphragm and accessory respiratory muscles. Neuromuscular respiratory weakness typically leads to hypercarbic respiratory failure, so the lack of hypoxia on monitoring should not be taken as a reassuring sign, and continuous capnometry should be used when available. There should be a low threshold to provide noninvasive and mechanical ventilation to a patient with MG in respiratory distress.

Approach/The Focused Examination

The typical clinical symptoms of MG include fatigable weakness, usually with associated ocular involvement causing impaired extraocular movements with diplopia and eyelid ptosis. Patients should be asked whether symptoms worsen at the end of the day or after exertional activities. Fatigable weakness can be tested on examination by having the patient repeatedly abduct the arm before retesting deltoid strength. Facial and bulbar weakness may be present and result in dysarthria and dysphagia. Neck extensor weakness is common and associated with respiratory muscle weakness; 15% of patients with MG have only eye symptoms, a subtype known as "ocular MG." Another characteristic historic finding is the exacerbation of symptoms with heat, for example, hot showers, high humidity, and with alcohol use.

In any patient presenting with ptosis or diplopia, MG should be considered on the differential diagnosis. Mimicking disorders include brainstem strokes, isolated cranial neuropathies, and multiple sclerosis. The physical examination finding of bilateral ptosis and extraocular movement abnormalities, however, should raise MG to the top of the diagnostic list, particularly if there is accompanying facial, bulbar, or generalized weakness.

Diagnosis of MG is made on the basis of typical clinical history and physical examination findings, together with serum antibody testing to AChR antibodies or other MG-associated antibodies, and electrodiagnostic testing. Because neuromuscular transmission improves with colder temperatures, a bedside "ice pack test" has good sensitivity for MG in patients with prominent ptosis. In this maneuver, baseline ptosis is assessed, an ice pack applied to the closed eyelids for 2 minutes, and then ptosis reexamined for improvement. IV edrophonium, or the "tensilon test," assessing for improvement in ocular symptoms, was historically performed to establish diagnosis, but is no longer routinely performed because of cardiac side effects and reduced availability of this medication.

Assessing and examining a patient with known MG should focus on signs of disease exacerbation and impending respiratory failure. Patients with bulbar and neck weakness are at greater risk for respiratory muscle weakness and should be monitored very closely for worsening respiratory function with frequent bedside spirometry. Bulbar weakness causing dysarthria and dysphagia should be assessed, and patients should not eat if there is concern for dysphagia; nasogastric tube use for nutrition and medication administration is sometimes required.

Respiratory therapy should be involved, and check bedside spirometry measures frequently. A negative inspiratory force (NIF) below -30 cm H_2O or a vital capacity of less than 15 to 20 mL/kg is concerning and may warrant noninvasive ventilation or elective intubation. An arterial blood gas may be helpful at this point in clinical decision-making. These measurements should always be placed in the context of clinical examination and other factors (eg, facial weakness) that may affect the ability of the patient to participate in testing.

As described in the following section, treatments that suppress or modulate the immune system are key to the treatment in the majority of patients with MG. As such, these patients are at increased risk for complications related to their treatments. Any patient with MG on immune-suppressing medication, whether it be corticosteroid or steroid-sparing immunosuppression, is at increased risk for infection. When presenting in the emergency setting, there should be a high index of suspicion for infectious complication. Patients receiving IVIG are at risk for thromboembolic complications of this therapy, including deep vein thrombosis (DVT), pulmonary embolism, and arterial thrombotic events including myocardial infarction and acute ischemic stroke. Patients getting plasmapheresis typically require indwelling central venous catheter or port and are at risk for line infections and associated DVT. Frequent plasmapheresis also increases risk of bleeding complications. When evaluating a patient on treatment for MG in the emergency setting, it is critical to consider what immunomodulating therapies the patient has been receiving and the potential complications related to those treatments.

Management

The treatment of MG includes both short- and long-term strategies. The first-line, symptomatic treatment for MG is acetylcholinesterase inhibitor drugs, primarily pyridostigmine. These medications work by preventing the enzymatic degradation of acetylcholine in the neuromuscular junction, giving the neurotransmitter more time to exert effect on the postsynaptic neuromuscular membrane. Most patients have some improvement with pyridostigmine, but often the improvement is not sufficient to be sole therapy. Side effects from acetylcholinesterase inhibitors, primarily GI cramping and diarrhea, limit dose escalation, and rarely very high doses can result in cholinergic toxicity.

Most patients, despite partial improvement with pyridostigmine, will require further treatment with immunomodulating medications to suppress the underlying autoimmune pathophysiology of the disease. Corticosteroids, as discussed subsequently, can be used both acutely and long term to treat MG, but are limited by side effects long term. IVIG and plasmapheresis are quick acting and used often for acute exacerbations, but have short-lived effects. For long-term disease control, many patients require steroid-sparing immune-suppressing medications.

Corticosteroids are often the first medication prescribed for MG when there is insufficient improvement with pyridostigmine. Prednisone is typically used, but other oral corticosteroids are occasionally prescribed. Dosing strategies for prednisone vary, with some neurologists starting with high doses (60-80 mg daily) and then slowly tapering over weeks to months; others start at lower doses (10-20 mg daily) and increase over weeks before starting to taper. IV corticosteroids are sometimes given in the setting of acute MG exacerbation in a patient already on oral corticosteroid therapy at home. Caution must be taken, however, when initiating oral or IV corticosteroid treatment in a patient with MG, because there is often transient worsening of weakness that occurs for days to weeks after first starting corticosteroids in MG. Any patient with MG presenting in the emergency setting with worsened weakness after recent initiation of corticosteroids must be monitored closely; admission to the observation unit or hospital should be considered if there is bulbar or respiratory weakness or severe generalized limb weakness.

Treatment for an acute exacerbation of weakness from MG or a severe initial presentation of the disease includes IVIG or plasmapheresis. The exact mechanism of IVIG is unknown, but it is thought to facilitate the clearance of pathogenic autoantibodies. Plasmapheresis similarly removes pathogenic IgGs. These therapies typically have the most rapid effect to improve weakness in MG, but the response is transient, lasting typically 1 to 4 weeks before IgGs are reconstituted. Long-term immunotherapy must be added or adjusted in follow-up to IVIG or plasmapheresis treatment, or in some cases maintenance treatments with IVIG or plasmapheresis are arranged.

Long-term immunotherapy for MG typically requires use of an oral steroid–sparing immune-suppressing medication to prevent the chronic side effects of corticosteroid use. These therapies include mycophenolate, azathioprine, and, less often, cyclosporine, tacrolimus, or methotrexate. Eculizumab is a recently approved treatment for AChR antibody–positive MG that targets the complement-mediated destruction of the receptors on the postsynaptic membrane; it is also used in the long-term treatment of patients with refractory MG. MuSK MG, which is an IgG4-mediated disease, responds better to rituximab than to the other mentioned therapies, and this medication is considered first-line treatment in this subclass of MG.

Patients with thymoma underlying their MG must undergo thymectomy, and in some cases additional chemotherapy or radiation treatment. In patients with autoimmune but non-thymomatous MG, there is evidence that thymectomy results in improved treatment outcomes; thus, some patients with MG will undergo elective thymectomy as part of their disease management.

One of the most critical issues in the management of patients with MG in the emergency setting is being aware of medications that must be avoided because they can cause acute worsening of MG symptoms or even precipitate myasthenic crisis. The most frequent offenders for iatrogenic MG exacerbation include IV magnesium, neuromuscular blocking agents for anesthesia, IV β-blockers and calcium channel blockers, and certain antibiotic agents. A list of medications to avoid in MG is maintained by the Myasthenia Gravis Foundation of America (MGFA) and available on their website. An adapted list is shown in Table 7.5. These are relative contraindications, and it ultimately is at the discretion of the treating physician to weigh the risks and benefits of giving any of these medications in a patient with MG, but caution and monitoring are recommended when administering any agent that has a known risk of precipitating MG exacerbation.

Supportive measures may be needed in patients presenting with acute exacerbation of bulbar and respiratory weakness. Patients with severe dysphagia may require short-term nasogastric tube placement to receive medication and nutrition. Patients with myasthenic crisis causing respiratory failure from neuromuscular weakness may require noninvasive ventilation or intubation and mechanical ventilation. In patients requiring mechanical ventilation or noninvasive ventilation, pyridostigmine is typically temporarily held to reduce respiratory secretions. Neuromuscular blocking agents may be used in rapid sequence intubation (RSI) in patients with MG, but the effects may be prolonged and patients with MG may take longer to recover from these agents. Doses may need to be adjusted for patients with MG: depolarizing neuromuscular blocking agents (succinylcholine) require higher doses, and for non-depolarizing neuromuscular blocking agents (rocuronium or vecuronium), lower doses are recommended.

Pediatric Issues

The onset of MG is bimodal—with an increased incidence in young adults in the second to third decade and then increasing incidence in the sixth to eighth decade. Onset of MG before the age of 15 is termed *juvenile myasthenia gravis*. Treatment of juvenile MG is similar to that in adults, except that thymectomy is more often recommended and risks of long-term corticosteroid or steroid-sparing immunosuppressants would strongly be weighed against their benefits.

Congenital MG is a group of rare genetic disorders affecting proteins involved with neuromuscular transmission. Fatigable weakness, with ocular, bulbar, and respiratory involvement occurs similarly to autoimmune MG, usually in infancy or early childhood. Treatment is with acetylcholinesterase inhibitors, but there is no role for immunotherapy. For acute exacerbation of congenital MG, treatment is primarily supportive. Avoiding medications that adversely affect the neuromuscular junction, as noted earlier, is similarly critical.

Neonatal MG refers to the transient myasthenic syndrome in a baby born to a mother with autoimmune MG because of the transplacental transfer of maternal antibodies. Symptoms typically last only a few weeks and treatment is supportive.

LAMBERT-EATON MYASTHENIC SYNDROME

LEMS is a rarer autoimmune disorder affecting the presynaptic neuromuscular junction, which presents with overlapping symptoms to MG. Patients develop antibodies to the voltage-gated calcium channel (VGCC), resulting in impaired acetylcholine release into the neuromuscular junction. Half of LEMS is paraneoplastic, primarily in association with small cell lung cancer, so cancer screening is critical in association with this diagnosis. The other half of patients has a primary autoimmune cause to the disease.

Symptoms of LEMS have more overlap with myopathies than MG, typically presenting with slowly progressive proximal muscle weakness. Ocular and bulbar symptoms, similar to MG, can occur. As opposed to the typical fatigability of MG, patients with LEMS often have improved strength after brief periods of exercise, although more prolonged activity subsequently leads to postexercise exhaustion. Autonomic symptoms commonly accompany the weakness in LEMS, but do not predominate the clinical picture. Typical physical examination findings raising suspicion for LEMS include proximal muscle weakness that improves after brief exercise, minor ocular and bulbar weakness, and absent or reduced deep tendon reflexes that improve after brief exercise. Respiratory muscle weakness in LEMS is rare, but can occur.

LEMS is diagnosed using a combination of history and physical examination findings, laboratory testing for P/Q-type calcium channel antibodies, and short-exercise and repetitive nerve stimulation electrodiagnostic testing.

Treatment of LEMS first consists of evaluating for underlying small cell lung cancer. In patients with associated malignancy, treatment of the cancer must come first if the neuromuscular disorder is to improve. In most patients with LEMS, initial treatment is with pyridostigmine (30-120 mg q 4-8 hours), often in combination with 3,4-diaminopyridine (3,4-DAP). Some patients who do not sufficiently improve with pyridostigmine and 3,4-DAP are then treated with immunotherapy agents similar to those used for MG, including IVIG, plasmapheresis, corticosteroids, and other oral steroid–sparing medications.

As with MG, avoidance of medications that adversely affect neuromuscular junction function should be avoided in patients with LEMS, because they can result in exacerbation of weakness.

BOTULISM

Botulism is a neuromuscular disorder seen in both infants and adults resulting from exposure to toxin from the bacteria *Clostridium botulinum*. *C. botulinum* is naturally occurring anaerobic organism present in fruits and vegetables, in seafood and in soil. When the bacterial spores are in favorable environmental conditions, they germinate, producing bacteria that create botulinum toxin.

Botulinum toxin causes weakness through presynaptic neuromuscular junction blockade. The toxin is taken up into the presynaptic nerve terminal and then interferes with proteins necessary for release of acetylcholine into the neuromuscular junction, resulting in weakness, and in severe cases, life-threatening paralysis.

Infant botulism occurs when *C. botulinum* spores are ingested, colonize the child's GI tract, and then develop into toxin-forming bacteria. In current times, this most often occurs from exposure to spore-containing dust or dirt. Historically, cases were associated with infant ingestion of raw honey, but this appears to be a minor source of new cases. Rarely, GI colonization by *C. botulinum* in adult patients can occur, typically with a history of GI surgery, preexisting GI disease, and immune suppression.

Foodborne botulism occurs with the ingestion of a food that has been contaminated by the preformed botulinum toxin. In most cases, this has occurred in association with home-canned foods.

Wound botulism can occur when *C. botulinum* infects a wound and then produces botulinum toxin. Typical wounds that favor *C. botulinum* infection are harboring anaerobic infections (puncture and deep and subcutaneous locations). An association has been reported with subcutaneous heroin injection.

The typical clinical features of foodborne botulism usually begin within 2 days of ingestion of the toxin, often starting with nausea and vomiting and then developing neurologic symptoms. Cranial neuropathies are generally the first of these symptoms, particularly loss of pupillary reflexes causing blurry vision, and then impaired eye movements, facial and bulbar weakness, followed by descending symmetric weakness. Mental status is normal. Autonomic symptoms may be present. Respiratory muscle involvement is common, and may require mechanical ventilation. Wound botulism presents similarly to foodborne botulism, but without the preceding GI symptoms and may have a longer delay in symptom development.

Infant botulism typically presents with constipation, generalized weakness and difficulty with feeding, and crying. Respiratory failure requiring mechanical ventilation can occur. This diagnosis should be considered in any infant presenting with acute hypotonia.

The diagnosis of botulism is confirmed by identifying the toxin in stool, blood, or other body fluid specimens, or by testing a suspected food source. Physicians should contact their state health department or the U.S. Centers for Disease Control and Prevention (CDC) for guidance on local testing procedures. Electrodiagnostic testing can be helpful in uncertain cases.

Treatment for botulism starts with close clinical monitoring, particularly for respiratory muscle involvement, and mechanical ventilation when needed. When the diagnosis of botulism is suspected, antitoxin should be administered, even before confirmatory tests have resulted. The state health department must be involved to facilitate testing and obtain antitoxin treatment. The dose of heptavalent botulinum antitoxin (HBAT) in adults is one vial given intravenously. Children receive a smaller percentage of the adult dose, guided by consultation with the CDC. Botulism immune globulin intravenous (BIG-IV) is also administered for infants younger than 1 year of age.

Antibiotics are not currently indicated for infant botulism or adult GI botulism, because of concern that antibiotic treatment can increase the amount of toxin released into the system. Wound botulism is additionally treated with debridement of the infected site. Antibiotics are often indicated in cases of wound botulism in conjunction with infectious disease consultation.

TICK PARALYSIS

Tick paralysis is an acute neuromuscular disorder caused by neurotoxins released by the bite of a number of tick species. The exact mechanism of tick paralysis is not well established, but involves slowing of nerve conduction responses and interference in neuromuscular junction transmission. Symptoms begin with paresthesias and generalized fatigue, and then progress to more weakness of the cranial and limb muscles. Diagnosis depends on finding the attached tick; thus, a thorough examination of the skin is necessary. Most patients improve quickly after removal of the tick.

TIPS AND PEARLS

- The diagnosis of MG should be considered in any patient with diplopia, ptosis, or bulbar weakness, particularly if there is a fatigable element to these symptoms.
- Any patient with known or suspected MG presenting with exacerbation of weakness should be closely monitored for neuromuscular respiratory weakness. Bulbar and neck weakness are associated with respiratory compromise, and these patients may require noninvasive or mechanical ventilation.
- Medications that can worsen neuromuscular junction function should be avoided in patients with MG, if possible. If these medications must be used, patients should be closely monitored for MG symptom worsening.
- Patients with MG on immune suppressing medications, IVIG, or plasmapheresis may present with infectious or thrombotic complications of these treatments.
- Botulism should be considered in patients presenting with cranial neuropathies followed by rapidly progressive descending weakness without fever or alteration of mental status.
- Infant botulism should be considered in a floppy infant.
- When clinically suspected, treatment for botulism with antitoxin should be initiated as soon as possible.

EVIDENCE

Is there evidence to support the superiority of IVIG or plasmapheresis in treating patients with MG?

There have been no large randomized controlled trials of IVIG or plasmapheresis in the treatment of MG, but smaller noncontrolled studies have shown benefit and one head-to-head study of the two showed equal efficacy.[7-11] In most centers, IVIG is more accessible than is plasmapheresis and thus is used more often, but some patients may have cardiac or thrombotic contraindications to IVIG therapy.

Does thymectomy improve outcomes for patients with non-thymomatous MG?

There has been a large randomized trial of thymectomy for AChR antibody–positive, non-thymomatous, generalized MG that showed improved clinical outcomes over a 3-year period in the thymectomy group.[12] Thymectomy is typically recommended in younger patients and those with medically refractory MG.

Does administration of antitoxin improve outcomes in patients with botulism?

There are limited studies on the use of antitoxin in patients with botulism. One meta-analysis of studies and case reports did show a reduction in mortality in patients treated with antitoxin therapy. There is a suggestion that treatment earlier in the disease course improves outcomes.[13,14]

References

1. Drake LA, Dinehart SM, Farmer ER, et al. Guidelines of care for dermatomyositis. American Academy of Dermatology. *J Am Acad Dermatol*. 1996;34(5 Pt 1):824-829.

2. Joffe MM, Love LA, Leff RL, et al. Drug therapy of the idiopathic inflammatory myopathies: predictors of response to prednisone, azathioprine, and methotrexate and a comparison of their efficacy. *Am J Med*. 1993;94(4):379-387.

3. Marie I, Menard J-F, Hatron PY, et al. Intravenous immunoglobulins for steroid-refractory esophageal involvement related to polymyositis and dermatomyositis: a series of 73 patients. *Arthritis Care Res (Hoboken)*. 2010;62(12):1748-1755.

4. Odeh M. The role of reperfusion-induced injury in the pathogenesis of the crush syndrome. *N Engl J Med*. 1991;324(20):1417-1422.

5. Bosch X, Poch E, Grau JM. Rhabdomyolysis and acute kidney injury. *N Engl J Med*. 2009;361(1):62-72.

6. Narayanaswami P, Weiss M, Selcen D, et al. Evidence-based guideline summary: diagnosis and treatment of limb-girdle and distal dystrophies: report of the guideline development subcommittee of the American Academy of Neurology and the practice issues review panel of the American Association of Neuromuscular & Electrodiagnostic Medicine. *Neurology*. 2014;83(16):1453-1463.

7. Barth D, Nabavi Nouri M, Ng E, Nwe P, Bril V. Comparison of IVIg and PLEX in patients with myasthenia gravis. *Neurology*. 2011;76(23):2017-2023.

8. Gajdos P, Chevret S, Toyka K. Plasma exchange for myasthenia gravis. *Cochrane Database Syst Rev*. 2002;(4):CD002275.

9. Gajdos P, Chevret S, Toyka KV. Intravenous immunoglobulin for myasthenia gravis. *Cochrane Database Syst Rev*. 2012;(12):CD002277.

10. Qureshi AI, Choudhry MA, Akbar MS, et al. Plasma exchange versus intravenous immunoglobulin treatment in myasthenic crisis. *Neurology*. 1999;52(3):629-632.

11. Sanders DB, Wolfe GI, Benatar M, et al. International consensus guidance for management of myasthenia gravis: executive summary. *Neurology*. 2016;87(4):419-425.

12. Wolfe GI, Kaminski HJ, Aban IB, et al. Randomized trial of thymectomy in myasthenia gravis. *N Engl J Med*. 2016;375(6):511-522.

13. O'Horo JC, Harper EP, El Rafei A, et al. Efficacy of antitoxin therapy in treating patients with foodborne botulism: a systematic review and meta-analysis of cases, 1923-2016. *Clin Infect Dis*. 2017;66(suppl 1):S43-S56.

14. Yu PA, Lin NH, Mahon BE, et al. Safety and improved clinical outcomes in patients treated with new equine-derived heptavalent botulinum antitoxin. *Clin Infect Dis*. 2017;66(suppl 1):S57-S64.

Suggested Readings

1. Barber BJ, Andrews JG, Lu Z, et al. Oral corticosteroids and onset of cardiomyopathy in Duchenne muscular dystrophy. *J Pediatr*. 2013;163(4):1080-1084.e1.

2. Chatham-Stephens K, Fleck-Derderian S, Johnson SD, Sobel J, Rao AK, Meaney-Delman D. Clinical features of foodborne and wound botulism: a systematic review of the literature, 1932-2015. *Clin Infect Dis*. 2017;66(suppl 1):S11-S16.

3. Danieli MG, Gelardi C, Guerra F, Cardinaletti P, Pedini V, Gabrielli A. Cardiac involvement in polymyositis and dermatomyositis. *Autoimmun Rev*. 2016;15(5):462-465.

4. Gilhus NE. Myasthenia gravis. *N Engl J Med*. 2016;375(26):2570-2581.

5. Howard JF, Utsugisawa K, Benatar M, et al. Safety and efficacy of eculizumab in anti-acetylcholine receptor antibody-positive refractory generalised myasthenia gravis (REGAIN): a phase 3, randomised, double-blind, placebo-controlled, multicentre study. *Lancet Neurol*. 2017;16(12):976-986.

6. Ionita CM, Acsadi G. Management of juvenile myasthenia gravis. *Pediatr Neurol*. 2013;48(2):95-104.

7. Mehndiratta MM, Pandey S, Kuntzer T. Acetylcholinesterase inhibitor treatment for myasthenia gravis. *Cochrane Database Syst Rev*. 2014;(10):CD006986.

8. Nicolle MW. Myasthenia gravis and Lambert-Eaton myasthenic syndrome. *Continuum (Minneap Minn)*. 2016;22(6, Muscle and Neuromuscular Junction Disorders):1978-2005.

9. Rao AK, Lin NH, Griese SE, Chatham-Stephens K, Badell ML, Sobel J. Clinical criteria to trigger suspicion for botulism: an evidence-based tool to facilitate timely recognition of suspected cases during sporadic events and outbreaks. *Clin Infect Dis*. 2017;66(suppl 1):S38-S42.

10. Sanders DB, Guptill JT. Myasthenia gravis and Lambert-Eaton myasthenic syndrome. *Continuum (Minneap Minn)*. 2014;20(5 Peripheral Nervous System Disorders):1413-1425.

11. Sieb JP, Gillessen T. Iatrogenic and toxic myopathies. *Muscle Nerve*. 2003;27(2):142-156.

12. Silvestri NJ, Wolfe GI. Myasthenia gravis. *Semin Neurol*. 2012;32(3):215-226.

13. Venance SL, Cannon SC, Fialho D. The primary periodic paralyses: diagnosis, pathogenesis and treatment. *Brain*. 2006;129(Pt 1):8.

14. Warren JD, Blumbergs PC, Thompson PD. Rhabdomyolysis: a review. *Muscle Nerve*. 2002;25(3):332-347.

The Neuropathies

Ethan Abbott

Although the neuropathies represent a broad, complex, and heterogeneous group of disorders, this chapter presents several distinct and commonly evaluated neurologic emergencies encountered by the acute care provider: Bell's palsy, Guillain-Barré syndrome (GBS), and the peripheral neuropathies with a focus on distal symmetric polyneuropathy (DSPN). With evolving evidence and questions regarding the efficacy of medications and timing of acute interventions for several of these conditions, this chapter helps guide the clinician with a focused approach based on the best available evidence.

BELL'S PALSY
THE CLINICAL CHALLENGE

Bell's palsy is an idiopathic, cranial nerve VII (facial) paralysis and the most common cause of unilateral facial nerve weakness or paralysis. The etiology is thought to be viral-mediated, but the pathophysiology is controversial. Management focuses on protecting the eye from injury and minimizing long-term sequelae.

Bell's palsy typically presents as an acute-onset, unilateral facial palsy peaking at 48 to 72 hours after the start of symptoms; the average age for presentation is 40. The clinical challenge with a facial palsy is to determine whether it is central or peripheral in origin. There are potential pitfalls that can occur, leading to missed or delayed diagnosis that may contribute to increased morbidity. It is estimated that up to 30% of patients will have a delayed or incomplete recovery of full function, resulting in permanent disability.[1] Bell's palsy is commonly seen in patients with diabetes, hypertension, a recent upper respiratory infection, or in late-term pregnancy. **Table 8.1** presents the differential diagnosis for unilateral facial nerve palsy.

PATHOPHYSIOLOGY

Understanding of the facial nerve anatomy and innervation is essential to differentiating central from peripheral causes of facial nerve palsy. The facial nerve innervates the muscles of facial expression, including the orbicularis oculi, frontalis, orbicularis oris, and the stapedius. It supplies sensation to the anterior two-thirds of the tongue, and the parasympathetic fibers of the lacrimal and submandibular glands. Because the cells of the facial nucleus that innervate the upper face receive fibers from bilateral hemispheres, a patient with the ability to move the forehead muscles should raise concern for a central etiology. Thus, in a patient with a peripheral facial nerve palsy such as Bell's, complete weakness of the ipsilateral facial nerve involves the entire forehead. Bilateral symptoms are uncommon, and should trigger considerations for an alternative diagnosis such as Lyme disease.

TABLE 8.1	Etiologies and Clinical Features of Facial Paralysis		
	Condition	Etiologic Agent	Distinguishing Factors
Autoimmune	Guillain-Barré	Autoimmune/infectious	Acute polyneuropathy; ascending paralysis; weakness of hands, feet progressing to the trunk
	Melkersson-Rosenthal syndrome	Unknown	Recurrent facial paralysis, swelling of face/lips, and fissures or folds in tongue
	Multiple sclerosis	Unknown	Abnormal neurologic examination with intermittent symptoms
	Sarcoidosis	Unknown	May be bilateral; laboratory abnormalities including angiotensin-converting enzyme level
Congenital	Mobius syndrome	Possibly viral	Age (young), bilateral in nature, unable to move face or eyes laterally
Endocrine	Diabetes	Microvascular disease	Other signs and symptoms of diabetes, laboratory testing
Idiopathic	Acute facial nerve paresis/paralysis	Unknown	Classic Bell's palsy with other etiologies excluded
Infectious	Encephalitis/meningitis	Fungal, viral, or bacterial	Headache, stiff neck, cerebrospinal fluid abnormalities
	Herpes simplex	Herpes simplex virus along axons of nerve residing in the geniculate ganglion	Fever, malaise
	Human immunodeficiency virus (HIV)	HIV	Fever, malaise, CD4 count
	Lyme disease	Spirochete *Borrelia burgdorferi*	May be bilateral, rash, arthralgias
	Mononucleosis	Epstein-Barr virus	Malaise, difficult to distinguish
	Otitis media	Bacterial pathogens	Gradual onset, ear pain, fever, hearing loss
	Ramsay-Hunt syndrome	Herpes zoster virus	Pronounced prodrome of pain, vesicular eruption in ear canal or pharynx
Inherited	Syphilis Heritable disorders	*Treponema pallidum* Autosomal dominant inheritance	Other neurologic and cutaneous manifestations Family history as high as 4%, may have other neurologic disorders
Neoplastic	Facial nerve tumor, skin cancer, parotid tumors	Multiple carcinomas of the head and neck	May involve only select branches of the facial nerve or other cranial nerves and present as multiple cranial neuropathies

TABLE 8.1	Etiologies and Clinical Features of Facial Paralysis (*continued*)		
	Condition	**Etiologic Agent**	**Distinguishing Factors**
Neurovascular	Stroke	Ischemia, hemorrhage	Forehead sparing most often, extremities often involved
Traumatic	Injury to facial nerve	Trauma, including forceps delivery	Timing of injury coincides with trauma

From Baugh RF, Basura GJ, Ishii LE, et al. Clinical practice guideline: Bell's palsy. *Otolaryngol Head Neck Surg.* 2013;149(3 suppl):S1-S27.

The facial nerve travels through the narrow fallopian canal within the temporal bone. Its anatomic course predisposes it to compression from inflammation, edema, or trauma. The most commonly accepted mechanism is reactivation of the herpes simplex virus 1 (HSV-1) originating from the geniculate ganglion, resulting in edema and swelling of the facial nerve with consequent compromise. This theory has been supported by the isolation of HSV-1 in the endoneurial fluid of the facial nerve in patients with Bell palsy. Edema has also been observed on magnetic resonance imaging (MRI) and seen in those patients surgically managed with a decompression procedure. Despite this, the relative association of HSV-1 within the facial nerve does not provide the definitive evidence for the etiology of Bell palsy, and there is still uncertainty regarding its pathophysiology.

PREHOSPITAL CONCERNS

The challenge for prehospital providers is when to activate the stroke protocol. Televideo resources such as those used in community paramedicine initiatives may be helpful. When there is doubt, emergency medical service (EMS) systems are best advised to transport to a stroke center.

APPROACH TO THE PATIENT WITH BELL PALSY

The diagnosis of Bell palsy is driven by clinical examination and history, and occurs when no other explanation for the cause of facial weakness has been determined. There is typically little role for imaging or laboratory testing. The examination should include careful assessment of the ability to move the forehead. Forehead movement or sparing suggests a central etiology; however, mild cases of Bell palsy may appear to spare the forehead. Examination of the oropharynx, external canal, and tympanic membranes should be performed to determine whether vesicular lesions are present. The presence of these lesions, which can also be accompanied by sensorineural hearing loss, represents the Ramsay-Hunt syndrome. The chorda tympani nerve, a sensory branch of the facial nerve that courses through the middle ear and supplies taste to the anterior two-thirds of the tongue is also seen in patients with Ramsay-Hunt syndrome.

Patients can present with a constellation of symptoms that vary in severity. Because of inability to close the affected eye, patients may have an ipsilateral dry eye and decreased tear production due to parasympathetic lacrimal gland involvement. Changes in the ability to taste and dry mouth can occur, and patients may have difficulty with handling food and secretions and demonstrate drooling or excessive tearing while eating. Facial and postauricular pain may also be present, often occurring before the onset of facial weakness. Hyperacusis, although less commonly seen, occurs because of loss of function of the stapedius muscle that typically mitigates vibrations in the inner ear and results in sound perceived as unusually loud on the affected side.

The differential diagnosis is divided into multiple etiologies: congenital, endocrine, infectious, traumatic, neoplastic, inherited, neurovascular, idiopathic, and autoimmune categories (see Table 8.1).

Other diagnostic testing, although not routinely recommended on initial presentation, includes the use of CT or MRI to assess the facial nerve, electromyography (EMG), electroneuronography (ENoG), and serologic testing for infectious etiologies.

MANAGEMENT

An algorithmic approach to management is seen in **Figure 8.1**. The natural history of Bell's palsy is such that symptoms improve (even without any medical treatment) within 3 to 4 weeks of initial presentation, and complete resolution occurs by 3 months. Patients with prolonged symptoms, although less commonly seen in the acute care setting, should undergo further testing and consideration for an alternative diagnosis. The severity of the paralysis in Bell's palsy will often determine potential for complete recovery and can be objectively assessed using the House-Brackmann scale, which incorporates visual inspection and motor testing to determine the grade of dysfunction. However, the House-Brackmann scale was not intended for use in the initial evaluation of paralysis in patients with suspected Bell's palsy, and thus will be of little aid to the emergency clinician.[2]

The mainstay of treatment in Bell's palsy is a short course of oral glucocorticoids often as monotherapy, or in combination with antivirals. Antivirals prescribed alone are not recommended. The use of combination therapy is controversial, and the evidence is not clear-cut. We recommend

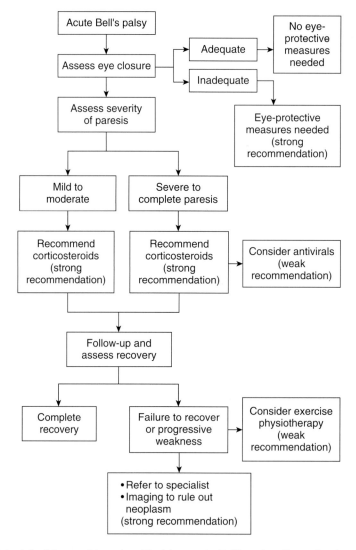

Figure 8.1: Clinical decision-making algorithm for acute Bell's palsy. From de Almeida JR, Guyatt GH, Sud S, et al. Bell Palsy Working Group, Canadian Society of Otolaryngology—Head and Neck Surgery and Canadian Neurological Sciences Federation. Management of Bell's palsy: clinical practice guideline. *CMAJ*. 2014;186(12):917-922.

prednisone, 60 mg/d, for 7 days without a taper. If antivirals are also given, we recommend either valacyclovir, 1000 mg three times a day, or acyclovir, 400 mg five times a day for 7 days. The greatest benefit demonstrated in studies is the administration of glucocorticoids within 72 hours of onset of symptoms, although there is evidence that recovery is improved if medications are started at 48 hours.[3] Rates of recovery and reduction of long-term sequelae have been found with the use of steroids alone. The combination of antivirals and steroids as a treatment regimen for Bell's palsy lacks consensus in the literature.

We recommend offering combination therapy to patients presenting within 72 hours of symptoms or in cases of severe facial nerve dysfunction. Providers should also counsel patients on the current evidence regarding antivirals so there is clear understanding of the uncertainty of their role in treatment of Bell's palsy. Other proposed treatments such as surgical decompression, physical therapy, and acupuncture have not demonstrated improved outcomes.[4,5]

Management of associated symptoms and potential sequalae is an important part of the management strategy. With the inability to fully close the eyelid, eye care is required to prevent corneal abrasion, ulceration, or keratitis. Patients should be prescribed artificial tears or eye lubricants and protection with an eye patch while sleeping. These patients will need urgent specialty follow-up with ophthalmology and otolaryngology.

TIPS AND PEARLS

- Up to 30% of patients with a Bell's palsy will have a delayed recovery or not recover full facial function.
- Bell's palsy is more commonly seen in patients with a history of diabetes, hypertension, and in late-term pregnancy. The pathophysiologic mechanisms are thought to be virally mediated.
- Bilateral Bell's palsy is uncommon, and should prompt a workup for other etiologies including Lyme disease, GBS, or sarcoidosis.
- Corticosteroids are the mainstay of treatment; and the use of combination therapy with antivirals may be beneficial for long-term sequelae, but lacks strong evidence.

EVIDENCE

Is there an advantage of combination treatment with steroids and antivirals versus steroids alone in the treatment of Bell's palsy?

The American Academy of Neurology (AAN) evidence-based guidelines in 2012 reviewed the role of steroids and antivirals in the treatment of Bell's palsy.[6] The authors examined the prior 12 years of literature and determined that for patients with new-onset Bell's palsy, the addition of antivirals might be offered to increase the likelihood of facial nerve recovery (Level C), but that a benefit has not been established. The authors did conclude that oral steroids should be offered, with a high likelihood of improving recovery of facial nerve function (Level A).

The American Academy of Otolaryngology published *Clinical Practice Guideline: Bell's Palsy in 2013* and recommended that antivirals may be offered in addition to steroids if given within 72 hours or for symptoms with Grade B.[2] The authors report that this conclusion is not supported by high-quality trials and that a "small benefit cannot be excluded" in light of the low risk of use of antivirals.

The Canadian Society of Otolaryngology published *Management of Bell's Palsy: Clinical Practice Guideline* in 2014 and recommended the addition of antiviral therapy to corticosteroids based on severity of the presentation of Bell's palsy.[7] For mild to moderate severity, the authors strongly recommend against the addition of antivirals, and for severe to complete paresis, they recommend the use of combined therapy, but both of these are weak recommendations based on the available evidence.

A Cochrane review from 2019, *Antiviral Treatment for Bell's Palsy* examined the role of combination therapy versus corticosteroids alone or combined with placebo.[8] The authors included 14 randomized controlled trials (RCTs) in their meta-analysis with a total of 2488 study subjects. The measured outcome criterion in the studies was recovery of facial function based on a scoring system such as House-Brackmann. The conclusions were that combination therapy with antivirals and corticosteroids may have "little or no effect on rates of incomplete recovery in comparison to corticosteroids alone, and there may be no clear difference with the combination therapy compared to corticosteroids alone." They did report that combination therapy could probably reduce late sequalae of the disease compared with monotherapy with corticosteroids.

Is there a role for surgical decompression in the treatment of Bell's palsy?

Surgical decompression is a controversial treatment and of questionable benefit for refractory patients, those with poor results from nerve conduction studies, or advanced disease as determined by an assessment using the House-Brackmann scale. Because of the natural history of the disease and spontaneous recovery without treatment, most likely there are limited patients who are surgical candidates.

A Cochrane review from 2013 examined the role of surgical decompression in Bell's palsy and found only two studies that met criteria for inclusion.[4] The authors incorporated two non-blinded RCTs with a total of 69 participants from both studies into the meta-analysis. The outcome was recovery of facial nerve palsy at 12 months. One study evaluated surgery with steroids versus surgery without and demonstrated similar rates of recovery at 9 months. The second study compared surgery versus no treatment and found no differences in recovery at 1 year. The authors concluded both studies were underpowered to detect a difference, and thus there is limited evidence to decide if surgical decompression is safe or harmful in Bell's palsy.

The American Academy of Otolaryngology published clinical guidelines for the management of Bell's palsy and provides no recommendation because of the paucity of literature and potential risks of surgery.[2]

What is the risk of misdiagnosing a central etiology as a Bell palsy and vice versa?

Because Bell's palsy is a clinical diagnosis with typically no role for invasive testing or imaging, there may be a concern for missing a more dangerous or life-threating diagnosis such as a stroke, subarachnoid hemorrhage, or other life-threatening condition on initial evaluation (**Table 8.2**).

TABLE 8.2	**Clinical Presentation of Bell's Palsy versus Acute Stroke**	
	Bell's Palsy	**Acute Stroke**
Age, years	30-50	Usually >60
Symptom time	Progressive; over	Sudden; over
Course	Hours or days	Seconds
Unilateral facial paralysis	Yes	Yes
Upper face	Always affected	Usually not affected
Lower face	Always affected	Affected
Ability to close eye on symptomatic side	Not likely	Likely
Ear or temporomandibular joint area pain	Likely	Not likely
Hyperacusis	Likely	Not likely
Decreased lacrimation, salivation or change in taste	Likely	Not likely
Pupils affected	Not likely	Sometimes
Arm or leg weakness	Not likely	Likely
Speech or vision affected	Not likely	Likely

From Induruwa I, Holland N, Gregory R, Khadjooi K. The impact of misdiagnosing Bell's palsy as acute stroke. *Clin Med (Lond)*. 2019;19(6):494-498.

There is a paucity of literature in this area, but a study from 2014 examined 6 years of administrative claims data from California to determine the incidence and risk factors that might lead clinicians in the emergency department (ED) to make an incorrect diagnosis of Bell's palsy.[9] The outcome measure was a change in the index diagnosis of Bell's palsy in the ED to a more serious International Classification of Diseases Ninth Revision (*ICD-9*) discharge or inpatient diagnosis code that included ischemic stroke, intracranial hemorrhage, brain tumor, or other, seen within 90 days of the initial visit. The study identified 365 patients who received one of the alternative diagnoses (0.8%) within 90 days; and when the authors limited this to life-threatening diagnoses, they found a total of 127 patients (0.3%). Patients who were assigned a more serious diagnosis were more likely to have more number of comorbidities, and underwent imaging on initial presentation. Ischemic stroke was the most commonly assigned serious diagnosis, representing 27.5% of the patients, with otitis media or mastoiditis representing 24% and herpes zoster 23.2%. The study was limited because it did not examine granular-level chart data and did not link outpatient visits where another diagnosis could have been assigned. The authors concluded that there is a low rate of misdiagnosis of Bell's palsy, but emergency clinicians should pay close attention to elderly patients with diabetes.

GUILLAIN-BARRÉ
THE CLINICAL CHALLENGE

GBS is an acute demyelinating polyneuropathy and the most common cause of flaccid paralysis worldwide. It is an autoimmune disorder of variable presentation that is typically triggered by an antecedent acute respiratory or gastrointestinal infection manifesting in symmetrical, ascending weakness, paralysis, and loss or decreased deep tendon reflexes (DTRs) and cranial nerve involvement, although the presentation does not always conform to these findings. There is an increasing incidence with age and a predilection for males.[10]

Although the severity of the disease is highly variable from mild weakness to complete respiratory failure, GBS should be treated as a true emergent condition because mortality from respiratory complications and autonomic dysfunction ranges from 3% to 7%. Weakness of diaphragmatic musculature can lead to respiratory compromise, which can affect up to 30% of patients.[11]

The clinical challenge for the practitioner in a patient with suspected GBS is anticipating which patients will progress to respiratory failure and need mechanical ventilation (MV) and those who can be closely monitored. Those who do require MV are at an increased risk for complications including hospital-acquired pneumonia and sepsis, the most common causes of death among patients with GBS. Adding further complexity is the potential for autonomic instability leading to cardiac arrhythmias and erratic blood pressures. Because of variants in the disease that deviate from the pure sensorimotor form, the clinician may miss the initial presentation leading to an early opportunity to protect the airway and provide definitive treatment.

GBS is primarily a clinical diagnosis, and there are no readily available assays or biomarkers to confirm the diagnosis in the acute care setting. Owing to the inherent complexity and challenges with GBS, many patients will require intensive monitoring to ensure adequate ventilatory and hemodynamic support.

PATHOPHYSIOLOGY

The pathogenesis of GBS is thought to occur through a mechanism of molecular mimicry between the epitopes of viral or bacterial proteins and peripheral nerves, resulting in an aberrant autoimmune response. This autoimmune response is targeted toward gangliosides in plasma membranes of the peripheral nerves, specifically the axonal or myelin structures, and produce the symptomatology associated with the several known subtypes of GBS.

Patients will report a respiratory or gastrointestinal illness up to 4 weeks before onset of symptoms. The autoimmune response targets peripheral nerves and their associated spinal roots, resulting in an ascending limb weakness, sensory deficits, and cranial nerve involvement, but will vary among the subtypes of the disease. *Campylobacter jejuni* is the most commonly reported infection, seen in 25% to 50% of cases.[12] Other bacterial and viral agents have been identified and include Cytomegalovirus, Epstein-Barr virus, measles, *Haemophilus influenzae*, *Mycoplasma pneumoniae*, influenza A virus, hepatitis E, and more recently Zika virus. GBS can, however, present in a more insidious way, with a subclinical trigger, and without evidence of a prior infection.

GBS is a heterogeneous disorder with several subtypes. The pathogenesis of acute inflammatory demyelinating polyradiculopathy (AIDP), most commonly seen in North America and Europe, represents 90% of cases seen in the United States. It is the result of injury to myelin sheaths and Schwann cells. This is in contrast to the axonal form, acute motor axonal neuropathy (AMAN), which typically has no sensory involvement, and is more commonly seen in China, Japan, and Mexico, and is the result of injury to membranes of nerve axons. Additional subtypes less commonly seen include acute motor sensory axonal neuropathy (AMSAN) and Miller-Fisher syndrome. Miller-Fisher syndrome will present with the triad of ophthalmoplegia, ataxia, and areflexia, but can have overlap with other variants of GBS.

PREHOSPITAL CONCERNS

Because of the potential for acute decompensation and respiratory failure, as well as autonomic instability, providers in the prehospital environment should be prepared for potential intubation and hemodynamic support. If long transport times from a hospital to a tertiary care center are anticipated, early and elective intubation may be necessary. Patients may fatigue quickly, are at high risk for aspiration, and may not demonstrate overt signs such as tachypnea or retractions on initial presentation as seen in other emergent conditions. These patients will require close monitoring, including waveform capnography, and IV access in anticipation of this potential for rapid decompensation, and emergent intubation.

APPROACH TO THE PATIENT WITH GBS

Any patient presenting to the ED with acute or rapid development of an ascending, symmetrical, bilateral extremity sensory loss progressing to weakness, typically starting in the lower limbs, should be evaluated for GBS. **Table 8.3** presents the differential diagnosis. Because of the potential for rapid progression to respiratory failure, this is an emergent condition that must be quickly recognized. There is often, but not always, a history of a preceding gastrointestinal or respiratory illness 4 weeks within onset of symptoms.

The sensorimotor form of GBS, or AIDP, more commonly seen in North America, presents with pain, paresthesias, and distal sensory loss, progressing to weakness in the lower extremities, with hyporeflexia or areflexia, then upper extremities, and then with cranial nerve involvement in some cases. Weakness of facial muscles and muscles of the oropharynx can affect respiratory effort and speech, and can be seen as the initial presentation. Although the presentation is variable and can progress rapidly, the disease reaches its peak at 2 weeks from onset of symptoms. GBS can additionally affect the autonomic nervous system, leading to heart and blood pressure instability in the form of tachycardia, bradycardias, and orthostatic hypotension. Labile blood pressures and tachycardia can mislead the clinician to suspect an occult infection or early sepsis. Bowel and bladder dysfunction can also be present, but is less common.

Clinicians should be alert to the variants of GBS and aware of atypical presentations. Although symptoms will be bilateral, there can be asymmetrical presentations, initially normal reflexes, and findings in the upper and lower limbs simultaneously. Early in the disease course, there may also be complaints of musculoskeletal pain, paresthesias, radicular symptoms, or ataxia, further confounding the diagnosis. The differential diagnosis can include other disease states such as Lyme, botulism, transverse myelitis, Lambert-Eaton syndrome, and myasthenia gravis, but these can often be ruled out by clinical examination, neuroimaging, and laboratory testing.

GBS is a clinical diagnosis that is supported by the cerebrospinal fluid (CSF) findings on lumbar puncture (LP). Although nerve conduction studies (NCS) and EMG will aid in confirmation of the diagnosis and may help elucidate possible variants or mimics, these tests are unlikely to be available in the ED and may also be normal in the first week of the disease. If performed, NCS in the AIDP variant would demonstrate prolonged distal motor latency and reduced nerve conduction velocity.

TABLE 8.3	Differential Diagnosis of Rapidly Progressive Limb Weakness[a]

Central Nervous System

Encephalitis, acute disseminated encephalomyelitis, transverse myelitis, brainstem or myelum compression, leptomeningeal malignancy

Motor Neurons

Poliomyelitis, West Nile virus anterior myelitis, amyotrophic lateral sclerosis, progressive spinal muscular atrophy

Plexus

Neuralgic amyotrophia, diabetes mellitus

Nerve Roots

Guillain-Barré syndrome, acute-onset chronic inflammatory demyelinating neuropathy, Lyme disease, cytomegalovirus-related radiculitis, HIV-related radiculitis, leptomeningeal malignancy

Peripheral Nerves

Guillain-Barré syndrome, acute-onset chronic inflammatory demyelinating neuropathy, iatrogenic, toxic, critical illness myopathy-neuropathy, vasculitis, diphtheria, porphyria, thiamine deficiency, Lyme disease, metabolic or electrolyte disorders (hypokalemia, phosphatemia or magnesemia, hypoglycemia)

Neuromuscular Junction

Myasthenia gravis, botulism, intoxication

Muscles

Critical illness myopathy-neuropathy, mitochondrial disease, acute rhabdomyolysis, polymyositis, dermatomyositis

[a]With or without respiratory failure.
From Willison HJ, Jacobs BC, van Doorn PA. Guillain-Barré syndrome. *Lancet.* 2016;388(10045):717-727.

LP should be performed to not only confirm the diagnosis but also to evaluate for other potential etiologies, such as neoplasm or infection.[13] Analysis of the CSF from LP will demonstrate elevated protein and a mild pleocytosis, known as "albuminocytologic dissociation," often described as a classic finding in GBS. However, early on in the course of the disease, often in the first 1 to 2 weeks, CSF findings can be normal; thus, a normal CSF finding does not eliminate the diagnosis. Other ancillary tests such as neuroimaging with MRI or antibody testing can be performed, but will be of limited utility in making a rapid diagnosis in the acute care setting.

MANAGEMENT

Patients with suspected GBS should be carefully evaluated to determine the potential for respiratory decompensation and risk stratification to determine the optimal level of care within the hospital setting. Nearly 25% of patients may require MV within the first week, although this may not be apparent on initial presentation and evaluation. Patients with facial or bulbar weakness on examination and rapid progression of weakness are more likely to require intubation.[14] Careful bedside evaluation of vital signs and respiratory status should be performed early because delayed intubation can result in aspiration and other complications. An arterial blood gas (ABG) should be obtained in patients with paradoxic respirations. Respiratory function testing will help elucidate which patients may need intubation and MV, versus those who can be closely observed in an intensive care setting.

The three main modalities—forced vital capacity (FVC), maximal inspiratory pressure (MIP; also referred to as negative inspiratory force [NIF]), and maximal expiratory pressure (MEP)—provide a quantitative assessment of respiratory status at the bedside. An FVC of less than 20 mL/kg predicts the need for intubation, a drop in MIP to -30 cm H_2O, and a MEP decrease to 40 cm

H_2O likely warrant intubation. A validated risk stratification score, the Erasmus GBS Respiratory Insufficiency Score (EGRIS) uses these three parameters and calculates the probability of MV in the first week at hospital admission; however, it may not be useful in the ED when evaluating the need for emergent intubation. ABGs trending increases in Pco_2 are also helpful in assessing the potential for respiratory compromise, although they should be interpreted in conjunction with the overall clinical presentation.

Plasma exchange (PE) and intravenous immunoglobulin (IVIG) are the mainstays of treatment for GBS. IVIG is given at a dose of 0.4 g/kg/d for 5 days in conjunction with expert consultation. Although there are no randomized placebo-controlled trials evaluating IVIG in GBS, evidence has demonstrated improved recovery from GBS, when compared to supportive care alone.[15] PE may not be as readily available as IVIG, but there are data to support its usage. A recent systematic review found that there was a shortened time to ambulate, improved disability scores, and decreased MV time when compared to supportive care.[16]

TIPS AND PEARLS

- GBS is a complex autoimmune disorder of variable presentation from mild weakness to complete respiratory failure, with 25% of patients requiring MV in the first week.
- AIDP is the most common subtype found in North America, and represents up to 90% of cases.
- Patients will typically present with an antecedent respiratory or gastrointestinal illness, with *Campylobacter jejuni* being the most commonly reported infection.
- The diagnosis is clinical, but supported by findings on CSF of elevated protein and a mild pleocytosis; however, the CSF findings can be normal in the first week of the disease.
- All patients with suspected GBS should undergo pulmonary function testing to provide quantitative assessment of respiratory status and determine the need for intubation and level of care within the hospital.
- IVIg and PE are the cornerstones of treatment. There is no role for corticosteroids in the treatment of GBS.
- Pain may be a feature of both GBS and Bell palsy.

EVIDENCE

Is there a role for corticosteroids in the management of GBS?

Because of the underlying pathophysiology and inflammatory nature of GBS, corticosteroids might intuitively seem like a potentially efficacious treatment option or adjunct to the current standard of IVIG or PE. A meta-analysis from 2016 reviewed the current literature on corticosteroids, examining their role in shortening recovery times and morbidity in GBS.[17] The studies included trials of both oral and intravenous (IV) steroids, and because of this, there was significant heterogeneity among the studies. To address the primary outcome measure, for example, mean improvement in disability grade after randomization at 4 weeks, the authors incorporated six of the eight studies for a total of 587 participants. The overall trend was no significant difference, but with several caveats: Four of the trials utilized oral steroids and two utilized IV. Among the oral steroid group, there was less improvement in the treatment groups than that in the controls. In the IV groups, there was a nonsignificant trend toward benefit in the treatment groups, although in one of the trials IVIg was not utilized, which does not reflect the current standard of care. The overall conclusions of the authors were, based on moderate quality of evidence, that corticosteroids do not increase recovery time or improve long-term outcomes, and that oral steroids, based on lower quality studies, may delay recovery and the combination of IV steroids and IVIg might hasten recovery.

What are the predictors for MV in patients with GBS?

Beyond the clinical examination and pulmonary function testing, it is challenging to predict which patients will decompensate and need MV. Several older studies examined this question in detail: One study from France looked at the primary outcome of the need for MV on the basis of baseline labs and clinical characteristics of a multicenter RCT utilizing a total of 722 patients.[18] This study found that from onset time to admission of less than 7 days, inability to lift elbows above the bed, inability to stand or lift the head, ineffective coughing, and elevated liver enzymes were predictive of the need for MV. Those patients with available vital capacity (VC) data, time from GBS onset to admission of less than 7 days, inability to lift the head, and a VC of less than 60% were independent predictors of the need for MV. The study did not examine elapsed time to MV.

A recent 2018 Australian systematic review examined the clinical and electrophysiologic predictors for MV in patients with GBS and included at total of 34 studies for final review.[19] There was significant heterogeneity among the studies. The authors found among 13 studies that underwent multivariable analysis, two independent variables were consistently found to be predictors for MV: short time from onset of symptoms and bulbar weakness. Neck weakness was also a predictor for MV among three of six studies. Interestingly, facial nerve involvement and autonomic dysfunction were not found predictive. The authors also examined the EGRIS tool and found it to have good predictive ability to help identify patients early on who will need MV. The NSB score (**N**eck weakness, **S**ingle breath count, and **B**ulbar weakness) is a weighted score and was found to have good discriminatory ability with a sensitivity of 100% and a specificity of 83.3% for predicting MV.

THE PERIPHERAL NEUROPATHIES
THE CLINICAL CHALLENGE

Peripheral neuropathy is a broad term encompassing a heterogeneous group of nervous system disorders. Among these, the subgroup of the DSPNs is the most common, with diabetes the leading cause. It has a high prevalence among patients with diabetes, human immunodeficiency virus (HIV), alcohol abuse, dysproteinemias, chronic kidney disease, and those undergoing treatment with chemotherapeutic agents; see **Table 8.4**. Even after a full evaluation, one quarter of cases will be classified as idiopathic.

Patients with DSPN present with paresthesia and or pain, typically distal and symmetrical, often described as "burning," starting in the lower extremities at the feet and toes and moving more proximally. The pattern and distribution are described classically as "stocking-glove." Loss of DTR, weakness, and motor changes are later findings. The presentation of DSPN can be inconsistent, and atypical presentations with more proximal symptoms and motor involvement can occur. Life-threatening central nervous system (CNS) conditions can mimic some of the symptoms found in DSPN, and the presentation can be further complicated in those patients with multiple comorbidities and use of polypharmacy.

Patients with DSPN are at high risk for falls, fractures, and lower extremity ulcers. Although occurring more insidiously, diabetics are at high risk for ulcers of the lower extremities, occurring in up to 10% of this population. The more common etiologies for a polyneuropathy include alcohol abuse, B_{12} deficiency, HIV, toxic and metabolic causes, chemotherapeutic agents, amyloidosis, and autoimmune disorders.

PATHOPHYSIOLOGY

Diabetic DSPN is the most well-studied model. At a global level, its pathophysiology involves damage to neurons, and occurs through hyperglycemia and hyperlipidemia in the setting of underlying metabolic derangements and poor glucose control. Many diabetics, despite rigorous glucose control, still develop neuropathy, suggesting that other pathophysiologic mechanisms are involved. The disease affects the myelinated and unmyelinated axons, targeting the long axons innervating the distal extremities first. Microvascular changes and decreases in perfusion to peripheral nerves contribute to further exacerbation of the disease. At the cellular level, excess lipids and glucose target receptors on neurons and endothelial cells, leading to disruption

TABLE 8.4	Common Etiologies of Distal Symmetric Polyneuropathy

Autoimmune
  Connective tissue disease
  Vasculitis
  Inflammatory bowel disease
  Sarcoidosis
  Celiac disease
Cancer Associated
  Paraprotein associated
    Monoclonal gammopathy of unknown
      significance
    Multiple myeloma
    Waldenstrom macroglobulinemia
    Lymphoma
  Primary amyloidosis
  Paraneoplastic
Endocrine/Metabolic
  Diabetes mellitus
  Prediabetes
  Hypothyroidism/hyperthyroidism
  Chronic renal failure
  Liver disease
Infectious
  Human immunodeficiency virus
  Human T-cell leukemia virus type 1
  Leprosy
Inherited
  Charcot-Marie-Tooth disease
  Familial amyloidosis
Nutritional
  Vitamin B12 deficiency
  Vitamin B1 deficiency
  Vitamin B6 deficiency or toxicity
  Vitamin E deficiency
  Copper deficiency
  Postgastric bypass

Toxic
  Ethanol
  Heavy metals
  Organic solvents
Medications
  Chemotherapy
    Ado-trastuzumab emtansine
    Brentuximab vedotin
    Eribulin
    Etoposide
    Ifosfamide
    Platinums
    Proteasome inhibitors (eg, bortezomib)
    Taxanes
    Thalidomide, lenalidomide, pomalidomide
    Vincristine
  Amiodarone
  Chloroquine
  Colchicine
  Disulfiram
  Ethambutol
  Hydralazine
  Isoniazid
  Leflunomide
  Metronidazole
  Nitronidazole
  Nucleoside reverse transcriptase inhibitors
  Phenytoin

From Doughty CT, Seyedsadjadi R. Approach to peripheral neuropathy for the primary care clinician. *Am J Med*. 2018;131(9):1010-1016.

of mitochondrial pathways with increased oxidative stress and neuronal injury. The pathophysiology of the neuropathic pain in painful diabetic neuropathy is thought to occur through both central and peripherally mediated pathways. Among the peripheral mechanisms, this includes changes in sodium channel distribution and expression, altered neuropeptide expression, loss of spinal inhibitory control, altered peripheral blood flow, and axonal atrophy, degeneration, and regeneration. Some central mechanisms include increased central sensitization and increased thalamic vascularity.

The pathophysiology of alcohol-induced polyneuropathy is associated with the quantity of alcohol and duration of abuse, and occurs through both direct and indirect pathways. This includes the direct toxic effects of ethanol and its metabolites on neurons, as well as the associated indirect effects on nutritional status and absorption of nutrients and vitamins. In chronic alcoholics, poor absorption and depletion of thiamine stores and B vitamins, as well as insufficient intake of micronutrients are major contributors. Ethanol and its toxic metabolites, especially acetaldehyde, further affect the metabolism at the neuronal level, interfering with metabolic pathways and leading to degeneration. The end result is injury to axons and demyelination of the motor and sensory fibers and the pathologic features of the disease.

PREHOSPITAL CONCERNS

In the prehospital environment, providers are likely to encounter patients with complaints related to peripheral neuropathy and may be required to manage pain, assist with ambulation or unsteady gait, and help manage fractures or infected ulcers in patients with chronic disease. Neuropathic pain will be challenging to treat, and caution should be exercised with the use of available prehospital medications because many patients will have underlying renal insufficiency, comorbidities, and potential for drug-drug interactions. The use of opioids to treat neuropathic pain in peripheral neuropathy is not recommended by current guidelines. Peripheral neuropathy can also mimic CNS conditions and there is potential for missed opportunities if patients are not evaluated and treated appropriately in the field.

APPROACH TO THE PATIENT WITH PERIPHERAL NEUROPATHY

The presentation in patients with signs of DSPN will certainly be variable and etiology dependent, but the findings will generally follow a pattern of distal lower extremity sensory changes, typically starting in the feet, symmetrical, and occurring in a "stocking-glove" distribution. Both small and large fibers are affected in the majority of cases, leading to changes in pain and temperature sensation as well as vibration and proprioception.

Symptoms are categorized as either negative or positive. Negative symptoms include a loss of sensation and positive symptoms include "burning" or "tingling" and will occur before the onset of motor weakness. The symptoms progress from distal to proximal, starting in the toes and feet; uncommonly the upper limbs are affected early on in the disease process. Because sensory changes occur and reach the level of the knees, the fingertips will start to be affected. Although a later feature, patients may present with concomitant autonomic symptoms such as impotence, orthostatic hypotension, early satiety, and gastroparesis. With disease progression, weakness, loss of DTRs, and changes in proprioception will start to occur, along with autonomic symptoms. Among the red flags that should prompt an alternative diagnosis and may require more complex evaluation are rapid onset of symptoms, an asymmetrical distribution, pure motor symptoms, bowel or bladder dysfunction, and low back pain with radicular signs.

The diagnostic approach includes a detailed history, neurologic examination, and, depending on suspected etiology, ancillary laboratory testing. Laboratory testing should be judicious and tailored depending on the suspected cause. The last update of the AAN Guidelines for evaluation of DSPN found the highest yield tests include blood glucose, serum B_{12}, and serum protein immunofixation electrophoresis.[20] An initial screening should also include a complete blood count (CBC), a comprehensive metabolic panel, a thyroid-stimulating hormone (TSH), and a hemoglobin A_{1c} (HbA_{1c}), and or an oral glucose tolerance test if available. Electrodiagnostic tests such as EMG and nerve conduction studies can help confirm the diagnosis and be helpful in equivocal or unclear cases, but will likely not be available in the ED for timely diagnosis.

HIV-associated DSPN is the most prevalent sensory neuropathy among patients diagnosed with HIV, affecting up to 57% of patients. The signs and symptoms and distribution of sensory changes follow a pattern similar to that of other etiologies. However, there is a higher prevalence of patients with HIV who have asymptomatic DSPN, and patients are at increased risk if recently treated, or actively being treated, for tuberculosis.

MANAGEMENT

For diabetic DSPN, tight glycemic control is the most important aspect of disease management. Patients with risk factors for DSPN include elevated HbA_{1c}, duration time of disease, smoking status, and cholesterol. Lowering the HbA_{1c} changes the prevalence of DSPN.

Several studies have demonstrated that intensive glucose control is effective in reducing the incidence of DSPN among type 1 diabetics and less efficacious among type 2 diabetics. Because of the potential for the development of lower extremity ulcers and fractures and increased risk of falls, patients will need close follow-up and long-term management that will extend beyond the acute care setting.

For neuropathic pain, however, tight glycemic control does not improve symptoms. Pharmacologic approaches focus on symptomatic treatment and generally do not address the underlying pathophysiologic mechanisms. Patients may have preexisting comorbidities or renal disease, further limiting the options for treatment. Guidelines and society recommendations regarding treatment of neuropathic pain are based on weak evidence and consensus. Many of the recommend medications require careful titration and consideration given to interactions with other medications.

Among the options for treatment of neuropathic pain in diabetes, pregabalin, duloxetine, and tapentadol are all approved by the U.S. Food and Drug Administration (FDA), with duloxetine and pregabalin preferred on the basis of available evidence and supported by a 2017 position statement by the American Diabetes Association (ADA) for the treatment of diabetic neuropathy.[21] The authors provide a Level A recommendation for the use of pregabalin or duloxetine as the initial drug for treatment of neuropathic pain. Pregabalin, starting at low doses such as 25 to 75 mg/d one to three times a day, should be carefully titrated upward over several days with close outpatient follow-up to reach the therapeutic range of 300 to 600 mg/d. Gabapentin, a drug with a mechanism of action similar to that of pregabalin, can be started at 100 to 300 mg/d one to three times a day. Gabapentin requires even more careful titration and is effective at doses from 1800 to 3600 mg—it has a Level B recommendation from the ADA. Pregabalin has an advantage over gabapentin, in that it has a more rapid onset of action and a linear dose-response profile. Both pregabalin and gabapentin are renally cleared. Caution should be exercised in elderly patients because of potential side effects including headache, dry mouth, somnolence, and dizziness.

Duloxetine is a selective norepinephrine and serotonin norepinephrine reuptake inhibitor (SNRI) that is effective at doses of 60 and 120 mg/d. The most common side effect is nausea, and also requires careful titration and monitoring for adverse drug events in the elderly population. Tapentadol extended release is a centrally acting opioid analgesic that is approved for use at a dose of 100 to 250 mg daily. Tramadol is a centrally acting, weak opioid analgesic, but given increased risk and potential for addiction, both tapentadol and tramadol are not recommended as a first-line treatment for diabetic DSPN.

Other classes of medications such as the monoamine reuptake inhibitors (MAOs) and tricyclic antidepressants (TCAs) have been supported by data from several randomized placebo-controlled trials for the treatment of diabetic DSPN, but are not FDA approved, are not considered first line, and have higher risk side effect profiles. Other nonsystemic options to treat localized symptoms include capsaicin creams and patches and lidocaine patches. Lidocaine (5%) patches have been evaluated as a treatment option and can be applied up to four times a day. Capsaicin cream (0.025%-0.075%) and high-concentration capsaicin patches (8%) are options, with the AAN giving lidocaine patches a Level C recommendation for diabetic neuropathy.

The treatment of HIV-associated DSPN is even more challenging for the clinician in that clinical trials for neuropathic pain have not demonstrated superiority to placebo. First-line agents that have shown efficacy for diabetic neuropathy have not demonstrated the same result among patients with HIV neuropathy. Several studies have shown the potential for the use of amitriptyline, gabapentin, and pregabalin, but these are not considered of high quality and there is weak evidence to support their use.

The treatment of alcoholic DSPN focuses on cessation and abstinence as well as dietary and nutritional supplementation. Several classes of these medications including amitriptyline and gabapentin can be tried, but evidence supporting them is lacking.

TIPS AND PEARLS

- Diabetic DSPN is the most common peripheral neuropathy, affecting up to 50% of patients with diabetes.
- Patients with peripheral neuropathy are at high risk for falls, fractures, and lower extremity ulcers, and will require careful outpatient follow-up for management.
- AAN guidelines report that the highest yield tests include blood glucose, serum B_{12}, and serum protein immunofixation electrophoresis.

- The approach to the patient with peripheral neuropathy will be etiology dependent, but the initial workup should include a CBC, comprehensive metabolic panel, HbA_{1c}, and TSH.
- Tight glycemic control is the mainstay of treatment for diabetic DSPN.
- Pregabalin and duloxetine are considered first-line treatment for diabetic DSPN (Level A) as well as gabapentin (Level B) with MAOs and TCAs as other available options.
- Trials of medications for neuropathic pain in HIV have not yielded options that are superior to placebo, limiting options for this patient population.

EVIDENCE

What is the current evidence for the treatment of diabetic and HIV peripheral neuropathy with pregabalin?

A Cochrane review from 2019 examined the evidence to support the use of pregabalin for neuropathic pain in adults.[22] The authors studied the use pregabalin in several specific disease states including painful diabetic neuropathy and HIV neuropathy. Because many studies can utilize a mixed population of varying types of neuropathic pain, the authors only utilized studies where 80% of the population shared the same condition.

For diabetic neuropathy, the authors included 20 studies with 5943 participants: 15 of the 20 studies utilized placebo for evaluation and the others compared medications such as TCAs SNRIs, and several other classes of medications. The pregabalin dose range was wide, from 75 to 600 mg, given at two to three times daily, but several of the studies utilized a more flexible dosing regimen. Patients were reported to have moderate pain of at least 3 months' duration.

For HIV neuropathy, two double-blind, placebo-controlled studies with 639 participants were used in the analysis. The pregabalin was dosed at 600 mg daily divided doses that were flexible and then titrated to a fixed dose for 14 weeks. The primary outcome measure included a 50% or greater reduction in pain.

With moderate quality of evidence, the authors found that daily oral doses of pregabalin at 300 to 600 mg provided good pain relief for patients with pain in diabetic neuropathy. On the basis of a moderate quality of evidence, pregabalin was not effective for HIV neuropathy at 600 mg when compared to placebo.

References

1. Masterson L, Vallis M, Quinlivan R, Prinsley P. Assessment and management of facial nerve palsy. *BMJ*. 2015;351:h3725.

2. Baugh RF, Basura GJ, Ishii LE, et al. Clinical practice guideline: Bell's palsy. *Otolaryngol Head Neck Surg*. 2013;149(3 suppl):S1-S27.

3. Axelsson S, Berg T, Jonsson L, et al., Prednisolone in Bell's palsy related to treatment start and age. *Otol Neurotol*. 2011;32(1):141-146.

4. McAllister K, Walker D, Donnan PT, Swan I. Surgical interventions for the early management of Bell's palsy. *Cochrane Database Syst Rev*. 2013;(10):CD007468.

5. Patel DK, Levin KH. Bell palsy: clinical examination and management. *Cleve Clin J Med*. 2015;82(7):419-426.

6. Gronseth GS, Paduga R, American Academy of Neurology. Evidence-based guideline update: steroids and antivirals for Bell palsy: report of the Guideline Development Subcommittee of the American Academy of Neurology. *Neurology*. 2012;79(22):2209-2213.

7. de Almeida JR, Guyatt GH, Sud S, et al., Management of Bell palsy: clinical practice guideline. *CMAJ*. 2014;186(12):917-922.

8. Gagyor I, Madhok VB, Daly F, et al. Antiviral treatment for Bell's palsy (idiopathic facial paralysis). *Cochrane Database Syst Rev*. 2015;(11):CD001869.

9. Fahimi J, Navi BB, Kamel H. Potential misdiagnoses of Bell's palsy in the emergency department. *Ann Emerg Med*. 2014;63(4):428-434.

10. Sejvar JJ, Baughman AL, Wise M, Morgan OW. Population incidence of Guillain-Barré syndrome: a systematic review and meta-analysis. *Neuroepidemiology*. 2011;36(2):123-133.

11. Willison HJ, Jacobs BC, van Doorn PA. Guillain-Barré syndrome. *Lancet*. 2016;388(10045):717-727.

12. Esposito S, Longo MR. Guillain-Barré syndrome. *Autoimmun Rev*. 2017;16(1):96-101.

13. Bourque PR, Brooks J, Warman-Chardon J, Breiner A. Cerebrospinal fluid total protein in Guillain-Barré syndrome variants: correlations with clinical category, severity, and electrophysiology. *J Neurol*. 2020;267(3):746-751.

14. Walgaard C, Lingsma HF, Ruts L, et al. Prediction of respiratory insufficiency in Guillain-Barré syndrome. *Ann Neurol*. 2010;67(6):781-787.

15. Hughes RA, Swan AV, van Doorn PA. Intravenous immunoglobulin for Guillain-Barré syndrome. *Cochrane Database Syst Rev*. 2014;(9):CD002063.

16. Chevret S, Hughes RA, Annane D. Plasma exchange for Guillain-Barré syndrome. *Cochrane Database Syst Rev*. 2017;(2):CD001798.

17. Hughes RA, Brassington R, Gunn AA, van Doorn PA. Corticosteroids for Guillain-Barré syndrome. *Cochrane Database Syst Rev*. 2016;(10):CD001446.

18. Sharshar T, Chevret S, Bourdain F, Raphaël JC; French Cooperative Group on Plasma Exchange in Guillain-Barré Syndrome. Early predictors of mechanical ventilation in Guillain-Barré syndrome. *Crit Care Med*. 2003;31(1):278-283.

19. Green C, Baker T, Subramaniam A. Predictors of respiratory failure in patients with Guillain-Barré syndrome: a systematic review and meta-analysis. *Med J Aust*. 2018;208(4):181-188.

20. England JD, Gronseth GS, Franklin G, et al., Practice parameter: the evaluation of distal symmetric polyneuropathy: the role of laboratory and genetic testing (an evidence-based review). Report of the American Academy of Neurology, the American Association of Neuromuscular and Electrodiagnostic Medicine, and the American Academy of Physical Medicine and Rehabilitation. *Neurology*. 2009;72(2):177-184.

21. Pop-Busui R, Boulton AJ, Feldman EL, et al. Diabetic neuropathy: a position statement by the American Diabetes Association. *Diabetes Care*. 2017;40(1):136-154.

22. Derry S, Bell RF, Straube S, Wiffen PJ, Aldington D, Moore RA. Pregabalin for neuropathic pain in adults. *Cochrane Database Syst Rev*, 2019;(1):CD007076.

Acute Presentations in Chronic Neurologic Conditions

Jeremy Rose

THE CLINICAL CHALLENGE

Neurologic conditions are typically diagnosed and managed in the outpatient setting. Many of the diagnostic tests that are staples of neurologic practice are difficult to access or simply not accessible in the emergency department (ED). Although magnetic resonance imaging (MRI) is becoming more available, it is time-consuming, often not appropriate in stable chronic complaints, and unsuitable for an unstable patient. Electroencephalogram (EEG), neuromuscular testing, and much of the autoimmune-focused blood work are generally not available in a timely fashion. Nevertheless, patients with neurologic conditions frequently present to the ED with an exacerbation or progression of their disease; thus, the emergency clinician must be familiar with stabilization strategies. Even if the diagnosis is beyond the purview of the emergency clinician, discovering and documenting neurologic deficits can greatly assist clinicians in the future in establishing symptom chronicity and correlating progress with diagnostic testing and treatments.

INFLAMMATORY CONDITIONS

Multiple Sclerosis (MS)

MS is the most common inflammatory neurologic condition seen in the ED. The current prevalence of MS in the United States is 149 per 100,000 individuals and is 3 times more common in women. Optic neuritis is, by far, the most common initial presentation, occurring in roughly half of patients with MS. That said, optic neuritis can occur in isolation and only half of the patients with optic neuritis will develop MS within 15 years of initial presentation.[1] Painful vision loss, though, tends to be a motivation to seek an emergent evaluation; thus, optic neuritis often brings patients to the ED rather than to an outpatient clinic. MS can also present as isolated motor deficits or vague sensory disturbances; its relapsing-remitting nature can make it hard to diagnose on an initial evaluation.

Advanced MS and its complications frequently present to the ED with problems that are not specifically neurologic. Depending on the degree of involvement and areas of the brain affected, MS-related symptoms can include sensory disturbances, bowel/bladder dysfunction, visual symptoms, muscle spasticity, and pain. Urinary dysfunction and paroxysmal motor weakness tend to present earlier in the disease course, whereas cognitive impairment and sensory alterations tend to be features of advanced disease. Some patients with advanced illness may become partially insensate, placing them at risk for injuries and prone to pressure ulcers.

The criteria for diagnosing MS rely on clinical deficits separated by space and time; however, characteristic white matter lesions on MRI can be highly suggestive of the disease. Although the cause of MS is unknown, it is characterized by inflammatory central nervous system (CNS) lesions that cause nerve demyelination and cell death. This inflammation appears to be the end result of an autoimmune cascade with genetic and environmental triggers.[2] Accordingly, treatment is aimed at reducing this inflammation.

The usual treatment for optic neuritis, regardless of the presence of MS, is intravenous (IV) methylprednisolone 1000 mg/day for 3 days followed by 11 days of oral prednisone.[3] Several randomized controlled trials (RCTs) have compared IV methylprednisolone to high-dose PO prednisone and found that symptoms resolve faster with IV medication, but the ultimate outcome remains unchanged. A 2015 meta-analysis concluded that the role of high-dose steroids in the acute setting is to speed up recovery rather than affect the long-term prognosis.[4] Regarding muscle spasticity and pain, see **Table 9.1** for a list of helpful medications.

TRANSVERSE MYELITIS

Transverse myelitis is a poorly understood condition characterized by acute spinal cord dysfunction below the level of a spinal cord lesion. Given its location and chronicity, transverse myelitis can mimic a compressive spinal cord lesion. Although transverse myelitis is thought to be inflammatory, it is unclear whether the trigger is autoimmune, infectious, or paraneoplastic. More likely, it is a heterogeneous syndrome with multiple possible etiologies.[5] Diagnosis is usually made with MRI, and treatment is aimed at addressing the underlying inflammation, with corticosteroids being the mainstay of acute management.[6]

POST STROKE SYNDROMES

Although stroke in the ED is typically considered in the context of acute presentation, there is an equally concerning chronic component. Brain tissue damaged in a stroke does not heal. Once infarcted, the tissue dies and becomes nonfunctional; even in the absence of revascularization, stroke deficits can improve or completely resolve. The process of overcoming these deficits requires the brain to adjust for the lost function rather than replace it. Neurologic function is transferred to other cells, and this "rewiring" can allow the deficit to improve.

The importance of this rewiring comes in the face of a second, often nonneurologic insult. When faced with another challenge, such as infection or sleep deprivation, the brain can decompensate and allow the stroke deficit to emerge again or worsen. Termed *recrudescence*, the

TABLE 9.1	Common Drugs Used to Treat Spasticity		
Drug	**Class**	**Usual Dose Range**	**Common Side Effects**
Baclofen	GABA-B antagonist	5-10 mg tid	Nausea, confusion, headache, weakness, dizziness
Tizanidine	Central acting α-2 agonist	2 mg qhs	Drowsiness, hypotension, dry mouth
Diazepam	GABA agonist	2 mg bid	Drowsiness
Dantrolene	Inhibition of Ca release in peripheral muscle cells	25 mg daily-tid	Flushing, drowsiness, headache
Methocarbamol	Skeletal muscle relaxant	500 mg qid	Drowsiness

bid, twice a day; Ca, calcium; GABA, gamma-aminobutyric acid; qhs, every night at bedtime; qid, 4 times a day; tid, 3 times a day.

recapitulation of old stroke deficits should prompt the clinician to look beyond stroke. Indeed, it is unlikely that the patient has a new infarct that exactly matches the neuroanatomy compensating for the old deficit. It is more likely that another process, such as occult infection, is causing the patient's brain to re-exhibit the old stroke pattern. Recrudescence must be differentiated from an acute stroke, and treatment should be focused on the acute process rather than anchoring on the neurologic deficit.

In addition to recrudescence, many patients present with complications of stroke-related disability. Weakness can precipitate falls. Swallowing impairment can lead to aspiration. Patients with strokes sometimes present with pain that is thought to be a centrally mediated variant of complex regional pain syndrome (CRPS; see section that follows).[7]

POST SPINAL CORD INJURY

Emergency clinicians are familiar with the acute management of spinal cord trauma. However, many clinicians are less familiar with the chronic complications of the same injuries. Patients with spinal cord injuries face numerous chronic problems associated with the repercussions of spinal cord injury and paralysis. In the weeks and months following spinal cord injury, blood pressure often drops and orthostasis is common. This is likely a result of muscle atrophy and paralysis. These symptoms usually level off as unused muscles become spastic and systemic circulation adjusts.

Coronary artery disease is an often-underappreciated component of spinal cord injury. It may be 3 times higher in patients with spinal cord injury than in the general population.[8] This is likely caused by poor mobility and reduced capacity for aerobic exercise. Accordingly, spinal cord injury should be viewed as an independent risk factor when evaluating a patient with chest pain.

Immobility can become even more pronounced as patients with spinal cord injury become older. Beyond the usual changes associated with aging, such as osteoarthritis, patients with spinal cord injury are far more likely to develop heterotopic bone formation, further limiting joint motion. Some degree of heterotopic ossification is seen in 20% of patients with traumatic brain injury/spinal cord injury.[9] It can exacerbate the direct consequences of paralysis and further disable the patient.

Spinal cord injury above the diaphragm can impair ventilation by weakening the chest wall and accessory muscles. This likely contributes to the development of atelectasis and pneumonia. A long-term study that followed patients up to 20 years post injury found that pneumonia was the third most common complication after pressure ulcers and autonomic dysreflexia.[10] Spasticity with pain is a frequent complication of spinal cord injury. It is likely the consequence of reduced inhibitory neurostimulation. Although the result is often painful muscle contraction, spasticity also helps increase venous return and maintain blood pressure in a paralyzed patient. Table 9.1 provides a list of medications used to treat spasticity and the acute discomfort it causes.

Most patients with spinal cord injury, even those with incomplete injuries, have some degree of bladder impairment. Lesions that are lower in the cord or cauda equina tend to produce bladder flaccidity, and these patients have trouble with voiding. Higher lesions may result in bladder spasms resulting in ongoing discomfort and difficulties with continence. Sphincter dysfunction can also impair bladder emptying. Patients with spinal cord injury may be unable to sense when their bladders are full, and in rare cases, this can produce a profound vagal reaction and hypotension.

The tools used to treat bladder dysfunction carry their own risks. Many patients with spinal cord injury use catheter devices either intermittently to facilitate continence or as chronic indwelling devices for ease of care. As with any introduction of a foreign body into a sterile space, these devices carry a higher risk of infection. Urosepsis should be high on the differential for a post–spinal cord injury patient presenting with shock.

COMPLEX REGIONAL PAIN SYNDROME

CRPS is a disorder that is characterized by chronic localized pain out of proportion to, or in the absence of, an inciting event. CRPS is divided into two main categories: CRPS type 1 encompasses cases without an obvious peripheral nerve injury (roughly 85% of cases) and CRPS type 2 is defined as CRPS with a clear mechanism for peripheral injury such as a crush injury or operation (15% of cases).[11]

The primary manifestation of CRPS is chronic, often extreme pain more commonly found in a patient's upper extremity. Sensory disturbances in a peripheral nerve distribution may also be present. Roughly two-thirds of CRPS patients have functional motor weakness related to pain. Autonomic symptoms, such as skin color changes, skin temperature changes, or sweat production may also be present. The cause of CRPS is unknown. Historically, theories have focused on nerve injury and the potential for a "short circuit" in nerve conduction. This type of explanation seems less probable, given that many CRPS patients have no inciting injury. More recent research has found elevated levels of inflammatory cytokines in CRPS patients, leading to the hypothesis that local release of pain mediating peptides may be the underlying etiology.[12]

Although no curative treatment exists for CRPS, rehabilitation and analgesia are the mainstays of management. In the acute setting, a patient may present with pain out of proportion to any physical findings. There is no diagnostic test for CRPS; thus, acute management is focused on ruling out correctable causes, for example, necrotizing fasciitis, compartment syndrome, and acute limb ischemia, all of which can present with extreme pain in a relatively normal-appearing limb. In a patient with known CRPS, management of acute pain should focus on providing analgesia, encouraging motor function, and ensuring follow-up that provides both physical therapy and chronic pain treatment (see evidence section).

NEUROMUSCULAR DISORDERS

Neuromuscular disorders are covered in more detail in **Chapter 7: Myopathies and Neuromuscular Junction Disorders**; patients with chronic neuromuscular disorders can decompensate and become acutely ill. These exacerbations can be life-threatening when the muscular weakness impairs ventilation.

Myasthenia Gravis (MG)

MG is the most common chronic neuromuscular disorder that may present to the ED. Most importantly, a myasthenic crisis can impair a patient's ventilation. This impairment can be subtle and easy to miss if a clinician is not attuned to the possibility. Because this is fundamentally a problem of ventilation, not oxygenation, pulse oximetry may be normal. An easy bedside test is to simply ask the patient to inhale and then count out loudly using a single breath. The clinician can do this too and observe how long it takes the patient to stop counting and breathe. Tests that measure CO_2, that is, blood gases and CO_2 capnography, are recommended. Additionally, the measurement of forced vital capacity (FVC) or negative inspiratory force (NIF) is relatively easy to do. A NIF of <20 mm H_2O is indicative of a respiratory compromise.[13]

The second component of treating a patient with MG is avoiding therapies that could inadvertently trigger a myasthenic crisis. Commonly used medications such as macrolides, quinolones, and even prednisone have been implicated. Because most of these data come from case reports, it is difficult to ascertain the risk of prescribing for any given patient. Nevertheless, these drugs should be avoided if at all possible. See **Chapter 7: Myopathies and Neuromuscular Junction Disorders** for a discussion on managing a myasthenic crisis.

PARKINSON DISEASE

First described >200 years ago, Parkinson disease remains a common cause of morbidity, especially in the aging population. The cardinal features of Parkinson are tremor, rigidity, and bradykinesia. Many symptoms of Parkinson are caused by the loss of dopamine production in the basal ganglia, although the underlying cause of this change remains unknown. Roughly 40% of patients with Parkinson will develop dementia.[14]

Although rarely the immediate cause of a patient's ED presentation, Parkinson is a frequent comorbidity in ED patients. Movement impairment can lead to falls, and a host of care problems arise when a Parkinson patient develops dementia. Facial muscle rigidity can lead to swallowing impairment, making Parkinson patients especially prone to aspiration. Furthermore, Parkinson patients tend to be elderly, and although they may come to the ED for other reasons, managing their Parkinson disease impacts ED care. Special care should be taken when discharging a patient with Parkinson to ensure that their disease is well managed and that the patient has adequate support.

Monoamine oxidase type B inhibitors are often used for mild disease. Anticholinergic agents can be helpful for tremor. The mainstay of treatment for moderate to advanced disease is levodopa. Levodopa is usually combined with carbidopa to prevent the conversion of the drug to dopamine in the peripheral circulation. Unfortunately, many patients develop dyskinesia and treatment regimens may vary with respect to dosing and timing of the medication. In patients who tend to cycle rapidly from dyskinesia to rigidity, a G-tube can be placed to permit continuous administration of a levodopa compound via pump. Sudden withdrawal from levodopa is ill advised as it can result in a variant of neuroleptic malignant syndrome known as Parkinsonism hyperpyrexia.[15]

The rapid fluctuation of Parkinson symptoms presents the most challenging component of caring for the patient with Parkinson in the ED. Simply put, ***don't miss the meds*** (Table 9.2). Patients rarely receive their home medications while in the ED because most home medications can be safely delayed; levodopa is a notable exception to this practice. Missing even one dose can destabilize a patient or invite a period of rigidity that could have serious implications. Parkinson patients have regimented timing and dosing, especially for levodopa compounds, and the ED care plan should ensure there is no delay in medication administration.

DISORDERS OF ELEVATED INTRACRANIAL PRESSURE

Idiopathic Intracranial Hypertension (Pseudotumor Cerebri)

This disorder, formerly called benign intracranial hypertension, is defined by elevated cerebral pressures in the absence of a tumor or other obstructive lesions. Classically affecting obese, premenopausal female patients, idiopathic intracranial hypertension (IIH) can present in a subacute manner. The most common presenting symptom is headache often with associated nausea and vomiting.[16] Transient visual changes can also accompany the headache, making it difficult to distinguish from chronic migraine. Computed tomography (CT) and MRI are not diagnostic but can show certain characteristic features such as distension of the perioptic subarachnoid space. Papilledema can guide the clinician to making this diagnosis, but the gold standard test remains a lumbar puncture that demonstrates an elevated opening pressure of >200 mm H_2O. Although the presentation can be subacute, immediate intervention is needed in that if left unchecked for several weeks, IIH can result in permanent vision loss.

Weight loss and sodium reduction are effective interventions in obese patients with IIH. The first-line treatment for IIH is acetazolamide—initially 500 mg bid, increased up to 4 g/day. Furosemide (20-40 mg/day) can be added as an adjunct. Many patients continue to experience severe

TABLE 9.2	**Medications Used in the Treatment of Parkinson Disease**		
Class	**Drug**	**Usual Dose Range**	**Common Side Effects**
MAOI	Selegiline	5 mg bid	Headache, dizziness, nausea
MAOI	Rasagiline	1 mg daily	Headache
MAOI	Safinamide	50-100 mg daily	Dyskinesia
Dopamine agonist	Amantadine	129-233 mg daily	Orthostatic hypotension, dizziness, presyncope, hallucinations, delusions, paranoia, constipation
Anticholinergic	Trihexyphenidyl	6-10 mg tid or qid	Tachycardia, agitation
Anticholinergic	Benztropine	0.5-1 mg daily	Tachycardia, confusion
Dopamine agonist	Carbidopa-levodopa	12.5/50 mg bid-tid–200 mg/2 g daily[a]	Orthostatic hypotension, constipation, nausea, depression, dizziness, headache, dyskinesia

[a]Frequency can vary; extended-release formulas also available.
bid, twice a day; MAOI, monoamine oxidase inhibitor; qid, 4 times a day; tid, 3 times a day.

headaches despite medical management. Many of the antiepileptic drugs used for migraine pro-phylaxis may have a role in IIH treatment. Topiramate inhibits carbonic anhydrase and causes weight loss, which may provide an additional benefit. Valproate and tricyclic antidepressants are also used. Steroids are not recommended as a long-term treatment because they can cause weight gain; however, they may be used as a temporizing measure for patients awaiting surgical interven-tion. Surgical management is generally accomplished with a ventriculoperitoneal (VP) or lum-boperitoneal (LP) shunt. Although this tends to stabilize vision loss, headaches often persist. In patients with a known diagnosis, presenting to the ED with ongoing pain, it is best to consider the patient's pain control regimen. Overuse of analgesia can result in rebound headaches and should be discouraged. Ketorolac and acetaminophen are useful first-line treatments in the ED.

NORMAL PRESSURE HYDROCEPHALUS (NPH)

NPH occurs from an excess of cerebrospinal fluid (CSF) in the brain either by increased production or by decreased absorption. Often, the exact cause of hydrocephalus is never identified. In contrast to IIH, LP opening pressures are normal, whereas imaging demonstrates ventriculomegaly. The classic clinical triad of NPH is dementia, gait instability, and urinary incontinence. Definitive treat-ment is accomplished with the placement of a VP shunt.

A VP shunt is a one-way flow device that diverts excess CSF. The most common complication of VP shunting is overdrainage. This usually presents as headaches that may be constant or aggra-vated by position. Other complications include shunt infection; seizures; abdominal complications, such as ascites or peritonitis; and mechanical disruption. If shunt disruption is suspected, a radio-graphic shunt series can be performed to evaluate the shunt along its entire length. A normal CT head does not exclude the possibility of shunt malfunction. If shunt infection is suspected, diagnosis may require tapping the shunt to obtain a sample of the CSF. Complications of this procedure include permanent damage to the shunt and the introduction of infection into the shunt CSF. It is best to coordinate care with neurosurgery.

EVIDENCE

Does the diagnosis of optic neuritis indicate that the patient has MS?

Optic neuritis is one of the most common presenting signs of MS. However, the diagnosis of MS is by no means certain in a patient with optic neuritis (**Figure 9.1**). A 15-year longitudinal study found that only half (50%) of patients with isolated optic neuritis developed MS.[17] Additionally, the visual prognosis of optic neuritis is relatively good with approximately 72% of affected eyes recovering 20/20 vision.[18] The mainstay of treatment is steroids. IV methylprednisolone for 3 days (250 mg

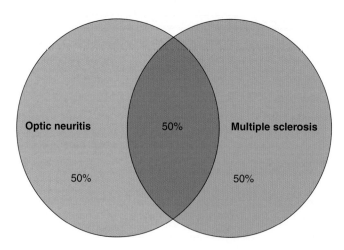

Figure 9.1: Optic neuritis versus multiple sclerosis.

4 times a day [qid]) followed by oral prednisone for 11 days (1 mg/kg with a 4-day taper) was found to achieve earlier symptom resolution than oral prednisone alone. Longer term recovery was similar in both groups.[19]

What is the most accurate bedside test for predicting respiratory compromise in a patient with MG?

Both NIF and FVC can be easily measured at bedside. As the name implies, NIF measures the negative force a patient generates. FVC, on the other hand, measures the **volume** of air expelled during the patient's exhalation (**Figure 9.2**). This volume gives a more accurate picture of the entire respiratory cycle. Respiratory volumes are also routinely considered by emergency clinicians when performing ventilator management, so FVC is a parameter they are more familiar with. This logic has been validated in several studies that show FVC to be at least as good as, if not better than,

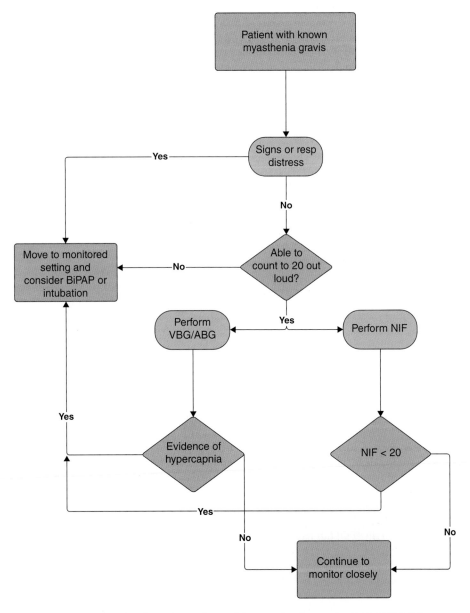

Figure 9.2: Respiratory evaluation of a patient with myasthenia gravis. ABG; NIF; VBG

NIF.[20,21] Predicted FVC decreases with age, but an FVC of <20 mL/kg (roughly 25%-30% of predicted) is indicative of potential respiratory failure.

Does bilevel positive airway pressure (BiPAP) have a role in the management of decompensated neuromuscular disorders?

Intubation is always a clinical decision based on a combination of factors. Many patients with MG, for example, can maintain their airways despite not being able to ventilate adequately. This makes noninvasive forms of ventilation an alternative to intubation in some patients. Noninvasive ventilation is associated with shorter periods of mechanical ventilation.[22] Early use of noninvasive ventilation can potentially stave off hypercarbia and the resulting altered mental status that might jeopardize the patient's airway.

What is the best approach to managing acute pain and spasticity in an ED patient with MS?

Spasticity with pain is a common feature of many neurologic conditions. This can exacerbate disability and the discomfort associated with the underlying neurologic condition. The first-line treatment for chronic spasticity is cyclobenzaprine[23] (starting at 5 mg daily and creasing to 5 mg 3 times a day [tid]) or tizanidine (starting at 2 mg every night at bedtime [qhs] and titrating up to mx 36 mg/day in 3-4 doses). The presumed mechanism of cyclobenzaprine is the inhibition of the reflex arc at the level of the spinal cord by binding at gamma-aminobutyric acid (GABA) receptor sites. With a half-life of 6 hours, oral cyclobenzaprine may take days to become therapeutic. Adverse effects such as nausea and dizziness are common. Tizanidine is an α-2 agonist. The most common side effects are dry mouth and drowsiness because of which it is typically administered qhs and titrated up. Multiple RCTs have found tizanidine and cyclobenzaprine to be equivalent in efficacy when used to treat spasticity. Dantrolene also has been trialed and found effective at relieving spasticity, but it is typically avoided because of its hepatotoxic effects.[24]

In the acute setting, muscle relaxants such as diazepam or methocarbamol can be more effective to address spasticity. Additionally, these medications are readily available in most ED settings and do not have the same adverse effects associated with cyclobenzaprine initiation. That being said, there is a paucity of evidence for these drugs and no high-quality RCTs conducted in an ED setting.

An oral spray cannabinol-based drug (Sativex) has been studied in MS patients with spasticity. RCTs on Sativex have shown spasticity reductions in 30% to 70% of patients when it is used in a prn fashion (mean daily dose < 7 sprays/day). Improvement in other MS symptoms, such as sleep disturbance, was also noted. This benefit appears durable without increasing the dose, and deleterious effects like cognitive impairment were not observed.[25] At present, Sativex is approved in Europe for the treatment of refractory spasticity, but it has not yet received U.S. Food and Drug Administration (FDA) approval in the United States.

What is the best analgesic for acute flares of chronic regional pain syndrome?

Chronic regional pain syndrome can be difficult to manage and acute flares can be especially problematic (**Figure 9.3**). The pathophysiology of CRPS is incompletely understood, but it appears to be a primarily neuropathic phenomenon with vasomotor, sensory, and trophic manifestations. Recent functional MRI studies have raised the possibility of CNS involvement because studies demonstrate reduced activation in cortical areas associated with limbs affected by CRPS.[26] However, this still may be a central reaction to a fundamentally peripheral nervous system disease.

Given the proposed pathophysiologic mechanism, neuropathic drugs like gabapentin have been proposed. To date, there are three RCTs which demonstrate that gabapentin (dose range 900-2400 mg orally [PO] tid) reduces pain in patients with CRPS. An additional RCT has shown that amitriptyline (10 mg qhs) can be as effective as gabapentin in children.[27] Pregabalin may also be effective, but it has only been shown to work in case reports, mostly in a pediatric subgroup. Carbamazepine (600 mg/day) has also been shown to be more effective than placebo and has also proven more effective than long-acting morphine (90 mg/day).[28] Oxcarbazepine may also be effective, but the evidence is limited to a single case report.[29] The evidence supports physical therapy for

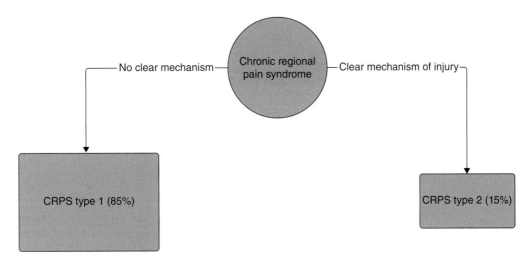

Figure 9.3: Chronic regional pain syndrome.

CRP type 1, and patients do best when adhering to a multimodal treatment regimen that addresses rehabilitation and the psychosocial components of chronic pain.[30]

Despite their efficacy, neuropathic drugs typically take weeks to yield a benefit. In the ED, nonsteroidal anti-inflammatories, such as Ibuprofen (400-800 mg PO) or ketorolac (30 mg intramuscularly [IM]/IV), are good choices for the treatment of acute CRPS pain exacerbations.[31] Topical analgesics, such as topical lidocaine cream, can also be an effective adjunct for acute flares.

There is little evidence for steroids in treating flares of CRPS, and they are not recommended for acute pain. Likewise, opiates lack supporting data for the treatment of acute pain in CRPS, and their use is discouraged. Subdissociative doses of ketamine have been proposed to manage CRPS, but there is insufficient evidence to support its use at present.

References

1. de Seze J. Inflammatory optic neuritis: from multiple sclerosis to neuromyelitis optica. *Neuroophthalmology*. 2013;37(4):141-145.

2. Ghasemi N, Razavi S, Nikzad E. Multiple sclerosis: pathogenesis, symptoms, diagnoses and cell-based therapy. *Cell J*. 2017;19(1):1-10.

3. Wilhelm H, Schabet M. The diagnosis and treatment of optic neuritis. *Dtsch Arztebl Int*. 2015;112(37):616-626.

4. Gal RL, Vedula SS, Beck R. Corticosteroids for treating optic neuritis. *Cochrane Database Syst Rev*. 2015;8(8):CD001430.

5. West TW. Transverse myelitis—a review of the presentation, diagnosis, and initial management. *Discov Med*. 2013;16(88):167-177.

6. Sá MJ. Acute transverse myelitis: a practical reappraisal. *Autoimmun Rev*. 2009;9(2):128-131. doi:10.1016/j.autrev.2009.04.005

7. Treister AK, Hatch MN, Cramer SC, Chang EY. Demystifying poststroke pain: from etiology to treatment. *PM R*. 2017;9(1):63-75.

8. Myers J. Cardiovascular disease in spinal cord injury: an overview of prevalence, risk, evaluation, and management. *Am J Phys Med Rehabil*. 2007;86(2):142-152.

9. Sullivan MP, Torres SJ, Mehta S, Ahn J. Heterotopic ossification after central nervous system trauma: a current review. *Bone Joint Res*. 2013;2(3):51-57.

10. McKinley WO. Long-term medical complications after traumatic spinal cord injury: a regional model systems analysis. *Arch Phy Med Rehabil*. 1999;80(11):1402-1410.

11. Guthmiller KB, Varacallo M. Complex regional pain syndrome (Reflex sympathetic dystrophy, CRPS, RSD) In: StatPearls [Internet]. StatPearls Publishing; 2020. Updated July 19, 2020. https://www.ncbi.nlm.nih.gov/books/NBK430719/

12. Munnikes RJ, Muis C, Boersma M, Heijmans-Antonissen C, Zijlstra FJ, Huygen FJ. Intermediate stage complex regional pain syndrome type 1 is unrelated to proinflammatory cytokines. *Mediators Inflamm*. 2005;2005(6):366-372.

13. Wendell LC, Levine JM. Myasthenic crisis. *Neurohospitalist*. 2011;1(1):16-22.

14. Svenningsson P, Westman E, Ballard C, Aarsland D. Cognitive impairment in patients with Parkinson's disease: diagnosis, biomarkers, and treatment. *Lancet Neurol*. 2012;11(8):697-707. doi:10.1016/S1474-4422(12)70152-7

15. Factor SA. Fatal parkinsonism-hyperpyrexia syndrome in a Parkinson's disease patient while actively treated with deep brain stimulation. *Mov Disord*. 2007;22(1):148-149. doi:10.1002/mds.21172

16. Wall M, Kupersmith MJ, Kieburtz KD, et al. The idiopathic intracranial hypertension treatment trial: clinical profile at baseline. *JAMA Neurol*. 2014;71(6):693-701.

17. Optic Neuritis Study Group. Multiple sclerosis risk after optic neuritis: final optic neuritis treatment trial follow-up. *Arch Neurol*. 2008;65(6):727-732. doi:10.1001/archneur.65.6.727

18. Optic Neuritis Study Group. Visual function 15 years after optic neuritis: a final follow-up report from the Optic Neuritis Treatment Trial. *Ophthalmology*. 2008;115(6):1079-1082.e5.

19. Beck RW, Cleary PA, Anderson MM Jr, et al. A randomized, controlled trial of corticosteroids in the treatment of acute optic neuritis. The Optic Neuritis Study Group. *N Engl J Med*. 1992;326(9):581-588.

20. Prigent H, Orlikowski D, Letilly N, et al. Vital capacity versus maximal inspiratory pressure in patients with Guillain-Barré syndrome and myasthenia gravis. *Neurocrit Care*. 2012;17(2):236-239.

21. Sharshar T, Chevret S, Bourdain F, Raphaël JC; French Cooperative Group on Plasma Exchange in Guillain-Barré Syndrome. Early predictors of mechanical ventilation in Guillain-Barré syndrome. *Crit Care Med*. 2003;31(1):278-283.

22. Seneviratne J, Mandrekar J, Wijdicks EF, Rabinstein AA. Noninvasive ventilation in myasthenic crisis. *Arch Neurol*. 2008;65(1):54-58. doi:10.1001/archneurol.2007.1

23. Ertzgaard P, Campo C, Calabrese A. Efficacy and safety of oral baclofen in the management of spasticity: A rationale for intrathecal baclofen. *J Rehabil Med*. 2017;49(3):193-203. doi:10.2340/16501977-2211

24. Chou R, Peterson K, Helfand M. Comparative efficacy and safety of skeletal muscle relaxants for spasticity and musculoskeletal conditions: a systematic review. *J Pain Symptom Manage*. 2004;28(2):140-175.

25. Pozzilli C. Advances in the management of multiple sclerosis spasticity: experiences from recent studies and everyday clinical practice. *Expert Rev Neurother*. 2013;13(suppl 12):49-54.

26. Palmer G. Complex regional pain syndrome. *Aust Prescr*. 2015;38(3):82-86. doi:10.18773/austprescr.2015.029

27. Brown S, Johnston B, Amaria K, et al. A randomized controlled trial of amitriptyline versus gabapentin for complex regional pain syndrome type I and neuropathic pain in children. *Scand J Pain*. 2016;13:156-163.

28. Harke H, Gretenkort P, Ladleif HU, Rahman S, Harke O. The response of neuropathic pain and pain in complex regional pain syndrome I to carbamazepine and sustained-release morphine in patients pretreated with spinal cord stimulation: a double-blinded randomized study. *Anesth Analg*. 2001;92(2):488-495.

29. Javed S, Abdi S. Use of anticonvulsants and antidepressants for treatment of complex regional pain syndrome: a literature review. *Pain Manag*. 2021;11(2):189-199.

30. Daly AE, Bialocerkowski AE. Does evidence support physiotherapy management of adult Complex Regional Pain Syndrome Type One? A systematic review. *Eur J Pain*. 2009;13(4):339-353.

31. Harden RN, Oaklander AL, Burton AW, et al. Complex regional pain syndrome: practical diagnostic and treatment guidelines, 4th edition. *Pain Med*. 2013;14(2):180-229.

Dizziness and Vertigo

Matthew S. Siket

Jonathan A. Edlow

THE CLINICAL CHALLENGE

Dizziness poses a conundrum for patients and health care providers. First, it is a common and nonspecific symptom accounting for over 4.3 million emergency department (ED) visits annually in the United States.[1] Although the vast majority of patients with dizziness are experiencing a benign process, approximately 15% of patients have a dangerous and potentially life-threatening underlying cause. Differentiating the dangerous from benign causes can be challenging, especially because more than half of all patients in the ED report having experienced the subjective sensation of dizziness within the preceding week.[2]

The term "dizziness" means different things to different people. Classic teaching used the diagnostic paradigm that separates dizziness into "lightheadedness" or "vertigo" or "disequilibrium." The value of this approach has been challenged and is currently being reassessed: In one study, patients were presented with a series of options to describe the "type" of dizziness experienced, and then reasked the same question with the same choices, but in a different sequence 6 minutes later. Concordance was less than 50%.[3] In the real world, not all patients with vestibular dysfunction report vertigo, and not all patients with cardiovascular dysfunction report lightheadedness. Relying on symptom description to guide the differential considerations is a setup for diagnostic error.

As an alternative, patients are much more consistent in reporting the timing and triggers of their symptoms. As part of a history and review of systems, providers should elucidate the context of the symptoms to individualize the differential diagnosis.

- Did the symptoms begin abruptly?
- Has the dizziness been persistent or episodic?
- Were there any precipitating triggers to provoke the dizziness?
- Were there associated symptoms such as focal neurologic deficits, palpitations, shortness of breath, ear pain, or tinnitus?

These are all reasonable questions to ask to gain a better understanding of precisely what the patient experienced and hone in on the underlying cause.

We recommend using the ATTEST mnemonic as a helpful way to systematically approach the chief complaint of dizziness and avoid misdiagnosis.[4,5] ATTEST stands for Associated symptoms, Timing, Triggers, Examination Signs, and Testing (**Figure 10.1**, **Table 10.1**). This approach focuses on key components of the history and examination to distinguish four different vestibular syndromes:

1. Acute spontaneous vestibular syndrome ($A_S VS$)
2. Acute triggered vestibular syndrome ($A_T VS$)
3. Episodic spontaneous vestibular syndrome ($E_S VS$)
4. Episodic triggered vestibular syndrome ($E_T VS$)

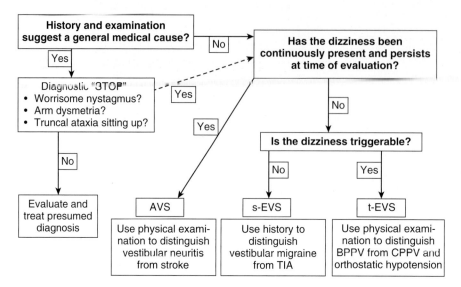

Figure 10.1: Diagnostic approach to the acutely dizzy patient. AVS, acute vestibular syndrome; BPPV, benign paroxysmal positional vertigo; CPPV, central paroxysmal positional vertigo; s-EVS spontaneous episodic vestibular syndrome; t-EVS, triggered episodic vestibular syndrome; TIA, transient ischemic attack.

TABLE 10.1	The ATTEST Mnemonic
Associated symptoms	
Timing	
Triggers	
Exam	
Signs	
Testing	

Each of these distinct vestibular syndromes is discussed in greater detail later in this chapter in **Approach/The Focused Examination** section.

ANATOMY AND PATHOPHYSIOLOGY

The sensation of dizziness typically occurs either after a loss of postural tone causing decreased cerebral perfusion, or dysfunction of the vestibular system. Having a basic knowledge of vestibular neurologic physiology provides a foundation on which a general diagnostic framework can be built.

The peripheral vestibular system includes the labyrinths and hair cells of each inner ear (**Figures 10.2 and 10.3**). Each labyrinth is composed of the cochlea (which controls hearing), the anterior, lateral, and posterior semicircular canals (SCCs) (which sense rotational motion), and the utricle and saccule (which sense linear motion). These structures are connected to one another and filled with endolymph fluid. Hair cells within the utricle and saccule sense movement of endolymph and displace the cupula, which triggers an electrical impulse via the vestibular nerve to the brainstem, causing the sensation of motion. The three paired SCCs, and each utricle and saccule collectively comprise each individual's vestibular apparatus, which is subject to dysregulation through a number of mechanisms (otolithic, inflammatory, infectious, traumatic, etc.). Vestibular apparatus dysfunction is typically unilateral, such as in vestibular neuritis, labyrinthitis, benign paroxysmal positional vertigo (BPPV), Meniere disease, and perilymphatic fistulas, each presented in more detail in **Table 10.2**.

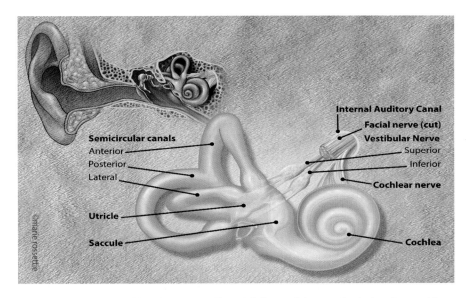

Figure 10.2: The anatomy of the inner ear. The eighth cranial nerve includes the cochlear nerve and the superior and inferior vestibular nerves, and it traverses the internal auditory canal with the facial nerve and labyrinthine artery. The semicircular canals, utricle, and saccule are innervated by the vestibular nerves, whereas the cochlea is supplied by the cochlear nerve. Courtesy of Dr. Jonathan A. Edlow and © Marie Rossettie, CMI.

The central vestibular system originates in the vestibular nuclei of the pons and upper medulla, which receive afferent input from the vestibular apparatus via the vestibular nerves (**Figure 10.4**). They relay connections to the cerebellum, oculomotor system, cerebral cortex, and spinal cord, orchestrating balance via intricate control of trunk and oppositional muscles, eye movements, and position sense. Both ablative (such as stroke) and irritative (such as migraine) phenomena can produce symptoms of central dizziness and vertigo, as outlined in **Table 10.3**.

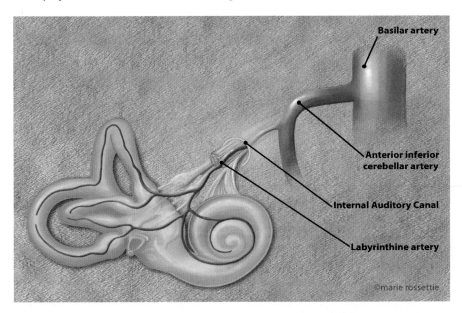

Figure 10.3: Vascular anatomy of the inner ear. The anterior inferior cerebellar artery (AICA) branches from the basilar artery and feeds the labyrinthine artery, which supplies the cochlea and vestibular apparatus. Courtesy of Dr. Jonathan A. Edlow and © Marie Rossettie, CMI.

TABLE 10.2	Partial List of Peripheral Vestibular Disorders	
Condition	Mechanism	Classic Presentation
BPPV	Canalolithiasis caused by oto-lithic debris within the SCCs (85% posterior)	Brief, but intense, episodes of dizziness and vertigo triggered by head turning associated with nausea and vomiting. Upward torsional nystagmus during episodes is pathognomonic
Vestibular neuritis	Unilateral vestibular hypo-function, usually from an inflammatory process of the vestibular nerve afferent signals	Acute-onset and sustained dizziness and vertigo without a trigger. May be postinfec-tious and is associated with horizontal and unidirectional nystagmus with the fast phase beating toward the unaffected ear
Labyrinthitis	Similar to vestibular neuritis, but affecting the cochlear nerve afferents as well	Similar to, but less common than, vestibular neuritis with associated hearing loss
Meniere disease	Overproduction or under-re-sorption of endolymph in the cochlea causing hydrops	Spontaneous episodic dizziness and vertigo, with a sensation of aural fullness as well as hearing loss and tinnitus
Perilymphatic fistula	Leakage of perilymphatic fluid into the middle ear, usually following a trauma	Subacute dizziness and vertigo with hearing loss or sensitivity, and aural fullness typically following head or barotrauma

BBPV, benign paroxysmal positional vertigo; SCC, semicircular canal.
Data from Jahn K. Vertigo and dizziness in children. Handb Clin Neurol. 2016;137:353-363. doi: 10.1016/
B978-0-444-63437-5.00025-X

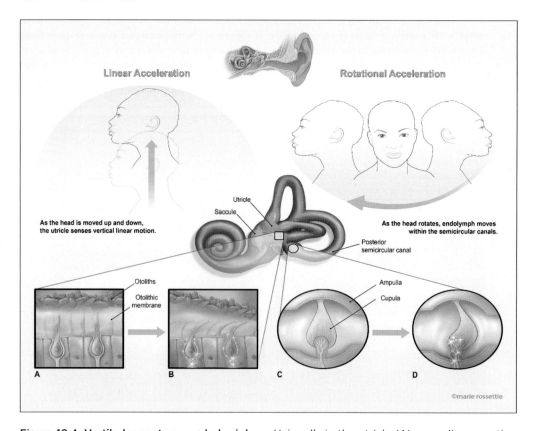

Figure 10.4: **Vestibular anatomy and physiology.** Hair cells in the utricle (A) sense linear motion such as gravitational force (B). The semicircular canals, specifically the cupola in the ampulla (C), sense rotational acceleration, such as being on a merry-go-round (D). Courtesy of Dr. Jonathan A. Edlow and © Marie Rossettie, CMI.

TABLE 10.3	Partial List of Central Vestibular Disorders	
Condition	Mechanism	Classic Presentation
Posterior circulation ischemia	Focal cerebral hypoperfusion from an occlusion (from an embolus or from atherosclerosis) or dissection along the vertebrobasilar circulation	Spontaneous and abrupt-onset dizziness, usually with additional focal neurologic deficits. May be transient (transient ischemic attack)
Vestibular migraine	Excitation along the trigeminovascular pathway	Episodic with or without an associated aura and/or headache

Posterior circulation stroke predominantly affects the cerebellum and brainstem and, although it is an infrequent cause of dizziness, it is among the most commonly misdiagnosed stroke syndromes.[3] Most will have measurable neurologic deficits, but of all patients with posterior stroke, approximately 10% had isolated dizziness on presentation. Among strokes affecting the cerebellum, dizziness was reported in 73% of cases.[6] Occlusion of the anterior inferior cerebellar artery (AICA) mimics labyrinthitis and causes vestibular dysfunction and hearing loss, whereas posterior inferior cerebellar artery (PICA) infarction resembles vestibular neuritis. Differentiating dangerous central lesions from benign peripheral causes is diagnostically challenging, but critically important because missed cerebellar strokes portend a high risk of long-term morbidity and mortality (~40%).

Special consideration should be given to toxic exposures and to acute and chronic medication, drug, or alcohol effects. Dizziness is a common symptom of carbon monoxide toxicity, which can also cause hearing loss due to damage to the cochlea, vestibular nerve, and central auditory pathways. Alcohol intoxication may alter endolymph density, causing dizziness and gait instability, whereas vestibular toxicity can be caused by chronic alcohol abuse, antiepileptic drugs, aminoglycoside antibiotics, and some chemotherapeutic agents.

PREHOSPITAL CONCERNS

Reliably differentiating benign from dangerous causes of dizziness and vertigo can be difficult from the field. Individuals experiencing debilitating dizziness seeking medical care should not attempt to drive themselves. Prehospital providers should do their best to determine the likelihood of posterior circulation stroke by knowing the warning signs and symptoms, following local emergency medical service (EMS) protocols, using validated stroke recognition/severity grading tools, and adhering to destination determination protocols. A finger-stick glucose test is easy to perform and generally indicated, and if stroke is suspected, obtaining a confirmed time last known well (LKW) is very important in screening eligibility for stroke reperfusion therapies. If able, an electrocardiogram (ECG) is often useful to screen for cardiac dysrhythmias in addition to a full set of vital signs. If the patient is ambulatory, an assessment of gait stability is very helpful as well.

APPROACH/THE FOCUSED EXAMINATION

Use ATTEST to help guide the history of present illness and review of systems and resist the urge to anchor your patient into either a "lightheadedness" or "vertigo" track. Spend a few moments reviewing associated symptoms to get a better sense as to whether the cause appears to be neurovestibular or cardiac in etiology or from an underlying medical cause. Commonly relevant associated symptoms are listed in **Table 10.4**.

Interpret historic data in conjunction with the patient's vital signs to determine whether a general medical cause should be pursued. Note that some patients with an underlying medical cause of their dizziness (such as hypotension) may have a central neurologic process as well, or have a stroke mimicking a general illness, so it is best to still perform a targeted neurologic examination in these patients. Next, determine the timing of symptoms and any precipitating triggers to differentiate A_SVS, A_TVS, E_SVS, and E_TVS, further described in **Table 10.5**.

TABLE 10.4	Partial List of Associated Symptoms Relevant in Dizziness
Infectious	Fever, chills, dysuria, cough, sinus congestion
Gastrointestinal	Abdominal pain, black or bloody stools, profuse diarrhea, heavy nonsteroidal anti-inflammatory use
Traumatic	Head or neck injury, whiplash, recent cervical manipulation
Reproductive	Lower abdominal pain, vaginal bleeding, positive pregnancy test
Medication related	New antihypertensive or other medication with dizziness as a side effect, potentially ototoxic medication use
Cardiovascular	Chest pain, palpitations, shortness of breath, dyspnea on exertion, orthopnea, syncope
Aortic	Chest/back/abdominal/flank pain, discrepant pulses, known aortic aneurysm
Neurologic	Visual loss, diplopia, ataxia, unilateral weakness, speech disturbance, loss of coordination, seizure

Acute Spontaneous Vestibular Syndrome

A_SVS should be considered in patients with abrupt-onset and persistent dizziness without a precipitating trigger that remains present during the time of evaluation. Some patients may have difficulty assessing whether symptoms have abated, because they may still feel nauseous or generally unwell. The key is to ascertain whether the patient is still experiencing the full extent of their dizziness at the time of the evaluation. If so, the patient should be presumed to have A_SVS and the ensuing physical examination should be targeted to differentiate central from peripheral causes. Nystagmus is one of the best tests to help discern central from peripheral causes and is an appropriate first test in the physical examination. We recommend testing for nystagmus first because it is easy for the patient, and if it is absent, it makes vestibular neuritis and labyrinthitis very unlikely diagnoses (it is almost always present in the first 2-3 days), and, furthermore, it informs using the Head Impulse Test (HIT), which has only been validated in patients with acute vestibular syndrome (AVS) with nystagmus.

Patients with peripheral A_SVS from vestibular neuritis or labyrinthitis should have a characteristic horizontal and unidirectional nystagmus. Nystagmus has a slow phase (when the eyes slowly move toward the side of the pathology) and a fast phase (when the eyes quickly jerk back). This is noted on neutral gaze (with patient staring straight ahead) and becomes more pronounced when the eyes look in the direction of the fast phase. When looking to the opposite side, unidirectional nystagmus should become less pronounced or extinguish altogether. Alternatively, if the fast phase of the nystagmus changes and begins beating in the other direction (eg, beats to the right when looking to the right and to the left when looking to the left), then that is bidirectional or direction-changing nystagmus and is concerning for a central cause, such as stroke.

To perform this test, simply have the patient open their eyes and look forward. Wearing Frenzel goggles will magnify the patient's eyes and overcome fixation (which can suppress nystagmus) through an illuminating light. However, these are seldom available in the ED, and are not necessary to detect the presence and type of nystagmus, which is usually easy to see. The direction of the fast phase of nystagmus points toward the unaffected ear in peripheral A_SVS. Approximately 50% of cerebellar strokes do not cause nystagmus, so if no nystagmus is seen in a patient who otherwise seems to have an ASVS, stroke is still a possible diagnosis. Patients with vertical, pendular, torsional, or direction-changing nystagmus have a central cause.

Nystagmus testing is one of the three components of the HINTS examination, which is a battery of three tests including the **H**ead **I**mpulse Test, **N**ystagmus, and **T**est of **S**kew. The HINTS examination was shown to outperform early diffusion-weighted magnetic resonance imaging (MRI), which is widely regarded as the gold standard for stroke diagnosis.[7] It should be noted that the HINTS examination was developed and validated by neuro-otologists, and performed only on patients with A_SVS with nystagmus, which is present in only half of patients with cerebellar stroke.[8] Although it is believed that emergency clinicians can accurately perform and interpret this examination, widespread adoption in EDs is low.[9] Furthermore, a recent meta-analysis found that HINTS, as performed by emergency physicians, lacked adequate diagnostic sensitivity.[10] HINTS

TABLE 10.5	Vestibular Syndromes Based on Timing and Triggers with Corresponding Differential Diagnosis and Key Examination Features			
Syndrome	Description	Dangerous Causes	Benign Causes	Key Examination Features
A$_S$VS	Acute, abrupt-onset and sustained dizziness and vertigo with nausea, vomiting, and unsteadiness[a]	Posterior circulation stroke	Vestibular neuritis, labyrinthitis	Assess for presence and type of nystagmus, Head Impulse Test and vertical skew deviation (**HINTS** examination, **see subsequent text**). Look for focal neurologic deficits and ataxia
A$_T$VS	Sustained or progressive dizziness and vertigo precipitated by a trigger such as trauma or toxic exposure	Vertebral artery dissection, temporal bone fracture, vestibular toxicity	Perilymphatic fistula, barotrauma	Assess for signs of skull fracture (raccoon eyes, battle sign, hemotympanum), tympanic membrane rupture, associated focal neurologic deficits
E$_S$VS	Episodic dizziness occurring spontaneously and without clear precipitating trigger. Episodes last minutes to hours	Posterior circulation TIA, cardiac arrhythmia, pulmonary embolism	Meniere disease, vestibular migraine	Thorough physical examination, assess for neurologic deficits, cardiac arrhythmia, etc. (examination often normal when symptoms resolved)
E$_T$VS	Episodic dizziness with a clear precipitating trigger such as standing up from a seated position or turning the head to one side	Shock	BPPV, orthostatic hypotension	Provocative maneuvers for BPPV (Dix-Hallpike, see Table 10.9) and orthostatic vital signs

A$_S$VS, acute spontaneous vestibular syndrome; A$_T$VS, acute triggered vestibular syndrome; BPPV, benign paroxysmal positional vertigo; E$_S$VS, episodic spontaneous vestibular syndrome; E$_T$VS, episodic triggered vestibular syndrome; HINTS, Head Impulse Test, Nystagmus, and Test of Skew; TIA, transient ischemic attack.
[a]Technically, nystagmus is a part of the definition of the acute vestibular syndrome (AVS). However, some patients, especially those with cerebellar strokes, have all the other elements of the AVS but no nystagmus. This has important implications in the differential diagnosis and interpretation of the physical examination (see 10.6).

should be performed in conjunction with a more complete neurologic examination including a targeted assessment of the posterior circulation (cranial nerves, assessment for dysmetria, dysdiadochokinesia, and gait).

The HIT assesses the vestibulo-ocular reflex (VOR), which was first described in 1988 and is currently the best way to test unilateral vestibular nerve dysfunction in awake patients.[11] The test is performed by having the sitting or reclined patient rest their head in the palms of the examiner's hands, who then performs a very rapid, passive head rotation 10 to 20 degrees to one side (either center-to-lateral or lateral-to-center) with the patient's eyes open and fixated on a central target (usually the tip of the examiner's nose; see **Figure 10.5**). It has only been validated in patients with an ASVS and nystagmus. Peripheral vestibular hypofunction is diagnosed when a catch-up saccade is noted, which occurs when the patient's eyes are unable to stay fixed on the target and instead "overshoots" and then corrects back. The corrective saccade is indicative of a peripheral lesion (ie, abnormal test suggests vestibular neuritis) with 93% sensitivity and 79% specificity. A normal (ie, no catch-up saccade) HIT in a patient who is acutely dizzy suggests a central lesion, although it can be falsely positive in certain lateral pontine infarcts. When appropriately applied, a normal HIT is 93% specific for a central cause with a likelihood ratio of 12. It is important to remember, however,

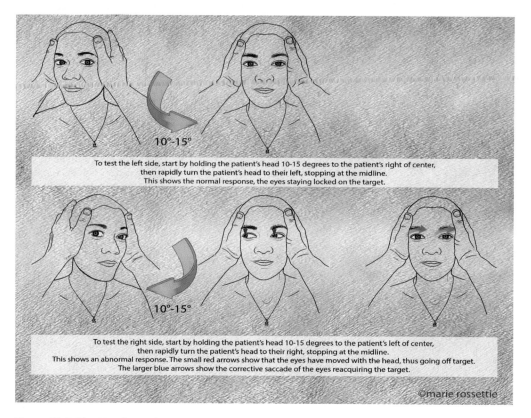

To test the left side, start by holding the patient's head 10-15 degrees to the patient's right of center, then rapidly turn the patient's head to their left, stopping at the midline. This shows the normal response, the eyes staying locked on the target.

To test the right side, start by holding the patient's head 10-15 degrees to the patient's left of center, then rapidly turn the patient's head to their right, stopping at the midline. This shows an abnormal response. The small red arrows show that the eyes have moved with the head, thus going off target. The larger blue arrows show the corrective saccade of the eyes reacquiring the target.

©marie rossettie

Figure 10.5: The Head Impulse Test. Courtesy of Dr. Jonathan A. Edlow and © Marie Rossettie, CMI.

that this test should **only** be performed in patients with acute and persistent dizziness for whom A_SVS is suspected. Inappropriate application to patients who are not actively dizzy will produce falsely concerning results, increasing confusion and unnecessary imaging utilization.

The test of skew assesses for a vertical refixation using the alternating cover test. The test is performed by again having the patient's eyes open and fixated on a central target (such as the tip of the examiner's nose). The examiner alternates, covering and uncovering each eye and looking for a hypertropia/hypotropia. If the eyes cannot stay fixed on the target and correct up and down, that is an abnormal test result, indicating a midbrain lesion (central cause). Patients with peripheral A_SVS should not exhibit an abnormal test of skew. Slight side-to-side horizontal correction is considered benign and presents with many forms of amblyopia.

To summarize, perform the HINTS examination only on patients suspected of having A_SVS with an otherwise normal neurologic examination (**Table 10.6**). When assessing the components of HINTS, begin with nystagmus, and, if horizontal unidirectional nystagmus is present, then proceed to assessing the VOR by performing the HIT. If catch-up saccades are observed on unilateral HIT testing, then proceed to the final step by checking for vertical refixation on alternating cover test, aka the test of skew. If the test of skew finding is normal, then patients are very likely to have a peripheral vestibulopathy (vestibular neuritis or labyrinthitis) and can be safely discharged home with a vestibular suppressant, as will be discussed further in the **Management** section. The HINTS examination is summarized in **Table 10.7**.

If any element of the HINTS examination is not consistent with a peripheral lesion, a central lesion should be assumed, and the patient needs further evaluation. The next step is to generally perform neuroimaging. Although computed tomography (CT) is the most common neuroimaging modality obtained in these patients, it has a very poor sensitivity for posterior circulation stroke and is a common cause of diagnostic error.[12] A CT should still be the initial test of choice if the patient is being considered for intravenous (IV) thrombolysis with tissue plasminogen activator (t-PA), because the priority in these patients is to exclude contraindications to treatment (intracranial hemorrhage,

TABLE 10.6	A Targeted Posterior Circulation Neurologic Examination	
Area Being Tested	Name of Test	Description
Cerebellar vermis	Truncal ataxia	Sit the patient upright and have him/her maintain posture without assistance
	Gait ataxia	Observe for steady ambulation and normal coordination
Cerebellar hemispheres	Dysmetria	Have patients perform finger-to-nose and heel-to-shin testing. This ataxia must be out of proportion to weakness and is often in the horizontal plane
	Dysdiadochokinesia	Assess rapid alternating movements using opposi-tional muscles. Examples include flipping one hand in the palm of the other, mimicking playing the pi-ano, etc.
Brainstem	Cranial nerves (CN)	CN I is usually not tested. CN II-XII can be tested quickly. See **Chapter 2: The Neurologic Examination** for additional details
Occipital lobe, optic nerve, and retina	Visual fields	Assess all four quadrants of each eye individu-ally. While covering one eye, the patient identifies an object (such as number of fingers held up by examiner)

TABLE 10.7	The HINTS Examination			
Component	Description	How to Perform	How to Interpret	Pearl
Head **I**mpulse Test	Assesses the VOR to identify unilateral ves-tibular afferent hypofunction	Rapid, passive head rotation 10-15 degrees (can be center-to-lateral or lateral-to-cen-ter) with patient's eyes open and attempting to re-main fixated on a central target (ex-aminer's nose)	A positive test means a catch-up saccade is noted (eyes unable to stay fixated on a central target) and points to a peripheral lesion. The ear being tested is the one to-ward which the head is being turned	Movement needs to be passive, with the patient's neck relaxed. The faster the head is moved, the easier it is to see. Test can be falsely reassuring in AICA stroke
Nystagmus	Assesses for ab-normal eye move-ments that either occur sponta-neously or are gaze-evoked	Observe for nys-tagmus on direct forward gaze and then on lateral and vertical gaze	Horizontal, unidirec-tional nystagmus that suggests a peripheral lesion, but can occur with central causes. Direction-changing, vertical or torsional nystagmus means a central lesion	Can be over-come with fixation. Shin-ing a light into the eye or having the patient gaze at a blank piece of paper can overcome fixation
Test of **S**kew	Assesses for ver-tical refixation on alternating cover test	With the patient's eyes focused on a central target, alternate which eye is covered and look for up/down correction	A positive test finding means vertical refix-ation is seen noting a hypertropia/hypotro-pia and suggesting a central lesion in the midbrain	This uncom-mon finding is highly specific for a brain-stem lesion

AICA, anterior inferior cerebellar artery; HINTS, Head Impulse Test, Nystagmus, and Test of Skew.

large subacute stroke, etc.) as efficiently as possible. Although there is a lack of supporting clinical trial data showing efficacy of t-PA in patients with posterior stroke presenting with dizziness, it is reasonable to consider reperfusion treatment in patients with clearly disabling deficits. Otherwise, diffusion-weighted (DW) MRI should be considered as the diagnostic test of choice in patients with a suspected central cause of dizziness. The false-negative rate of diffusion-weighted imaging (DWI) is greater than 10% in patients with posterior circulation ischemia within the first 48 hours of onset.[13] Providers should trust their clinical judgment and physical examination aided by HINTS more than an MRI in these patients during the early phase of illness, recognizing that it takes some practice to learn how to perform and interpret the HINTS examination. This makes the timing of an MRI less clear in these patients, although it is generally thought that it should not be purposely delayed. When performed and interpreted correctly, the HINTS battery of tests outperforms DWI in the detection of posterior circulation stroke within the first 48 hours of onset (sensitivity of 100% versus 88%).[14]

Acute Triggered Vestibular Syndrome

A_TVS should be considered in the setting of trauma or toxic exposure. It should be approached similarly to A_SVS, and providers should avoid anchoring after identifying a potential trigger. Patients should still undergo a careful neurologic examination. Blunt head injury causing a traumatic vestibulopathy, barotrauma, chemical exposure such as carbon monoxide, and medications that cause dizziness such as benzodiazepines or antiepileptic drugs and ototoxic medication use are known potential triggers. Trauma patients presenting with acute dizziness should be assessed for signs of basilar skull fracture (see Table 10.5), as well as tympanic membrane rupture. In addition, vertebral artery dissection can initially present with subtle neurologic deficits and isolated dizziness,[15] and cervical vessel imaging should be obtained if clinically suspected.

Episodic Spontaneous Vestibular Syndrome

E_SVS is differentiated from A_SVS by resolution of symptoms between distinct episodes. As opposed to E_TVS, these episodes occur without provocation or an identifiable trigger. This subset of patients with resolved symptoms while in the ED can be among the most challenging for providers because patients are asymptomatic in the ED and the symptoms cannot be triggered. Thus, it is a careful history that is most important in these patients. Common causes include vestibular migraine, transient ischemic attack (TIA), and Meniere disease; and so elucidating whether symptoms were associated with a headache, focal neurologic deficits, or hearing loss and ear fullness can be particularly useful in formulating the differential diagnosis. All patients should still have a physical examination, including a targeted neurologic examination to exclude subtle abnormalities. In vestibular migraine, if nystagmus is present, it can be of a central type because migraine is a central phenomenon. Because cardiac dysrhythmias may cause episodic dizziness, a 12-lead ECG should be considered routine. Stuttering episodes should raise concern for a high-risk TIA. Half of patients with transient isolated brainstem symptoms experience no symptom other than dizziness or vertigo, and do not fit classic, traditional descriptions of TIAs.[14] Providers should maintain a high degree of suspicion in these patients, particularly if other cerebrovascular risk factors are present. Patients who are suspected of having a TIA should undergo brain and vessel imaging of the head and neck (see **Chapter 15: Acute Stroke**).

Episodic Triggered Vestibular Syndrome

E_TVS should be considered in patients with brief, but usually severely symptomatic, episodes of dizziness provoked by a clearly identifiable trigger, usually standing up from a seated position, suggesting orthostasis, or with head turning, as can be seen in BPPV (**Figure 10.6**) . Note that the provider should be sure to distinguish triggered episodes from persistent dizziness that merely exacerbates with movement. Bedside diagnostic maneuvers are generally indicated in these patients for diagnostic confirmation. If orthostatic hypotension is suspected, then formal assessment of orthostatic vital signs can be performed for confirmation. However, subjective worsening when upright without vital sign abnormalities is generally accepted as evidence of clinical orthostasis.

When BPPV is suspected, the Dix-Hallpike and Supine Roll tests can be performed. Approximately 85% of BPPV occurs in the posterior SCC, which is why the Dix-Hallpike test brings the head into extension, so as to isolate the posterior canal in the gravitational plane. The Supine Roll test assesses the horizontal canal, which accounts for the majority of the remaining 15% of BPPV

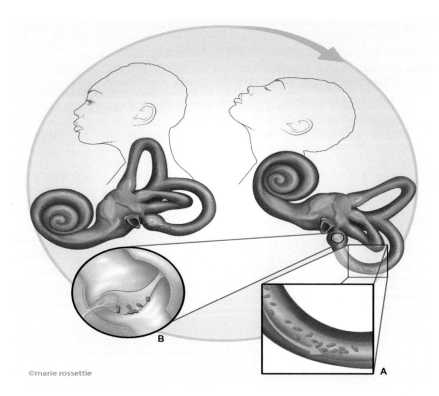

©marie rossettie

Figure 10.6: Benign paroxysmal positional vertigo mechanisms. Typical mechanism (A); cupuloli-thiasis (B). Courtesy of Dr. Jonathan A. Edlow and © Marie Rossettie, CMI.

cases. For this reason, we recommend that the Dix-Hallpike test be performed first, and if not con-firmatory, then the Supine Roll test be attempted. Both of these provocative maneuvers can be tran-sitioned into therapeutic canalith repositioning maneuvers with relative ease and performed over the course of a few minutes. The steps involved in performing these tests are outlined in **Table 10.8**.

MANAGEMENT

The goal of focusing on a systematic approach to identifying the underlying cause of dizziness is to make treatment and disposition decisions evident. First and foremost, patients with A_SVS thought to be from a central cause should not be discharged from the ED without consideration of poste-rior circulation stroke. Similarly, patients with E_SVS thought to be from a posterior circulation TIA should undergo an appropriate etiologic workup, which generally includes neuroimaging and vessel imaging of the head and neck.[16] High-risk patients, such as those with new-onset atrial fibrillation, stuttering symptoms, or significant cerebrovascular risk factors should be considered for hospital admission. Patients with an underlying medical cause for their dizziness should be approached individually and management decisions made specific to the underlying condition.

Patients with A_SVS from a unilateral peripheral vestibulopathy are typically experiencing a self-limited condition that can be safely managed as an outpatient with a vestibular suppressant. Pre-scribing a few days of an anti-vertiginous medication such as meclizine, dimenhydrinate, diphenhydr-amine, scopolamine, or a benzodiazepine is a reasonable approach, unless there are contraindications or if the patient is so symptomatic with nausea and vomiting that oral medications are unlikely to be tolerated. Patients should be cautioned about the sedating effects of most of these medications. Corti-costeroids are also often prescribed, because they offer a significant upside in their anti-inflammatory properties, without much downside. Although a Cochrane review failed to show evidence of efficacy of corticosteroids over vestibular physical therapy alone, we recommend a taper of an oral steroid such as prednisone. There is no universally agreed upon dose or duration, but we recommend the

TABLE 10.8	Diagnostic Maneuvers for BPPV			
Name of Test	**Description**	**How to Perform**	**How to Interpret**	**Pearls**
Dix-Hallpike	Assesses posterior canal BPPV	With the patient seated, turn the head 45 degrees to one side, then recline the patient to a supine position with the head hyperextended slightly. Hold this position for 30-45 s	A positive test finding will produce symptoms typically after a brief latency period, and pathognomonic upward torsional nystagmus will be observed in both eyes. If symptoms and nystagmus are not reproduced, attempt the other side	Ensure the head stays turned 45 degrees when the patient lies back. If finding is positive, then transition to the corresponding repositioning maneuver (Epley for posterior canal, or Lempert Roll for horizontal canal) discussed subsequently
Supine Roll	Assesses horizontal canal BPPV	Similar to the Dix-Hallpike, but the patient lays supine and the head is not hyperextended		

BPPV, benign paroxysmal positional vertigo.

following: 60 mg prednisone per day for 4 days, 40 mg for 4 days, 20 mg for 4 days, and then 10 mg for 2 days, each daily dose being administered once in the morning. Vestibular physical therapy can improve symptoms and expedite return to normal function, and we recommend it for patients who are significantly symptomatic.[17] Some patients with protracted and refractory symptoms may benefit from referral to an otolaryngologist (ear, nose, throat [ENT]) (**Figure 10.7**).

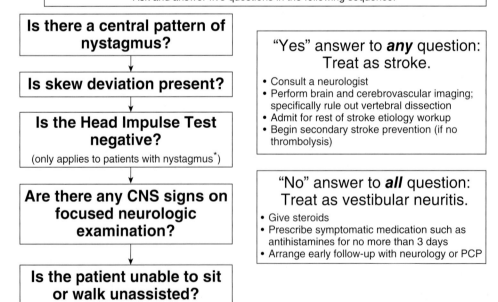

Diagnosis of patients with the acute-onset persistent dizziness
Ask and answer five questions in the following sequence:

Is there a central pattern of nystagmus?

Is skew deviation present?

Is the Head Impulse Test negative?
(only applies to patients with nystagmus*)

Are there any CNS signs on focused neurologic examination?

Is the patient unable to sit or walk unassisted?

"Yes" answer to *any* question: Treat as stroke.
- Consult a neurologist
- Perform brain and cerebrovascular imaging; specifically rule out vertebral dissection
- Admit for rest of stroke etiology workup
- Begin secondary stroke prevention (if no thrombolysis)

"No" answer to *all* question: Treat as vestibular neuritis.
- Give steroids
- Prescribe symptomatic medication such as antihistamines for no more than 3 days
- Arrange early follow-up with neurology or PCP

* In patients **without** nystagmus, the head impulse test may give misdealing results: the focused neurological exam and gait assessment become more important in this group (see text).

Figure 10.7: **Diagnostic and management algorithm for acute spontaneous vestibular syndrome (ASVS).** CNS, central nervous system; PCP, primary care physician.

With regard to E$_S$VS, a vestibular suppressant is also a reasonable initial consideration for the treatment of Meniere disease.[18] Patients should be referred to an ENT specialist, because additional therapies including dietary salt restriction, loop diuretic use, intratympanic medications, and surgical options may be offered.[19] Vestibular migraine can be challenging to both diagnose and treat, but should be managed similar to other migrainous conditions. We recommend an initial approach that includes an antidopaminergic antiemetic (such as prochlorperazine or metoclopramide 10 mg IV), anti-inflammatories (such as ketorolac 15-30 mg IV), volume repletion, and consideration for triptan or ergot (eg, Sumatriptan 6 mg subcutaneous [SC] or dihydroergotamine 0.25 mg SC or IV) unless contraindicated.

When BPPV is diagnosed, the clinician should spend a few extra minutes attempting canalith repositioning maneuvers instead of turning to a vestibular suppressant. There is good evidence to support this practice,[20] which makes intuitive sense, because the repositioning maneuvers are curative, and the vestibular suppressants merely mask the symptoms of the illness. The Epley maneuver and Lempert Roll are performed when a positive Dix-Hallpike or Supine Roll test reproduces the triggered vertiginous symptoms. The steps involved in performing these maneuvers are listed in **Table 10.9**. It is useful to review a video of these procedures (easy to find on the Internet) before doing it on a patient if one is not very familiar with it. The Semont maneuver is an alternative to Epley for posterior canal BPPV, and modified versions of both can be performed unassisted. Given

TABLE 10.9	Therapeutic Canalith Repositioning Maneuvers for BPPV	
Name of Test	**Description**	**How to Perform**
Epley maneuver	Follows Dix-Hallpike in treating posterior canal BPPV	After reproducing the upward torsional nystagmus and symptomatic vertigo with the head turned 45 degrees and the neck slightly hyperextended with the patient supine, hold this position for 40 s or so. The nystagmus should start to fatigue. Then, turn the patient's head 90 degrees toward the contralateral side with the nose upward. Hold this position for 40 s or so, then have the patient roll onto their side while turning the head another 90 degrees (the patient's eyes should now be looking at the floor). Hold this position for 40 s or so and then have the patient sit upright facing that side with their legs over the side of the bed (as if preparing to get out of bed)
Semont maneuver	Treats posterior canal BPPV and can be performed unassisted	The patient should sit on the side of a bed with their legs hanging over one side. The patient turns their head to one side and lies back resting the back of the head on the bed and looking up. After holding this position for several seconds, the patient then sits up and lies forward in one motion, maintaining the head in the same position relative to the body, now with the forehead resting on the foot of the bed (180 degrees from prior position)
Lempert Roll	Follows supine roll and used to treat horizontal canal BPPV	After reproducing the symptoms while lying supine with the head turned to one side, the patient rotates the head 90 degrees in the opposite direction (away from the affected side). This position is held for 20 s or so and then the patient rolls onto one side and rotates the head an additional 90 degrees, maintaining the head in the same position relative to the body. This position is held for another 20 s and then the body and head are advanced an additional 90 degrees. This is repeated again for a total of four steps until the patient rolls completely over 30 degrees and returns to the supine position

BPPV, benign paroxysmal positional vertigo.

the tendency for BPPV to recur over time, consider providing patients with instructions as to how to perform these exercises at home, which has been shown to be effective in resolving symptoms at 1 week the majority of the time.[21]

Although benign causes of dizziness such as BPPV and unilateral peripheral vestibulopathy can be reliably diagnosed at the bedside and without exhaustive laboratory or radiographic resource allocation, these conditions can still be severe and debilitating for some. Patients should be given a trial of symptomatic and/or curative treatment if able to, some patients will be too symptomatic and unsteady to be discharged home. Be sure to conclude all dizzy patient encounters with an ambulatory assessment. This ensures that a gait assessment is performed as part of the neurologic examination in patients who may have been too symptomatic to do so initially, as well as ensuring that the patient is safe for discharge.

PEDIATRIC ISSUES

Dizziness is a less common complaint in children, but the pathologies are generally the same. Over half of school-aged children with dizziness also report a headache.[22] Vestibular migraine, BPPV, and orthostasis are among the most common diagnoses. Although less common, more serious central causes should be considered; and pediatric patients also warrant a thoughtful neurologic assessment.

TIPS AND PEARLS

- Use the ATTEST mnemonic to focus on a timing and triggers approach rather than symptom quality. Spend a little extra time determining whether symptoms have been acute and persistent, or episodic and whether episodes occur spontaneously or are triggered. This will inform a much more specific differential diagnosis and targeted physical examination and diagnostic tests.
- Interpretation of the HINTS examination can be difficult to remember. The HINTS to INFARCT mnemonic can be a helpful tool to avoid confusion. It stands for **I**mpulse **N**ormal **F**ast-phase **A**lternating **R**efixation on **C**over **T**est, and reminds us when findings on the HINTS examination suggest a concerning central cause.[14]
- When feeling the need to obtain neuroimaging on a patient with concerning dizziness, resist the urge to obtain a noncontrast head CT, unless specifically looking for intracranial hemorrhage or considering t-PA. One study of patients discharged from ED with a diagnosis of peripheral vertigo found that patients who had a CT scan performed were twice as likely to have a stroke in 30 days compared to patients who did not have a CT performed.[12] This suggests that providers properly identified a higher risk group, but were falsely reassured by the CT. A DW-MRI is much more sensitive for the detection of posterior circulation stroke, although it too can be falsely negative within the first 48 hours of symptoms.
- BPPV is best managed with canalith repositioning maneuvers, rather than with vestibular suppressants. Although ED clinicians perform these maneuvers relatively infrequently, they are therapeutic and easy to learn.[23]

EVIDENCE

Does administration of t-PA improve clinical outcomes in patients with acute stroke presenting with isolated dizziness?

At present, there is a lack of clinical trial data studying the efficacy of t-PA specifically in patients with dizziness. Many of these patients will have a very low National Institutes of Health Stroke Scale (NIHSS). There is limited observational data suggesting a lower rate of symptomatic intracerebral hemorrhage following t-PA in patients with posterior circulation stroke compared to patients with anterior circulation stroke.[24] Current ischemic stroke treatment guidelines support the use of t-PA for disabling symptoms from an acute ischemic stroke less than 4.5 hours duration.[25] As to whether isolated dizziness is disabling is a matter of subjectivity, as opposed to ataxia and loss of coordination that are objectively measured and often quite disabling.

Does large vessel occlusion (LVO) stroke present with isolated dizziness?

Given the rapid evolution in clinical trial data supporting the efficacy of endovascular intervention with mechanical thrombectomy for patients with LVO stroke up to 24 hours of LKW,[26] consideration should be given as to whether occlusion of the basilar artery can present with mild symptoms such as isolated dizziness. Although LVO stroke is typically associated with more severe disability and higher baseline deficits on the NIHSS, approximately 5% of LVOs presenting within 3 hours of onset have an NIHSS less than 4.[27] The NIHSS is preferentially weighted toward the anterior circulation, and is poorly predictive of posterior circulation vessel occlusion.

Should BPPV be routinely treated with vestibular suppressants?

Because canalith repositioning maneuvers can easily be performed at the bedside and be curative, these should be prioritized over vestibular suppressant therapy, such as with a benzodiazepine or antihistamine. Although they may help abate the severity of symptoms, they are not curative and can be very sedating.

References

1. Saber Tehrani AS, Coughlan D, Hsieh YH, et al. Rising annual costs of dizziness presentations to U.S. emergency departments. *Acad Emerg Med*. 2013;20(7):689-696. doi: 10.1111/acem.12168

2. Newman-Toker DE, Cannon LM, Stofferahn ME, Rothman RE, Hsieh YH, Zee DS. Imprecision in patient reports of dizziness symptom quality: a cross-sectional study conducted in an acute care setting. *Mayo Clin Proc*. 2007;82(11):1329-1340.

3. Kerber KA, Brown DL, Lisabeth LD, Smith MA, Morgenstern LB. Stroke among patients with dizziness, vertigo, and imbalance in the emergency department: a population-based study. *Stroke*. 2006;37(10):2484-2487.

4. Edlow JA. A new approach to the diagnosis of acute dizziness in adult patients. *Emerg Med Clin North Am*. 2016;34(4):717-742. doi: 10.1016/j.emc.2016.06.004

5. Siket M, Edlow J. Vertigo and dizziness. In: Mattu A, Swadron S, eds. *CorePendium*. CorePendium, LLC; 2020.

6. Edlow JA, Newman-Toker DE, Savitz SI. Diagnosis and initial management of cerebellar infarction. *Lancet Neurol*. 2008;7(10):951-964. doi: 10.1016/S1474-4422(08)70216-3

7. Kattah JC, Talkad AV, Wang DZ, Hsieh YH, Newman-Toker DE. HINTS to diagnose stroke in the acute vestibular syndrome: three-step bedside oculomotor examination more sensitive than early MRI diffusion-weighted imaging. *Stroke*. 2009;40(11):3504-3510. doi: 10.1161/STROKEAHA.109.551234

8. Edlow JA. Diagnosing dizziness: we are teaching the wrong paradigm! *Acad Emerg Med*. 2013;20(10):1064-1066. doi: 10.1111/acem.12234

9. Quimby AE, Kwok ESH, Lelli D, Johns P, Tse D. Usage of the HINTS exam and neuroimaging in the assessment of peripheral vertigo in the emergency department. *J Otolaryngol Head Neck Surg*. 2018;47(1):54. doi: 10.1186/s40463-018-0305-8

10. Ohle R, Montpellier RA, Marchadier V, et al. Can emergency physicians accurately rule out a central cause of vertigo using the HINTS examination? A systematic review and meta-analysis. *Acad Emerg Med*. 2020;27(9):887-896. doi: 10.1111/acem.13960

11. Halmagyi GM, Curthoys IS. A clinical sign of canal paresis. *Arch Neurol*. 1988;45(7):737-739.

12. Grewal K, Austin PC, Kapral MK, Lu H, Atzema CL. Missed strokes using computed tomography imaging in patients with vertigo: population-based cohort study. *Stroke*. 2015;46(1):108-113. doi: 10.1161/STROKEAHA.114.007087

13. Tarnutzer AA, Berkowitz AL, Robinson KA et al. Does my dizzy patient have a stroke? A systematic review od bedside diagnosis in acute vestibular syndrome. CMAJ 2011;183(9):E571-E592. https://www.ncbi.nlm.nih.gov/pmc/articles/PMC3114934/

14. Paul NL, Simoni M, Rothwell PM, Oxford Vascular Study. Transient isolated brainstem symptoms preceding posterior circulation stroke: a population-based study. *Lancet Neurol*. 2013;12(1):65-71. doi: 10.1016/S1474-4422(12)70299-5

15. Newman-Toker DE. Missed stroke in acute vertigo and dizziness: it is time for action, not debate. *Ann Neurol*. 2016;79(1):27-31. doi: 10.1002/ana.24532

16. Siket MS, Edlow JA. Transient ischemic attack: reviewing the evolution of the definition, diagnosis, risk stratification, and management for the emergency physician. *Emerg Med Clin North Am*. 2012;30(3):745-770. doi: 10.1016/j.emc.2012.05.001

17. Strupp M, Arbusow V. [Therapy of vertigo]. *Dtsch Med Wochenschr*. 1998;123(36):1041-1045.

18. Seemungal B, Kaski D, Lopez-Escamez JA. Early diagnosis and management of acute vertigo from vestibular migraine and Ménière's disease. *Neurol Clin*. 2015;33(3).619-628.ix. doi: 10.1016/j.ncl.2015.04.008

19. Strupp M, Zingler VC, Arbusow V, et al. Methylprednisolone, valacyclovir, or the combination for vestibular neuritis. *N Engl J Med*. 2004;351(4):354-361.

20. Bhattacharyya N, Baugh RF, Orvidas L, et al. Clinical practice guideline: benign paroxysmal positional vertigo. *Otolaryngol Head Neck Surg*. 2008;139(5 Suppl. 4):S47-S81. doi: 10.1016/j.otohns.2008.08.022

21. Radtke A, von Brevern M, Tiel-Wilck K, Mainz-Perchalla A, Neuhauser H, Lempert T. Self-treatment of benign paroxysmal positional vertigo: Semont maneuver vs Epley procedure. *Neurology*. 2004;63(1):150-152.

22. Jahn K. Vertigo and dizziness in children. *Handb Clin Neurol*. 2016;137:353-363. doi: 10.1016/B978-0-444-63437-5.00025-X

23. Kerber KA, Damschroder L, McLaughlin T, et al. Implementation of evidence-based practice for benign paroxysmal positional vertigo in the emergency department: a stepped-wedge randomized trial. *Ann Emerg Med*. 2020;75(4)459-470. doi: 10.1016/j.annemergmed.2019.09.017

24. Powers WJ, Rabinstein AA, Ackerson T, et al. Guidelines for the early management of patients with acute ischemic stroke: 2019 update to the 2018 guidelines for the early management of acute ischemic stroke: a guideline for healthcare professionals from the American Heart Association/American Stroke Association. *Stroke*. 2019;50(12):e344-e418. doi: 10.1161/STR.0000000000000211.

25. Powers WJ, Rabinstein AA, Ackerson T, et al. 2018 Guidelines for the early management of patients with acute ischemic stroke: a guideline for healthcare professionals from the American Heart Association/American Stroke Association. *Stroke*. 2018;49(3):e46-e110. doi: 10.1161/STR.0000000000000158

26. Mokin M, Ansari SA, McTaggart RA, et al. Indications for thrombectomy in acute ischemic stroke from emergent large vessel occlusion (ELVO): report of the SNIS Standards and Guidelines Committee. *J Neurointerv Surg*. 2019;11(3):215-220. doi: 10.1136/neurintsurg-2018-014640

27. Heldner MR, Zubler C, Mattle HP, et al. National Institutes of Health stroke scale score and vessel occlusion in 2152 patients with acute ischemic stroke. *Stroke*. 2013;44(4):1153-1157. doi: 10.1161/STROKEAHA.111.000604

Suggested Readings

1. Edlow JA. The timing-and-triggers approach to the patient with acute dizziness. *Emerg Med Pract*. 2019;21(12):1-24.

2. Herr RD, Zun L, Mathews JJ. A directed approach to the dizzy patient. *Ann Emerg Med*. 1989;18(6):664-672.

3. Kim JS, Zee DS. Clinical practice. Benign paroxysmal positional vertigo. *N Engl J Med*. 2014;370(12):1138-1147. doi: 10.1056/NEJMcp1309481

4. Newman-Toker DE, Hsieh YH, Camargo CA Jr, Pelletier AJ, Butchy GT, Edlow JA. Spectrum of dizziness visits to US emergency departments: cross-sectional analysis from a nationally representative sample. *Mayo Clin Proc*. 2008;83(7):765-775. doi: 10.4065/83.7.765

5. Oostema JA, Chassee T, Baer W, Edberg A, Reeves MJ. Brief educational intervention improves Emergency Medical Services stroke recognition. *Stroke*. 2019;50(5):1193-1200. doi: 10.1161/STROKEAHA.118.023885

6. Savitz SI, Caplan LR, Edlow JA. Pitfalls in the diagnosis of cerebellar infarction. *Acad Emerg Med*. 2007;14(1):63-68.

7. Seale B, Ahanger S, Hari C. Subacute carbon monoxide poisoning presenting as vertigo and fluctuating low frequency hearing loss. *J Surg Case Rep*. 2018;2018(8):rjy205. doi: 10.1093/jscr/rjy205

8. Tinetti ME, Williams CS, Gill TM. Health, functional, and psychological outcomes among older persons with chronic dizziness. *J Am Geriatr Soc*. 2000;48(4):417-421.

CHAPTER 11

Mild Traumatic Brain Injury and Concussion

Christopher Reverte

George Kramer

Andy S. Jagoda

THE CLINICAL CHALLENGE

Mild traumatic brain injury (mTBI) including concussion is the most common type of brain injury and can have long-term medical, behavioral, and financial effects on the life of the patient. Of all types of trauma, it may be the most underreported and underdiagnosed because the effect on the patient may not be immediate or clinically overt.

The Glasgow Coma Scale (GCS) was developed as a tool to describe level of consciousness after a traumatic brain injury (TBI) and to assist in prognosis (**Figure 11.1**). A score of 3 to 8, indicating a severe injury, is associated with coma; a score of 9 to 12, indicating a moderate injury, is associated with lethargy; and a score of 13 to 15, indicating a "mild" injury, is associated with an alert level of consciousness. GCS scores may change over time; and, therefore, a single score is not prognostic, whereas the score at 4 to 6 hours post the injury has a stronger correlation with outcome. Limitations of the GCS score are pronounced in the "mild" range, where 10% to 20% of patients will have a traumatic lesion on head computed tomography (CT), and approximately 1% will have a lesion requiring neurosurgical intervention. Unfortunately, the GCS score is one-dimensional, and when used alone is not a good predictor of injuries in patients.

Concussion is a subcategory of mTBI. A concussion results from direct or indirect biomechanical forces to the brain, resulting in a transient change in brain function. The external forces that lead to concussion may be from a direct impact, a rapid deceleration, a blast injury, or a pressure wave. The transient change in brain function may range from a loss of consciousness (LOC) to pre- and/or post-traumatic amnesia, to more subtle findings including feeling dazed or "foggy," loss of attention, or decreased reaction time. Patients may experience a brief impact seizure or have an episode of nausea and vomiting. By definition, if a head CT is performed in a patient with a concussion, the finding will be negative for acute intracranial bleeding or other traumatic pathology.

In that mTBIs are heterogeneous, clinical presentations and time course are highly variable. Risk stratification tools such as the New Orleans Head Injury Criteria[1] or the Canadian Head CT Rule[2] focus on identifying patients with lesions requiring neurosurgical interventions and provide limited value on the clinical course. These tools, however, are helpful in directing the diagnosis

<table>
<tr><td valign="top">

Best motor response (1-6)

- 6: Obeying commands
- 5: Localizing to pain
- 4: Withdrawing to pain
- 3: Flexor response to pain
- 2: Extensor response to pain
- 1: No response to pain

</td><td valign="top">

Best verbal response (1-5)

- 5: Oriented (time, place, person)
- 4: Confused conversation
- 3: Inappropriate speech
- 2: Incomprehensible sounds
- 1: None

</td></tr>
</table>

Eye opening (1-4)

- 4: Spontaneous
- 3: In response to speech
- 2: In response to pain
- 1: None

Figure 11.1: Glasgow Coma Scale (GCS), total score 3 to 15.

of a patient with an mTBI toward a diagnosis of a concussion. Currently, there is no universally accepted gold standard to confirm the diagnosis of concussion, for example, imaging, a biomarker, or neuropsychological test, although this is an area of intense research. Patients with a concussion may have a wide range of subjective symptoms such as headache, nausea, or fatigue, but these are neither sensitive nor specific for the diagnosis.

EPIDEMIOLOGY

In the United States alone, it is estimated that there are over 2.5 million cases of TBI treated in the emergency department (ED) annually, with most of those being classified as mild.[3] It is difficult to know the true incidence because many TBIs do not present for medical evaluation. Many symptoms are underreported, and many patients may underestimate the importance of their symptoms. Patients often seek medical evaluation when they sustain LOC, but may minimize the importance of less dramatic signs and symptoms; in fact, most patients who sustain a concussion do not have LOC. In general, children and young adults have the highest incidence of concussion.

Civilian injuries may be grouped into sports-related concussions (SRCs) and accidental and non-accidental trauma (**Table 11.1**). Sports commonly associated with TBIs include football, boxing, basketball, soccer, lacrosse, and hockey. It is estimated by the U.S. Centers for Disease Control and Prevention (CDC) that up to 15% of all contact sport, high school athletes suffer a concussion during a season.[4] Common accidental causes in young adults and children include falls and bicycle accidents. Elderly patients with limited mobility are at a higher risk of accidental falls. Car crashes and assaults are often associated with alcohol and substance intoxication. TBIs in the military are most commonly caused by a blast injury, often from an improvised explosive device (IED).

Concussions associated with sports have recently been identified as a major public health concern, particularly with football, leading to increased awareness and research in the field. Recent studies estimate the average college football player experiences 800 to 1000 hits to the head in a single season.[5,6] Although most patients with SRC will have a spontaneous resolution of symptoms, there exists a subset who experience at least one neurobehavioral symptom for up to 3 months after injury, most commonly a headache. Symptoms that persist longer than expected may be part of a post-concussive syndrome (PCS) that may require a multidisciplinary treatment strategy. There is some evidence suggesting that repeat concussions may result in chronic traumatic encephalopathy (CTE) and permanent neurocognitive damage.

TABLE 11.1	Common Injuries Associated with Head Injury
Patient Type	Activity
Civilian	• Sports • Football, hockey, soccer, lacrosse

	• Accidental trauma
	   • Falls
	   • Bicycle and skateboard accidents
	   • Motor vehicle accidents

	• Non-accidental trauma • Assault with blunt trauma
Military	• Blast injury

PATHOPHYSIOLOGY

Direct or indirect forces on the brain result in transmitted energies that create shearing forces on axons; these forces lead to subsequent injury and edema, with consequent neuronal and or axonal metabolic and cellular damage. Although there may be initial structural damage, the prevailing belief is that some amount of functional disturbance is caused by a combination of inflammatory cascades, disrupted neurotransmitters, abnormal cerebral blood flow, and metabolic mismatch. It is likely that there are some feedback loops contributing to subsequent damage and contributing to the development of post-concussive symptoms. The literature suggests a similar, but milder, form of a diffuse axonal injury due to axonal stretching. Distortion to the vasculature, abnormalities with glucose uptake and blood flow, and release of inflammatory mediators have also been implicated. This can cause tearing of neuronal connections and slow the transmission of information that may result in deficits in attention and reaction times, which are hallmarks of a concussion.

There is a growing interest in the role of an inflammatory process associated with a concussion. Following an injury, neutrophils and monocytes secrete inflammatory cytokines as part of an immunologic response. Proinflammatory molecules such as interleukin and tumor necrosis factor-alpha (TNF-α) are thought to be released, contributing to recovery after injury. A better understanding of this inflammatory process could lead to improved diagnostic, prognostic, and treatment modalities.

PREHOSPITAL CONCERNS

In patients suffering from head trauma, other traumatic injuries, including cervical spine injury, should be considered. The basic principles of first aid should still be followed. Patients with TBI who are alert in the field, that is, GCS > 12, are still at risk for deterioration, as classically seen with an epidural hematoma. Patients with a TBI are at high risk for vomiting, and therefore accommodation for emesis should be proactively made, especially in those patients with spinal immobilization. Patients who are intoxicated may have altered mental status and are in a higher risk category. Seizure precautions are also recommended. Whenever possible, only trained personnel should mobilize an injured player and remove protective equipment. Frequent reassessments and monitoring of patients should be conducted during transport, with a focus on the GCS. A broad differential should be considered in patients sustaining traumatic head injury, and common causes of altered mental status such as hypoglycemia should not be overlooked (**Table 11.2**).

APPROACH/THE FOCUSED EXAMINATION

A focused history and physical examination direct the need for additional diagnostic testing. Findings may be subtle. The history focuses on the events surrounding the injury, including the presence of LOC and of pre- or post-traumatic amnesia; these findings establish that at a minimum there was a concussion, but the absence of these findings does not eliminate the diagnosis. Patients should be evaluated for common symptoms associated with concussion such as headache,

TABLE 11.2	Differential Diagnosis of Alert Patient Who Sustained a Head Injury and Presents with a Somatic Complaint
Complaint	**Description**
Cerebral contusion	Multiple microhemorrhages of brain tissue
Epidural hematoma	Extradural bleed, may see LOC followed by lucid interval, then decompensation with repeated LOC
Subdural hematoma	Bleed between dura mater and arachnoid mater, often tearing from bridging veins in subdural space
Intraparenchymal/intracerebral hematoma	Bleeding within brain parenchyma and may lead to edema and herniation
Intraventricular hematoma	Bleeding into ventricular system and CSF, typically associated with poor outcomes
Subarachnoid hemorrhage	May be associated with skull fracture or intracerebral contusion
Diffuse axonal injury	Shearing of axons diffusely, often causes comatose or vegetative state, may not be evident on CT and may require MRI for diagnosis
Metabolic abnormality	Consider hypoglycemia, dehydration, hyponatremia
Postictal state	May have period of amnesia, confusion
Skull fracture	Not necessarily associated with brain injury or AMS; assess for CSF leak
Post-traumatic headache	May be present without other concussion signs or symptoms; may take up to 7 days to develop after injury
Intoxication	May contribute to altered mental status and abnormal neurologic findings; may predispose patient to concussion; may be mixed alcohol and other substances
Post-traumatic stress disorder	Some overlap with concussion; often associated with intrusive images and memories of injury
Cranial nerve praxis	Double vision—often subtle, but may cause headache or sense of being off balance
Cervical strain	May cause headache
Cupulolithiasis	Can lead to vertigo and may lead to misdiagnosis of concussion
Medication overuse	Headache, somnolence, decreased concentration, and slowed reflexes

AMS, altered mental state; CSF, cerebrospinal fluid; CT, computed tomography; LOC, loss of consciousness; MRI, magnetic resonance imaging (eg, Headache).

dizziness, fogginess, "feeling off" or imbalanced, blurred or double vision, or nausea/vomiting. These findings often occur rapidly after the injury, but may also develop hours to days after the injury (**Table 11.3**). The use of anticoagulant or antiplatelet medications should be assessed and may increase the likelihood of the patient having intracranial bleeding.

The physical examination includes a primary and secondary survey. Examination of the skull, face, neck, and shoulders should be completed, looking for signs of traumatic injury such as hematoma, ecchymosis, lacerations, deformity, and/or tenderness. The cervical spine should be examined for tenderness with direct midline palpation or pain with range of motion from flexion/extension or turning to the sides.

The neurologic and cognitive examinations are at the core of the evaluation, and may reveal critically important, yet subtle, abnormalities, for example, a neuropraxia or a recall deficit. A best practice is to have a standardized evaluation template, for example, Sports Concussion Assessment

TABLE 11.3	Signs and Symptoms Associated with a Concussion	
Signs	Symptoms	Examination Findings
Impact seizure	Headache	Amnesia
Fencing posturing	Nausea/vomiting	Cranial nerve abnormalities
LOC	Dizzy/imbalanced	Balance problems
Appears dazed/stunned	Blurred/double vision (CN)	Memory recall deficit
Gross motor instability	Irritable	Focal cranial nerve deficit
Confused or forgetful	Concentration/memory problems	Scalp hematoma
Slow to answer questions	Feels foggy/hazy/sluggish	
	Amnesia	
	Irritability/moody	
	Sleep disturbance	
	Loss of balance	
	Photophobia/phonophobia	

CN, cranial nerve; LOC, loss of consciousness.

Tool-5 (SCAT5; see **Tables 11.4** and **11.5**). Specific standardized concussion examinations have not been validated in the ED; however, aspects of published sports or military tools (discussed subsequently) provide a framework to work from.

The cranial nerve (CN) examination focuses on CN II, III, IV, and VI (of interest, retinal detachment is the most common injury in boxers, whereas subdural and intracranial bleeds are the most common cause of death); injury may lead to visual disturbances contributing to headaches and postural instability. Balance testing is a key component in the evaluation of the patient with an mTBI and a diagnostic criterion on sideline assessments. Although the evaluation of balance is formally assessed in the sports arena, there is no official technique validated for use in the ED. Tandem gait and coordination tests such as finger-to-nose have been shown to be a useful part of the examination.

Neurocognitive and psychological testing are used to measure changes in attention and higher level cognitive functioning, the hallmarks of mTBI. A brief, but appropriate, ED mental status examination should include orientation, immediate and delayed recall, concentration, attention span, mood, and speech and language skills. The testing of memory may be composed of both visual and verbal components. Reaction times and speed of processing may be assessed and may include problem-solving ability. Ideally, although not always practical, these results should be compared to baseline tests that are now standard during preseason assessments in sports.

Evaluation Tools

There are numerous assessment tools that have been developed to assess for a concussion, and should be considered when evaluating an injured person (**Table 11.4**). A limitation of many of these tools is the need to have an established baseline to compare performance to, which may not always be completed. Some of the tools include a physical examination component, and others known as neuropsychological tests are completely written or computerized. These tools may have a role in determining which patients with a head injury actually sustained a concussion.

SCAT5

The SCAT5[7] is a standardized, commonly used sideline screening tool, used by medical professionals, that was designed for use in athletes aged 13 and older. It takes approximately 10 to 15 minutes to complete, and is often conducted with the assistance of an electronic device. Preseason baseline scores are generally established. If there is concern for a potential brain injury during practice or play, the athlete is retested on the sideline or locker room, and the scores are compared. The examination includes evaluating cognitive function, a detailed neurologic examination

TABLE 11.4	Evaluation Tools for the Diagnosis of Concussions
Assessment Tool/Evaluation	**Description**
SCAT5: Sport Concussion Assessment Tool	See Table 11.5.
MACE[26]: Military Acute Concussion Evaluation (MACE)	The military uses the MACE tool that includes a concussion screening history, a cognitive examination, a neurologic examination, and symptom screening. Baseline testing is often not available for comparison. The MACE first screens to confirm a patient had a head injury event and had either self-reported or witnessed alteration of consciousness (including being dazed, stunned, or seeing stars), loss of consciousness, or post-traumatic amnesia. If positive, a Standardized Assessment of Concussion (SAC) is then used to evaluate for deficits in four cognitive domains including orientation, immediate memory, concentration, and delayed recall. A score of 0-30 is then calculated. The MACE tool is ideally performed within the first 24 hr of the event and can be completed in a matter of minutes.
ImPACT: Immediate Post-concussion Assessment and Cognitive Testing	ImPACT is a computerized neurocognitive testing tool with objective scoring that can be compared to a patient's baseline test results obtained preseason. It takes approximately 20-25 min, and is usually compared to baseline testing when available. There is no physical examination component to the ImPACT test, and it can be completed on a computer. It tests visual and verbal memory, attention span, reaction time, and visual and verbal problem-solving. ImPACT is used by many professional organizations including MLB, NHL, and many colleges and universities.
PCSI-2: Post-Concussion Symptom Inventory-2	PCSI-2 is a 5-min test that assesses physical, cognitive, emotional and sleep/fatigue symptoms to help manage treatment and guide a patient returning to activities.
K-D: King-Devick Test	This test takes 2 min and evaluates the speed of rapid number naming and captures impairment of eye movement, attention, and language that may correlate with identifying suboptimal brain function. It is a visual performance measure that captures saccadic eye movements, and is also commonly used in neurologic evaluations of nontraumatic patients.
ACE: Acute Concussion Evaluation	The ACE was released by the CDC as a free tool to standardize a symptom checklist to assess key elements including headache and visual symptoms, difficulty concentrating, fatigue, and irritability. There is no physical examination component. The tool also assesses risk factors for protracted recovery and helps guide a treatment and follow-up plan.

CDC, U.S. Centers for Disease Control and Prevention; MBL, Major League Basketball; NHL, National Hockey League.

including balance assessment, and symptom evaluation (**Table 11.5**). Currently, the SCAT is utilized by Fédération Internationale de Football Association (FIFA), National Football League (NFL), and some Olympic committees to help guide assessments, need for neuroimaging, and eligibility for return to play.

TABLE 11.5	Some Components of the SCAT5 Examination
	Components
GCS: Glasgow Coma Scale	Scored with a range of 3-15. Score may change over time.
Maddocks Questions	A series of short questions that can be modified to each sport and be used to evaluate recall and orientation. If an athlete is unable to answer any of the questions correctly, there is a high level of concern for a concussive event, and further investigation is warranted. Some examples of questions include "who scored last" and "did our team win the last game we played."
mBESS: Modified Balance Error Scoring System	A series of tests evaluating balance and postural control and is a component of the SCAT examination.
SAC: Standardized Assessment of Concussion (see Figure 11.2)	Used as a sideline measure of cognitive function. It assesses orientation, immediate memory, concentration, and delayed recall. It can be used by nonphysicians and may detect a concussion in the early stages post the injury.
CSSS: Concussion Symptom Severity Score	A subjective examination that the patient completes on their own. The written form is a list of symptoms that may be seen with a concussion diagnosis, with a numerical scale of 0-6 for each symptom. The examination can be repeated periodically after the initial injury to monitor for resolution and improvement of symptom severity.

SCAT, Sport Concussion Assessment Tool.

The SCAT5 examination components include the following:

1. Immediate or on-field assessment:
   a. GCS; memory assessment with Maddocks questions (see **Table 11.5**); observable signs; cervical spine assessment; red flags such as seizures, LOC, severe headache, and so on
2. Symptom assessment:

   a. Evaluation of symptoms such as headache, dizziness, confusion, drowsiness, and so on (Concussion Symptoms Severity Score)
3. Cognitive screening and concentration (Standardized Assessment of Concussion tool, see **Figure 11.2**):

   a. Cognitive screening: testing of orientation and immediate recall memory (recall of a list of words)
   b. Concentration: repeating digits in reverse order; listing of months in reverse order
4. Neurologic screening:

   a. Physical neurologic examination
   b. Balance testing using the Modified Balance Error Scoring System (mBESS) (see **Table 11.5**)
5. Delayed recall:

   a. Repeating the list of words used at least 5 minutes earlier for immediate recall memory testing
6. Final assessment:

   a. Review of results and comparison to baseline testing
   b. Diagnosis of concussion or possible need for neuroimaging, and eligibility to return to play

STANDARDIZED ASSESSMENT OF CONCUSSION—ER VERSION   *FORM A*

INTRODUCTION
I am going to ask you some questions.
Please listen carefully and give your best effort.

ORIENTATION

What Month is it?_____	0	1
What's the Date today?_____	0	1
What's the Day of Week?_____	0	1
What Year is it?_____	0	1
What Time is it right now? (within 1 hr.)_____	0	1

Award 1 point for each correct answer.

ORIENTATION TOTAL SCORE ➡	

IMMEDIATE MEMORY

I am going to test your memory. I will read you a
list of words and when I am done, repeat back as
many words as you can remember, in any order.

LIST	TRIAL I	TRIAL 2	TRIAL 3
FINGER	0 1	0 1	0 1
PENNY	0 1	0 1	0 1
BLANKET	0 1	0 1	0 1
LEMON	0 1	0 1	0 1
INSECT	0 1	0 1	0 1
TOTAL			

Trials 2 & 3: I am going to repeat that list again.
Repeat back as many words as you can remember
in any order, even if you said the word before.

Complete all 3 trials regardless of score on trial 1 & 2, 1 pt. for each
correct response. Total score equals sum across all 3 trials.
Do not inform the subject that delayed recall will be tested.

IMMEDIATE MEMORY TOTAL SCORE ➡	

GRADED SYMPTOM CHECKLIST

Tell me if you are currently experiencing or have
experienced any of the following symptoms <u>since
you were injured</u>. If so, rate the symptom as mild,
moderate, or severe.   Circle response for each item.

SYMPTOM	SEVERITY			
	NONE	MILD	MODERATE	SEVERE
Headache	0	1	2	3
Nausea	0	1	2	3
Vomiting	0	1	2	3
Dizziness	0	1	2	3
Poor balance	0	1	2	3
Blurred/Dbl vision	0	1	2	3
Sensitivity to light	0	1	2	3
Sensitivity to noise	0	1	2	3
Ringing in ears	0	1	2	3
Poor concentration	0	1	2	3
Memory problems	0	1	2	3
Not feeling "sharp"	0	1	2	3
Fatigue/sluggish	0	1	2	3
Sadness/depression	0	1	2	3
irritability	0	1	2	3

NEUROLOGIC SCREENING

POST-TRAUMATIC AMNESIA? Poor recall of events after injury	☐ No ☐ Yes Length:	
RETROGRADE AMNESIA? Poor recall of events before injury	☐ No ☐ Yes Length:	

	NORMAL	ABNORMAL
STRENGTH—		
Right Upper Extremity	☐	☐
Right Lower Extremity	☐	☐
Left Upper Extremity	☐	☐
Left Lower Extremity	☐	☐
SENSATION—examples: FINGER -TO-NOSE/ROMBERG	☐	☐
COORDINATION—examples: TANDEM WALK FINGER-NOSE-FINGER	☐	☐

CONCENTRATION

Digits Backward: I am going to read you a string of
numbers and when I am done, you repeat them
back to me backwards, in reverse order of how I
read them to you. For example, if I say 7-1-9, you
would say 9-1-7.
If correct, go to next string length. If incorrect, read trial 2. 1 pt.
possible for each string length. Stop after incorrect on both trials.

4-9-3	6-2-9	0 1
3-8-1-4	3-2-7-9	0 1
6-2-9-7-1	1-5-2-8-6	0 1
7-1-8-4-6-2	5-3-9-1-4-8	0 1

Months in Reverse Order: Now tell me the months
Of the year in reverse order. Start with the list
month and go backward. So you'll say December,
November...Go ahead.   1 pt. for entire sequence correct.

Dec-Nov-Oct-Sept-Aug-Jul-Jun-May-Apr-Mar-Feb-Jan   0   1

CONCENTRATION TOTAL SCORE ➡	

DELAYED RECALL

Do you remember that list of words I read a few
times earlier? Tell me as many words from the list
as you can remember in any order. Circle each word
correctly recalled. Total score equals number of words recalled.

   FINGER   PENNY   BLANKET   LEMON   INSECT

DELAYED RECALL TOTAL SCORE ➡	

SAC SCORING SUMMARY

Symptom Index & Neurologic Screening are important for
examination, but <u>not</u> incorporated into SAC Total Score.

ORIENTATION	/ 5
IMMEDIATE MEMORY	/ 15
CONCENTRATION	/ 5
DELAYED RECALL	/ 5
SAC TOTAL SCORE ➡	/30

© 1998 MCCREA, KELLY & RANDOLPH

Figure 11.2: Standardized Assessment of Concussion, Form A. From McCrea M, Kelly JP, Randolph C, et al. Standardized assessment of concussion (SAC): on-site mental status evaluation of the athlete. *J Head Trauma Rehabil.* 1998;13(2):27-35.

DIAGNOSTIC TESTING

Neuroimaging

The likelihood of a visible intracranial lesion on CT scan is inversely correlated with the GCS. The majority of patients with a concussion presents to the ED with a GCS of 15. The incidence of an abnormal head CT with acute findings in a patient with a GCS of 15 is about 6%, and may rise to over 20% with a GCS of 14. However, the need for a neurosurgical intervention is generally below 2% with all mTBIs, and less than 1% when the GCS is 15. Several decision tools, for example, Canadian Head CT Rule and the New Orleans Head Trauma Rule, have been developed and validated to safely obviate the need for neuroimaging in a stable patient who has sustained a head injury. Although there are small clinical differences in the sensitivity and specificity of the tools for finding any traumatic lesion, both work remarkably well in decreasing imaging while maintaining specificity for diagnosing intracranial injuries requiring acute intervention.

The American College of Emergency Physicians (ACEP) performed a systematic review of the literature including the Canadian and New Orleans Rules, synthesized the findings, and generated evidence-based recommendations regarding when to obtain a non-contrast head CT in the ED in a patient with mTBI[8,9] (**Table 11.6**). These guidelines do not provide insight into which patients are at risk for developing neurobehavioral sequelae from an mTBI, and therefore are not useful in prognosis. A diagnosis of concussion is dependent on either the patient not having inclusion criteria for neuroimaging or, if imaged, a negative head CT finding.

Magnetic resonance imaging (MRI) is more sensitive in diagnosing contusions, petechial hemorrhage, and white matter injury, and if performed, may offer a diagnosis other than concussion if other acute findings, such as axonal injury, are seen. Standard T1- and T2-weighted MRI imaging is not indicated in the routine evaluation for an mTBI/concussion. Other imaging modalities are being studied such as functional MRI looking at neuronal activation, and diffusion-weighted MRI to look at tissue architecture and microhemorrhaging.

Biomarkers

Brain-specific biomarkers offer a promising approach to determining the need for neuroimaging. Many patients seeking medical attention after an mTBI obtain unnecessary radiation from head

TABLE 11.6	**ACEP Guidelines for Which Patients with Mild TBI Should Have a Noncontrast Head CT Scan in the ED**
Level	Recommendation
Level A recommendation	• A noncontrast head CT is indicated in patients with head trauma with loss of consciousness or post-traumatic amnesia only if one or more of the following symptoms is present: • Headache, vomiting, age older than 60 years, drug or alcohol intoxication, deficits in short-term memory, physical evidence of trauma above the clavicle, post-traumatic seizure, GCS < 15, focal neurologic deficit, or coagulopathy
Level B recommendation	• A noncontrast head CT should be considered in patients with head trauma without loss of consciousness or post-traumatic amnesia only if one or more of the following symptoms is present: • A focal neurologic deficit, vomiting, severe headache, age older than 65 years, physical signs of basilar skull fracture, GCS < 15, coagulopathy, or a dangerous mechanism of injury ○ Dangerous mechanism of injury includes ejection from a motor vehicle, a pedestrian struck, and a fall from a height of more than 3 feet or 5 stairs

ACEP, American College of Emergency Physicians; CT, computed tomography; ED, emergency department; GCS, Glasgow Coma Scale; TBI, traumatic brain injury.

CTs and advances in biomarker serum testing may be able to decrease the use of head CTs. Proteins that have been studied as brain injury biomarkers include those derived from neuronal tissue such as ubiquitin C-terminal hydrolase (UCH-L1) and neuron-specific enolase (NSE) and those derived from glial cells such as S100B and glial fibrillary astrocytic protein (GFAP).[10-12]

S100B has a sensitivity of 97% in detecting CT-visualized intracranial hemorrhage and a specificity of 30% to 50%.[10,12] Although approved in other parts of the world, S100B is not U.S. Food and Drug Administration (FDA) approved, and thus not readily available in the United States; however, ACEP acknowledged the use of biomarkers in its 2008 Clinical Policy by giving the use of S100B a level C recommendation.[8]

With single markers showing promise, some studies have suggested that combining multiple biomarkers can lead to improved sensitivity and specificity in predicting CT-evident intracranial hemorrhage.[14] A combined test using UCH-L1 and GFAP is the first FDA-approved biomarker for TBI, with a sensitivity nearing 100% and specificity of 46%[15]; at this time, the test does not have a platform that enables a rapid turnaround. Some combination of clinical factors and biomarkers will likely be used in the future to better predict the need for advanced imaging.

MANAGEMENT

The diagnosis of an mTBI/concussion requires some signs or symptoms by history, for example, LOC, amnesia, headache, "seeing stars" or "feeling foggy," and/or a determination of altered neurologic function, for example, impaired memory recall, decreased reaction time, or altered balance. Symptoms alone, for example, headache or nausea, are generally not sufficient to confidently make a diagnosis of concussion because other injuries, for example, cervical strain or orthopedic injuries, can cause these same symptoms.

The 2008 ACEP Clinical Policy based on literature supports that those patients with an mTBI who have a negative CT finding can be safely discharged without concern of later deteriorating from a neurosurgical lesion[8]; however, a caveat is that the majority of patients in the studies used to generate this recommendation had delays of several hours before imaging was obtained, and therefore there it may be an advantage to delaying imaging for several hours in those patients arriving quickly to the ED after injury. Although data on non-anticoagulated patients are very limited, the literature suggests about a 1% to 3% delayed hemorrhage rate in anticoagulated patients. It is likely much lower in the younger patient with a sports-related injury, although the data are lacking.

Determining appropriate treatment plans for patients with mTBI/concussion is not always straightforward, and often requires a multidisciplinary approach and a customized strategy. Patients who sustain a concussion should receive careful counseling on post-concussive symptoms. Risk factors that may lead to delayed recovery include preexisting psychiatric conditions such as depression or post-traumatic stress disorder (PTSD), substance abuse, poor health, and general life stress. Longer periods of LOC or amnesia may also be associated with a slower return to baseline.

Because patients with an mTBI/concussion often have impaired attention, balance, and or reaction times, they are at risk for a second injury. In general, an athlete should not return to play on the same day that the diagnosis of concussion is made, and many committees advise a period of at least 24 to 48 hours of cognitive and physical rest following the incident. To help avoid second injuries, athletes should have a gradual and stepwise return to play and avoid full contact until symptoms have resolved and they have cleared a concussion protocol. Many different sports governing bodies have guidelines and protocols for athletes to follow before returning to play after a concussion is diagnosed (**Table 11.7**). If possible, soldiers should not return to activities that put them at risk for injury until their symptoms have resolved and they have been cleared by medical staff. Avoidance of alcohol and illicit drugs can minimize high-risk behaviors and decrease chances of accidental head trauma. Patients should be counseled on indications to seek emergency care, particularly if no head imaging was obtained.

Although pain is a common component of the presentation, it may often be left unaddressed in the ED. Because the pathophysiology of mTBI is complex, the best analgesia is unclear, with limited information available on treatment options. Generally, most guidelines, including the CDC, recommend offering nonopioid analgesia such as ibuprofen or acetaminophen to patients with painful headaches after acute mTBI, but also provide counseling regarding the risks of analgesic overuse, including rebound headache.

TABLE 11.7	Guidelines on Returning to School or Play[a]		
	RETURN TO SCHOOL		
Stage	Aim	Activity	Goal of Each Step
1	Daily activities at home that do not give the student symptoms	Typical activities during the day as long as they do not increase symptoms (ie, reading, texting, screen time). Start at 5-15 min at a time and gradually increase	Gradual return to typical activities
2	School activities	Homework, reading, or other cognitive activities outside of the classroom	Increase tolerance to cognitive work
3	Return to school part time	Gradual introduction of schoolwork. May need to start with a partial school day or increased breaks throughout the day	Increase academic activities
4	Return to school full time	Gradually progress	Return to full academic activities and catch up on missed work
	RETURN TO PLAY		
Stage	Aim	Activity	Goal of Each Step
1	Symptom-limiting activity	Daily activities that do not provoke symptoms	Gradual reintroduction of activities
2	Light aerobic activity	Walking or stationary cycling at slow to medium pace. No resistance training	Increase heart rate
3	Sport-specific exercise	Running or skating drills. No head impact activities	Add movement
4	Noncontact training drills	Harder training drills, that is, passing drills. May start progressive resistance training	Exercise, coordination, and increased thinking
5	Full contact practice	Following medical clearance	Restore confidence and assess functional skills by coaching staff
6	Return to sport	Normal game play	

[a]From Canadian guide or Berlin consensus.

Cognitive rest may come in the form of taking time off from school and/or work. Those affected may need a brief leave of absence, reduction in work, or longer time frames to complete required tasks. Patients are generally encouraged to adhere to healthy sleep schedules that may include daytime naps.

Although physical and cognitive rest has long been considered key components of recovery after a concussion, there is a lack of supportive literature showing this is helpful. An alternate hypothesis has emerged that physical and cognitive activity may be helpful, particularly in patients with symptoms persisting beyond 1 month after the head injury. It is possible that after an initial period of a few days of rest, early exercise may actually help speed up recovery times. A large pediatric study suggests that patients who resumed physical activity within 7 days of acute injury had reduced risk of persistent post-concussive symptoms at 28 days when compared to those who did not engage in physical activity within 7 days.[16] It is hypothesized that prolonged avoidance of regular mental and physical activities may contribute to the persistence of symptoms, and may even lead to secondary symptoms such as depression, anxiety, and physiologic deconditioning. Further research is required to elucidate best practices for treatment on concussions.

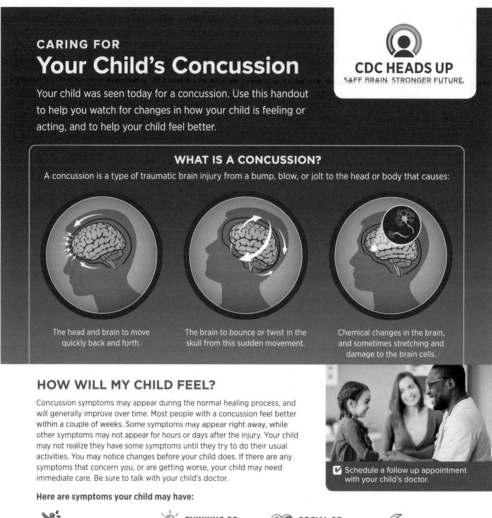

CARING FOR
Your Child's Concussion

CDC HEADS UP
SAFE BRAIN. STRONGER FUTURE.

Your child was seen today for a concussion. Use this handout to help you watch for changes in how your child is feeling or acting, and to help your child feel better.

WHAT IS A CONCUSSION?

A concussion is a type of traumatic brain injury from a bump, blow, or jolt to the head or body that causes:

The head and brain to move quickly back and forth.

The brain to bounce or twist in the skull from this sudden movement.

Chemical changes in the brain, and sometimes stretching and damage to the brain cells.

HOW WILL MY CHILD FEEL?

Concussion symptoms may appear during the normal healing process, and will generally improve over time. Most people with a concussion feel better within a couple of weeks. Some symptoms may appear right away, while other symptoms may not appear for hours or days after the injury. Your child may not realize they have some symptoms until they try to do their usual activities. You may notice changes before your child does. If there are any symptoms that concern you, or are getting worse, your child may need immediate care. Be sure to talk with your child's doctor.

☑ Schedule a follow up appointment with your child's doctor.

Here are symptoms your child may have:

PHYSICAL	THINKING OR REMEMBERING	SOCIAL OR EMOTIONAL	SLEEP
· Bothered by light or noise	· Attention or concentration problems	· Anxiety or nervousness	· Sleeping less than usual
· Dizziness or balance problems	· Feeling slowed down	· Irritability or easily angered	· Sleeping more than usual
· Feeling tired, no energy	· Foggy or groggy	· Feeling more emotional	· Trouble falling asleep
· Headaches	· Problems with short- or long-term memory	· Sadness	
· Nausea or vomiting (early on)	· Trouble thinking clearly		
· Vision problems			

Figure 11.3: U.S. Centers for Disease Control and Prevention (CDC) HEADS UP discharge instructions. Courtesy of the Centers for Disease Control and Prevention.

A key component to the discharge from the ED includes clear written and verbal discharge instructions to both the patient and family/friend, if available, along with clear instructions on when to follow up, and with who. The CDC has developed a series of educational initiatives known as HEADS UP, designed to increase awareness and protect against repeat injuries (www.cdc.gov/headsup).[17] HEADS UP offers many free resources for both health care providers and patients/parents that can easily be found on their website and utilized. Brochures highlighting discharge instructions can be printed out and given to parents on discharge from the ED; see **Figure 11.3**. Good education and guidance regarding concussion diagnosis and treatment/recovery plans have been shown to decrease patient stress regarding the diagnosis and lead to faster recovery, as demonstrated in several studies.

COMPLICATIONS/OUTCOMES

Patients with mTBI may endure persistent symptoms, most commonly headache, dizziness/fogginess, difficulty with concentration, and problems with balance. Symptoms may resolve within minutes to hours, and most commonly resolve within days. However, in some cases, a full recovery can take weeks to months. Headaches and/or dizziness are the most commonly reported post-concussive symptoms. Patients should be followed up by a specialist until all symptoms have fully resolved, and should be counseled on the risk of further head injuries. A multidisciplinary approach to follow-up and management of concussion-related complications is important and should be made available.

Post-Concussion Syndrome

In some circumstances, post-concussive symptoms may persist longer than 3 months in which case a diagnosis of PCS is considered. Symptoms may include headache, dizziness, fatigue, irritability, difficulty with concentration, insomnia, impairment of memory, and reduced tolerance to stress, alcohol, and emotional excitement. One study found that the median duration of symptoms in patients with PCS was 7 months with a range of up to 26 years.[18] It is thought that women and elderly patients are more likely to have PCS than do men and younger patients. PCS is often associated with multiple concussions, but in one sports study, 23% of players had PCS after only one concussion. It is also believed that lower economic status is associated with a greater risk for PCS. As with the concussion itself, it is unknown if PCS is caused by structural damage or psychological factors. Although there is no specific treatment, physical therapy and behavioral counseling are thought to aid in recovery. Fortunately, for most patients with PCS, the symptoms resolve completely. Patients should have a follow-up with a specialist experienced in TBI and may need to be accommodated to have more rest time and to alter their mental and physical activities.

Second-Impact Syndrome

Second-impact syndrome (SIS) is contested in the medical literature. The vast majority of cases occur in children younger than 16 years old. It is thought to occur when the brain suffers a new injury before it has fully healed from a previous one. An athlete with a history of previous concussion is more likely to have future concussive injuries than those with no history. One in 15 players may have additional concussions in the same playing season.[19] Sustaining a second concussion can be permanently debilitating, and in rare cases it is fatal. It is thought that the brain's vascular structures become damaged, leading to massive cerebral edema, increases in intracranial pressure (ICP), and can ultimately lead to herniation, profound disability, and, in some cases, death. For this reason, athletes suffering a concussion should be placed on a concussion recovery protocol and avoid further head injuries until all of their symptoms from the first concussion have resolved.

Chronic Traumatic Encephalopathy

CTE is a serious and irreversible condition that affects patients' neurologic and psychological health, and can lead to problems with mood, behavior, and judgment, and may also lead to memory loss and progressive dementia. It is thought that repetitive brain trauma including concussions is the main risk factor for developing CTE, although it is unclear what other risk factors or injuries may predispose a patient to developing CTE. It is possible that there is a genetic predisposition, but there is no definitive evidence to support this. CTE can only be diagnosed postmortem, making its true prevalence difficult to determine. Certain sports that predispose to repetitive head trauma such as boxing and football are likely to put athletes at a higher risk. A recent study of 111 former NFL players showed 99% had CTE[20]; however, selection bias and failure to account for comorbidities impact the finding. Although Tau protein damage is thought to be the dominant etiology of CTE, other contributing factors such as neuroinflammation and axonal damage may also play a role. Research into imaging techniques such as functional MRI and biomarkers including PET signals aimed at diagnosing CTE in living subjects is ongoing.

Despite all the possible related conditions associated with concussions such as PCS, SIS, CTE, and other conditions such as PTSD, most patients recover within days to weeks of the event and have good long-term outcomes. People who have suffered repetitive brain trauma and concussions, on the other hand, should focus on minimizing the risk of recurrent injuries to decrease the chances of having long-term effects and symptoms. Currently, there are no good predictors of which subset of patients suffering one or more concussions is at risk for developing more long-term symptoms such as those seen in PCS or CTE. Researchers are evaluating the possibility of a genetic predisposition putting a person at higher risk for developing such conditions after sustaining an mTBI.

TIPS AND PEARLS

- A concussion is a subcategory of mTBI that results from direct or indirect biomechanical forces to the brain, leading to a transient change in brain function with no evidence of injury on head CT (if one is obtained).
- Concussions are often underreported, but may have significant neurobehavioral sequelae that impact a patient's quality of life.
- Currently, there is no universally accepted gold standard to confirm the diagnosis of concussion, for example, imaging, a biomarker, or neuropsychological test. Evaluation tools can help standardize examination findings and aid in confirming a diagnosis.
- The most common symptoms associated with a concussion include headache, feeling "dizzy" or "foggy," or nausea/vomiting; however, none of these are specific or diagnostic.
- LOC and amnesia are diagnostic of concussion, but absence of these features does not eliminate diagnosis.
- If an athlete is suspected of having a concussion, they should immediately be removed from the activity for a formal evaluation. Avoidance of a secondary injury is critical.
- Use of serum biomarkers S-100B or GFAP + UCH-L1 can be used as a screening tool for which patients may require neuroimaging.
- Most patients with a concussion recover quickly, but some can have long-term sequelae; some may develop CTE, particularly if they experience repeat injuries.
- Education and clear discharge instructions should be arranged with patients after being evaluated for a concussion. Access to appropriate follow-up should also be arranged, and treatment may require a multidisciplinary approach.

EVIDENCE

Do computerized evaluation tools have a role in non–sports-related concussion assessment in the ED?

There are numerous evaluation tools available to aid in the diagnosis of concussion, most commonly used in sports medicine and in the military. The Military Acute Concussion Evaluation (MACE) tool is mostly utilized in the military, but is limited because baseline testing is often not available. Many other tools are utilized by different sports organizations and schools to help guide diagnosis and treatment. Some tools such as the SCAT5 are comprehensive and include a detailed neurologic examination, whereas others known as neuropsychological tests such as Immediate Post-concussion Assessment and Cognitive Testing (ImPACT) do not incorporate a physical examination component and are self-administered computer-based or pencil-and-paper–based modules.

Although many of these tools are commonly used on the sidelines and in locker rooms immediately after a minor head trauma, there may be a role for their use in the ED when used in conjunction with a thorough history and physical. Use of the ImPACT tool takes about 25 minutes to complete, and consists of six computerized modules testing verbal memory, reaction time, visual-motor speed, and visual-memory functioning, as well as a validity index to determine whether poor test results may reflect poor effort during baseline scoring. It is the most widely used neuropsychological computerized test, and is used by many professional sports organizations. One study of athletes reported a 91.4% sensitivity and 69.1% specificity for diagnosing concussion.[21]

Clinicians should consider using ImPACT to aid in the evaluation of the patient with an mTBI, but its use in the ED is not clearly defined, and no single test has proved sufficient for stand-alone use in the diagnosis of SRCs. There has not been standardization for age and no normative data sets to help interpret results. Owing to these limitations, its role is not clearly defined, but its use is likely helpful as one component of the concussion assessment.

Are decision rules useful in determining which mTBI patients need a head CT?

More than 2.5 million patients present annually to U.S. EDs for evaluation of head trauma. After a patient sustains a minor head injury, a structural injury that could require neurosurgical intervention should still be in the differential diagnosis. Some high-risk features such as persistently low or decreasing GCS, multiple episodes of vomiting or seizures, or use of anticoagulants are some factors that would clearly indicate the need for an emergent head CT. In less severe cases, the decision may not be so obvious, and overuse of CT imaging can lead to increased costs, prolonged length of visit, and radiation exposure to the patient.

Many tools are available to identify mTBI candidates for head CT, but two of the most commonly used and validated options in adults are the New Orleans Criteria (NOC) and the Canadian CT Head Rule (CCHR). One validation study comparing the two found that both had a sensitivity nearing 100%, for determining patients with clinically important brain injury and need for neurosurgical intervention.[22] CCHR has higher specificity than does NOC for both the need for neurosurgical intervention (76% vs 12%) and for clinically important brain injuries (51% vs 13%). The ACEP guidelines released in 2008 lists Level A and B recommendations for which patients who have had an mTBI require a head CT.[8,9] In those guidelines, patients are separated into those who experienced LOC and those who did not. In the pediatric population, Pediatric Emergency Care Applied Research Network (PECARN) reported a sensitivity approaching 100% in all age groups.[23] Use of these clinical decision tools may aid a physician in determining which patients suffering an mTBI require a head CT and may result in reduced imaging rates.

In patients with an mTBI, can serum biomarkers rule out the need for a CT?

S100B is one biomarker that is used in the international community to determine which patients with an mTBI required a CT. S100B is predominantly found in astrocytes and found mostly in cerebrospinal fluid (CSF; 18:1 ratio compared to serum); after a TBI, it may leak from the CNS and cross the blood-brain barrier (BBB) into the serum. Although not yet FDA approved in the United States and with limitations such as lack of access for testing in U.S. laboratories, ACEP acknowledged the use of biomarkers in its 2008 Clinical Policy by giving the use of S100B a level C recommendation.[8] Levels less than 0.1 µg/L measured within 4 hours of injury have a sensitivity of 96.8% for ruling out a neurosurgical lesion. Unfortunately, many patients often present greater than 4 hours from the time of injury. In addition, S100B is not specific to the CNS, and elevated levels are found in polytrauma and after strenuous physical activity.

In 2018, the FDA approved a panel of biomarkers, UCH-L1 and GFAP, based on a prospective multicenter study of patients older than 18 years of age who presented to EDs with blunt head trauma within 12 hours of injury, a GCS between 9 and 15, and who had a CT of the head.[24] Of 1959 patients, only 39 patients had a GCS of 9 to 13 and 31% of those had injuries. Among all participants, 66% tested biomarker positive. The test had a sensitivity of 97.6% and a negative predictive value (NPV) of 99.6% for injury. The positive predictive value (PPV) among patients with GCS 14 to 15 was only 8.8%. The study demonstrates high sensitivity and NPV for the combined use of UCH-L1 and GFAP biomarker testing.

Although many challenges exist before the routine use serum biomarkers are incorporated into clinical practice, there is a mounting body of evidence supporting their use. Evidence supports a role for use of multiple biomarkers in combination to improve sensitivity and specificity.[13] In the future, use of biomarker testing will likely assist in determining need for neuroimaging; their role in assisting determining prognosis is unclear.

Are signs and symptoms sufficient to diagnose a concussion?

Concussions present with many different clinical findings. Observed physiologic signs, subjective symptoms, and deficits of neurologic or cognitive function are used to help determine which patients may have experienced a concussion or a potential concussive event. The development of symptoms related to a concussion does not always occur immediately after an injury and may present within hours to days after the event. Some findings are common and often detected on a routine history and physical, whereas others may be more subtle and difficult to detect, for example, neurocognitive deficits. Complicating the diagnosis, many patients who have evidence of injury, for example, decreased reaction time or decreased attention, have none of the expected findings associated with concussion, for example, headache, nausea, or fogginess.

A comprehensive review of concussion literature funded by the Department of Defense and the Brain Trauma Foundation identified some prevalent signs and consistent indicators of concussion[25]:

- Observed and documented disorientation or confusion immediately after the event
- Impaired balance within 1 day of the injury
- Slower reaction time within 2 days of the injury
- Impaired verbal learning and memory within 2 days of the injury

This analysis of the literature found the most common symptoms for subjects with potential concussive events versus controls include headache (93% vs 18%), dizziness (64% vs 4%), blurred vision (75% vs 0%), and nausea (61% vs 7%). Patients may also commonly report amnesia or problems with memory and feeling loss of balance, fatigue, other visual symptoms, or changes in mood and sleeping habits.

There is a lack of distinction between which signs, symptoms, and deficits are specific to concussion versus other injuries or comorbidities. Recovery and time to resolution of symptoms also vary widely. Although one particular finding cannot independently rule in the diagnosis of concussion, the presence of the abovementioned listed signs in patients sustaining an mTBI may be an indicator of the underlying change in brain function used to identify that a concussion occurred.

References

1. Haydel MJ, Preston CA, Mills TJ, et al. Indications for computed tomography in patients with minor head injury. *N Engl J Med*. 2000;343(2):100-105. doi: 10.1056/NEJM200007133430204

2. Stiell IG, Wells GA, Vandemheen K, et al. The Canadian CT Head Rule for patients with minor head injury. *Lancet*. 2001;357(9266):1391-1396. doi: 10.1016/s0140-6736(00)04561-x

3. Taylor CA, Bell JM, Breiding MJ, Xu L. Traumatic brain injury–related emergency department visits, hospitalizations, and deaths — United States, 2007 and 2013. *MMWR Surveill Summ*. 2017;66(9):1-16. doi: 10.15585/mmwr.ss6609a1

4. Kann L, McManus T, Harris WA, et al. Youth risk behavior surveillance – United States, 2017. *MMWR Surveill Summ*. 2018;67(8):1-114. doi: 10.15585/mmwr.ss6708a1

5. Crisco JJ, Fiore R, Beckwith JG, et al. Frequency and location of head impact exposures in individual collegiate football players. *J Athl Train*. 2010;45(6):549-559. doi: 10.4085/1062-6050-45.6.549

6. Broglio SP, Eckner JT, Martini D, et al. Cumulative head impact burden in high school football. *J Neurotrauma*. 2011;28(10):2069-2078. doi: 10.1089/neu.2011.1825

7. Echemendia RJ, Meeuwisse W, McCrory P, et al. The Sport Concussion Assessment Tool 5th Edition (SCAT5): background and rationale. *Br J Sports Med*. 2017;51(11):848-850.

8. ACEP. https://www.acep.org/patient-care/clinical-policies/mild-traumatic-brain-injury2/

9. Jagoda AS, Bazarian JJ, Bruns JJ, et al. Clinical policy: neuroimaging and decision making in adult mild traumatic brain injury in the acute setting. *Ann Emerg Med*. 2008;52(6):714-748. doi: 10.1016/j.annemergmed.2008.08.021

10. Thelin EP, Nelson DW, Bellander B-M. A review of the clinical utility of serum S100B protein levels in the assessment of traumatic brain injury. *Acta Neurochir (Wien)*. 2017;159(2):209-225. doi: 10.1007/s00701-016-3046-3

11. Schulte S, Podlog LW, Hamson-Utley JJ, et al. A systematic review of the biomarker S100B: implications for sport-related concussion management. *J Athl Train*. 2014;49(6):830-850. doi: 10.4085/1062-6050-49.3.33

12. David A, Mari C, Vignaud F, et al. Evaluation of S100B blood level as a biomarker to avoid computed tomography in patients with mild head trauma under antithrombotic medication. *Diagn Interv Imaging*. 2017;98(7):551-556. doi: 10.1016/j.diii.2017.03.010

13. Undén J, Romner B. Can low serum levels of S100B predict normal CT findings after minor head injury in adults?: an evidence-based review and meta-analysis. *J Head Trauma Rehabil*. 2010;25(4):228-240. doi: 10.1097/HTR.0b013e3181e57e22

14. Diaz-Arrastia R, Wang KKW, Papa L, et al. Acute biomarkers of traumatic brain injury: relationship between plasma levels of ubiquitin C-terminal hydrolase-L1 and glial fibrillary acidic protein. *J Neurotrauma*. 2014;31(1):19-25. doi: 10.1089/neu.2013.3040

15. Lagerstedt L, Egea-Guerrero JJ, Bustamante A, et al. Combining H-FABP and GFAP increases the capacity to differentiate between CT-positive and CT-negative patients with mild traumatic brain injury. *PLoS One*. 2018;13(7). doi: 10.1371/journal.pone.0200394

16. Guthrie R. Physical activity following acute concussion and persistent postconcussive symptoms in children and adolescents. *Phys Sportsmed*. 2018;46(4):416-419. doi: 10.1080/00913847.2018.1516479

17. Centers for Disease Control and Prevention. Caring for your child's concussion: discharge instructions. 2020. https://www.cdc.gov/traumaticbraininjury/pdf/pediatricmtbiguidelineeducationaltools/2018-CDC_mTBI_Discharge-Instructions-508.pdf

18. Tator CH, Davis HS, Dufort PA, et al. Postconcussion syndrome: demographics and predictors in 221 patients. *J Neurosurg*. 2016;125(5):1206-1216. doi: 10.3171/2015.6.JNS15664

19. Guskiewicz KM, McCrea M, Marshall SW, et al. Cumulative effects associated with recurrent concussion in collegiate football players: the NCAA Concussion Study. *JAMA*. 2003;290(19):2549-2555. doi: 10.1001/jama.290.19.2549

20. Mez J, Daneshvar DH, Kiernan PT, et al. Clinicopathological evaluation of chronic traumatic encephalopathy in players of American football. *JAMA*. 2017;318(4):360-370. doi: 10.1001/jama.2017.8334

21. Schatz P, Sandel N. Sensitivity and specificity of the online version of ImPACT in high school and collegiate athletes. *Am J Sports Med*. 2013;41(2):321-326. doi: 10.1177/0363546512466038

22. Stiell IG, Clement CM, Rowe BH, et al. Comparison of the Canadian CT Head Rule and the New Orleans Criteria in patients with minor head injury. *JAMA*. 2005;294(12):1511-1518. doi: 10.1001/jama.294.12.1511

23. Kuppermann N, Holmes JF, Dayan PS, et al. Identification of children at very low risk of clinically-important brain injuries after head trauma: a prospective cohort study [published correction appears in *Lancet*. 2014;383(9914):308]. *Lancet*. 2009;374(9696):1160-1170. doi: 10.1016/S0140-6736(09)61558-0

24. Bazarian JJ, Biberthaler P, Welch RD, et al. Serum GFAP and UCH-L1 for prediction of absence of intracranial injuries on head CT (ALERT-TBI): a multicentre observational study. *Lancet Neurol*. 2018;17(9):782-789. doi: 10.1016/s1474-4422(18)30231-x

25. Carney N, Ghajar J, Jagoda A, et al. Concussion guidelines step 1: systematic review of prevalent indicators. *Neurosurgery*. 2014;75:(Suppl 1):S3-S15. doi: 10.1227/NEU.0000000000000433

26. French L, McCrea M, Baggett M. The Military Acute Concussion Evaluation (MACE). *J Spec Oper Med*. 2008;8(1):68-77.

Head Trauma (Severe)

Scott A. Goldberg

Cappi Lay

THE CLINICAL CHALLENGE

Management of severe traumatic brain injury (TBI) focuses not on reversing the initial insult but on minimizing sequelae and preventing secondary injury mediated by hypoxia, hypotension, hyperventilation, seizures, and increased bleeding. These secondary injuries, occurring after the initial insult, can have a profound impact on clinical course and patient outcomes.

Prehospital providers are tasked with the rapid identification of the brain-injured patient and the provision of expedient stabilization and transport to an appropriate facility for definitive care. Prehospital management focuses on the basics of stabilization and resuscitation, avoiding hypoxia, maintaining eucapnia, and identifying and correcting hypotension.

On arrival at the emergency department (ED), the patient should undergo an initial evaluation following the principles of trauma care. The airway should be secured, oxygenation and ventilation secured, and blood pressure optimized. The initial physical examination and brief neurologic examination should include an evaluation of mental status and calculation of a Glasgow Coma Scale (GCS) score, which should be frequently reassessed. In the setting of airway compromise necessitating endotracheal intubation, rapid sequence intubation (RSI) is the preferred technique, optimizing first-pass success. Preoxygenation is essential. Following intubation, the goals of ventilator management are to maintain normoxia and to avoid hyperventilation and hypocapnia. Blood pressure should be maintained with fluid resuscitation and the addition of vasopressors as necessary: Traditional mean arterial pressure (MAP) goals of 65 mm Hg may be insufficient to maintain cerebral perfusion pressure (CPP).

Patients who are anticoagulated should be expeditiously reversed with a goal international normalized ratio (INR) of <1.5. If the patient is taking antiplatelet agents, platelet transfusion may be considered, although existing literature is equivocal on its benefit. Tranexamic acid (TXA) should be administered if the patient presents within 3 hours of injury. Once the patient is stabilized, attention is turned toward management in the intensive care unit or surgical management with hematoma evacuation and cranial decompression.

PATHOPHYSIOLOGY

Anatomy and Intracranial Physiology

The brain is coated with three layers: the pia mater, adhered to the brain itself; the arachnoid mater; and the meningeal dura mater. The inner aspect of the skull is lined with periosteal dura, reflecting back on itself to form the meningeal dura that compartmentalizes the various components of the brain. In adults, the bones of the skull are fused, creating a chamber with a fixed volume. The internal components of this vault are the brain tissue, cerebrospinal fluid (CSF), and arterial and venous blood compartments.

All intracranial pressure (ICP) issues are intracranial volume issues. Owing to the rigid nature of the skull, the cumulative volume of intracranial contents must always equal the sum of the various components within it. As long as the cranium is intact, improving compliance requires the reduction of the volumes of one or more of these components. The CSF and venous blood compartments normally serve as a capacitor whose volumes can be extruded with little impact on neurologic function. However, because this capacitance is exhausted with the incursion of hemorrhage or edema, ICP rises rapidly.

Cerebral autoregulation also plays an important role in determining ICP. In the uninjured state, cerebral arterioles reflexively dilate and constrict in response to changes in systemic blood pressure, maintaining a constant cerebral blood flow (CBF). Increases in cerebral arteriolar diameter, even at constant flow, have the effect of increasing the intracranial blood volume. In the injured brain where intracranial compliance has been compromised, increases in arterial blood volume due to arteriolar dilation may lead to upward swings in ICP.

Injury Patterns

Primary brain injury occurs at the time of the initial insult. This may be the result of a direct force to the head or by an indirect force, such as in an acceleration-deceleration injury. Penetrating injuries may cause direct injury to the brain and surrounding tissues or indirect injury secondary to associated concussive forces. Both epidural hematoma (EDH) and subdural hematoma (SDH) can progress quickly owing to the high pressure of the arterial system. Traumatic subarachnoid hemorrhage (tSAH) is the most common pattern of severe TBI, resulting from shearing of the small subarachnoid vessels and leading to accumulation of blood in the subarachnoid space, within the CSF and meningeal intima. Unlike hemorrhagic lesions, traumatic axonal injury (TAI) results from stretching or tearing of axonal connections within the brain tissue. Intracerebral hematomas or contusions of the cerebrum or cerebellum may also occur.

Cerebral Herniation Syndromes

Herniation refers to the mechanical deformation of brain tissue caused by a mass lesion or cerebral swelling that destroys tissue architecture. Although herniation often occurs in the setting of increased total ICP, certain lesions may result in herniation syndromes and death at relatively low ICP as a result of their locations within the intracranial vault close to vital structures. The temporal lobe and cerebellum are examples of locations where lesions causing local swelling may rapidly result in neurologic deterioration and death due to their direct compression on the adjacent brainstem. Conversely, elevated ICP can cause diffuse neuronal injury even in the absence of frank herniation because of neuronal ischemia.

PREHOSPITAL CONCERNS

Field providers are an essential link between the point of injury and definitive care. Initial interventions provided on scene can impact morbidity and mortality; and prehospital providers are tasked with clinical decision-making, informing where, when, and how rapidly a patient is transported to hospital. Management in the field should be focused on the rapid identification of possible TBI and management of any other traumatic injuries. As with in-hospital management, prevention of secondary injury through the maintenance of blood pressure > 110 mm Hg systolic and oxygenation saturation > 90% is paramount. Continuous pulse oximetry monitoring and frequent assessment of blood pressure should be utilized. A clear algorithm for prehospital management focusing on adequate oxygenation, maintaining blood pressure, and avoiding hyperventilation should be developed and used by field providers.

Airway

Advanced airway management in the field is an inherently risky procedure, and every effort must be made to maximize first-pass success. Although it is clear that some patients require immediate endotracheal intubation in the field, this population is not well defined. Advanced airway management comes at the expense of prolonged transport times and may delay definitive in-hospital care, which adversely impacts patient outcomes. Conversely, failure of the patient to protect their own airway, persistent hypoxia despite supplemental oxygen administration, and CO_2 retention are all indications for advanced airway intervention.

Paralytic-assisted endotracheal intubation in the field should only be performed by skilled practitioners practicing in a system with a rigorous quality assurance program and continuous provider training. In systems with short transport times and in patients in whom an oxygen saturation > 90% can be maintained with supplemental oxygen, definitive airway management should be delayed until arrival in the ED. All advanced airway placement should be confirmed with quantitative end-tidal capnography ($ETCO_2$), which dramatically improves the detection of improperly placed airway devices and inadvertent hyperventilation by field providers.

Blood Pressure

Avoiding hypotension, and managing it when and if it does occur, is a critical element of the prehospital treatment of the head-injured patient.[1] As MAP falls, CPP follows, predisposing to tissue ischemia. Blood pressure should be monitored as frequently as possible with the most advanced means available.[2]

Although the concept of prehospital permissive hypotension may be beneficial in some trauma patients, it is detrimental in the setting of brain injury.[1] Hypotension should be immediately identified and aggressively managed. Any ongoing external hemorrhage should be expeditiously addressed and controlled. Scalp lacerations may bleed a large volume into a bulky dressing, and a less bulky dressing should be used with firm constant manual pressure applied to avoid excessive blood loss. Fluid resuscitation should be administered on the basis of local prehospital protocols, but generally consists of crystalloids. Hypertonic saline (HTS) has been suggested as a useful resuscitation solution for patients with TBI in the field, but clinical trials have consistently failed to show any benefit over standard resuscitation with crystalloid solution.[3,4]

Agitation

Severely head-injured patients may present agitated or combative. Transporting a patient in this condition is challenging, and may be unsafe for both patient and providers. Transporting an agitated patient who is fighting against physical restraints may exacerbate physical injury, cause an increase in ICP, and interfere with stabilization and management. The priority of the field provider mirrors that of in-hospital management, including rapidly identifying alternative etiologies of agitation such as hypoglycemia, hypoxia, or hypotension.

Options for management in the field may be limited, and will be based on local emergency medical service (EMS) protocols. Ketamine has a fast onset of action when administered by the intramuscular (IM) route, and may be a viable option for rapid sedation of the agitated patient if available to prehospital providers.[5] Concerns about neurotoxicity and transient increases in ICP following administration have historically limited its use in TBI, although recent studies have not demonstrated any harm when used as an induction agent.[6] Benzodiazepines including midazolam are also effective in the rapid sedation of an agitated patient, but the patient must be closely monitored for hypoventilation, hypoxia, and hypotension. Antipsychotics including droperidol, haloperidol, or olanzapine are infrequently carried by prehospital providers, but may be additional considerations if available.[7,8]

THE FOCUSED EXAMINATION

Initial Assessment

A thorough history and physical examination are important, but emergent stabilization must be prioritized in all patients with suspected TBI while minimizing secondary injury during the immediate resuscitation. A brief neurologic examination should be performed on all patients with suspected TBI if at all possible before the administration of sedatives or paralytics, and the neck should be evaluated for evidence of a cervical spine fracture. If the patient is unable to cooperate with a neurologic evaluation, a cervical collar should be placed and remain in place until a definitive neurologic examination can be performed.

Focused Neurologic Examination

Mental Status and Glasgow Coma Score

Evaluation of the patient's mental status is one of the most critical components of the neurologic evaluation of the patient with TBI. The GCS (**Table 12.1**) is one of the strongest predictors of outcome following TBI and should be calculated on all patients with suspected TBI. More important than the initial GCS, however, is the change in GCS over time. A declining GCS is a marker of poor prognosis, and a decline in GCS score of ≥ 2 should prompt immediate reevaluation.

A reliable total GCS score may be challenging to obtain in certain patient populations, such as intubated or intoxicated patients or those with other injuries affecting the eye opening or speech component of the GCS score. In these patients, evaluation of the motor component of the GCS score in isolation may still provide sufficient information in lieu of the total GCS (**Table 12.2**).[9]

Pupil Examination

Although a portion of the general population has anisocoria at baseline, pupil asymmetry, and specifically a change in the pupillary examination over time, indicates increasing ICP. Although pupil asymmetry in isolation is neither sensitive nor specific for intracranial pathology, a change in pupil asymmetry should raise concern of increasing ICP.

Motor Examination

The patient's acute motor examination should evaluate for symmetry of strength. A response to pressure is a reasonable surrogate in the comatose or otherwise uncooperative patient. Decorticate posturing (abnormal flexion) implies injury above the brainstem, whereas decerebrate posturing (abnormal extension) suggests an injury of the deeper brain areas and portends a poorer prognosis. Abnormal posturing on arrival at the ED strongly suggests increased ICP and should trigger immediate empiric treatment.

Invasive Monitoring

TBI outcomes are inversely related to the amount of time the patient spends with elevated ICP. Although invasive ICP monitor placement has the advantage of providing a numerical trigger for

TABLE 12.1	The Glasgow Coma Scale Score					
	1	2	3	4	5	6
Best motor response	None	Extension	Abnormal flexion	Normal flexion	Localizing	Obeys commands
Best verbal response	None	Sounds	Words	Confused	Oriented	
Eye opening	None	To pressure	To speech	Spontaneous		

Data from Teasdale G, Maas A, Lecky F, Manley G, Stocchetti N, Murray G: The Glasgow Coma Scale at 40 years: Standing the test of time. *Lancet Neurol* 13:844 -854, 2014 and Teasdale, G., & Jennett, B. (1974). Assessment of coma and impaired consciousness: a practical scale. *The Lancet*, 304(7872), 81-84.

TABLE 12.2	The mGCS Score and SMS					
	None	Extension	Abnormal Flexion	Normal Flexion	Localizing	Obeys Commands
tGCS	1	2	3	4	5	6
SMS	0				1	2
mGCS	Severe injury					Minor injury

mGCS, motor Glasgow Coma Scale score; SMS, Simplified Motor Score; tGCS, total Glasgow Coma Scale score.

delivering treatment, emergency clinicians will generally make decisions about ICP management in the absence of invasive ICP monitoring. Carefully monitoring the clinical examination and radiologic findings are a viable alternative to ICP monitoring, at least until such invasive monitoring is available.

Laboratory Testing

No specific laboratory tests that reliably diagnose TBI or predict outcomes have been identified. Laboratory evaluation in patients with TBI should follow standard practice for management of the trauma patient. The INR should be routinely evaluated, and although there are no clear guidelines for INR target, we recommend an INR < 1.5.[10] The direct oral anticoagulants (DOACs) are not reliably detected by routine coagulation testing, making the history essential in identifying patients who require reversal. The brain is a rich source of tissue thromboplastin that is released after injury, causing a consumptive coagulopathy with an elevated INR that is not related to oral anticoagulant use. An elevated INR in this case is a poor prognostic indicator.

Recent interest has shifted to the use of viscoelastic hemostatic assays in trauma such as thromboelastography (TEG) and rotational thromboelastometry (ROTEM) to better characterize the specific nature of the coagulopathy present and potentially guide treatments, providing information not only about the initiation of clotting but also about clot strength and fibrinolysis. Unfortunately, the standard TEG and ROTEM assays have inconsistent sensitivity for the presence of the newer DOACs such as dabigatran, rivaroxaban, and apixaban, as well as for antiplatelet medications such as aspirin and clopidogrel.

Radiography

The standard imaging modality in a patient with suspected TBI is non-contrast computed tomography (CT) scan of the head, which should be performed in any patient with head injury and a GCS of 14 or lower. CT imaging of the brain provides information about the likelihood of raised ICP, can demonstrate impending herniation, and guides the need for surgical intervention. The Marshall classification and the Rotterdam Score are CT grading scales developed for patients with TBI that have been shown to predict outcome. Both scoring systems have identified the presence of midline shift and compression or effacement of the basal cisterns as strongly predictive of mortality. Although hyperdense blood and obvious asymmetry are usually noticed on the CT, the loss of visible CSF spaces around the midbrain is more subtle and is an important clue to increased ICP and early herniation.

In healthy individuals, CT imaging of the brain normally demonstrates at least a thin margin of CSF outlining the midbrain (**Figure 12.1(B)**) , distinguishing it from the temporal lobes to either side. In the setting of uncal herniation, the ipsilateral temporal lobe is displaced medially, obliterating the CSF space on that side. In the setting of global cerebral edema that ultimately leads to downward transtentorial herniation, both cerebral hemispheres are displaced inferiorly, causing effacement of the cisterns bilaterally. Other CT findings that have been associated with worse outcome after TBI are the presence of midline shift >5 mm, and mass lesions >25 cm^3. All patients with TBI with cisternal effacement or significant midline shift on CT should be treated as having critically elevated ICP.

Repeated CT imaging may be useful in monitoring the evolution of TBI, and is warranted if the patient's condition changes. The utility of repeat CT scan in patients with stable neurologic examinations is less clear, and although a repeat scan 4 to 6 hours following an initial diagnostic scan is reasonable, it does not regularly change management.[11] CT angiogram may be considered in patients without a clear etiology of head trauma or in those with central subarachnoid hemorrhage, although it rarely changes management.[12,13]

Ultrasound may help identify patients at risk for intracranial hypertension by assessing optic nerve sheath diameter. The optic nerve sheath is in continuity with the dura and envelops the optic nerve with a thin intervening layer of CSF that expands under conditions of increased ICP. Nerve sheath diameter of >5.0 mm has been demonstrated to correlate with presence of intracranial hypertension with a sensitivity of 97% and a specificity of 86%.[14] Ultrasound thus has the potential to help the emergency provider expedite ICP lowering therapy in the first minutes after arrival before initial head imaging (see **Chapter 16: Headache**).

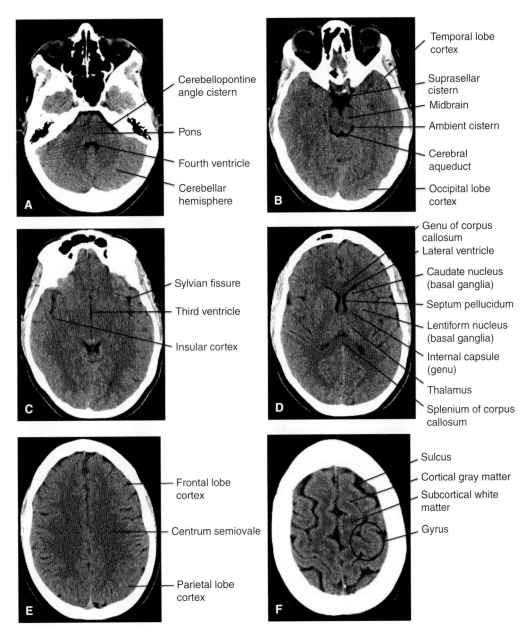

Figure 12.1: Normal computed tomography (CT) anatomy. A-F: Major brain structures of brainstem (medulla, pons, midbrain), cerebellum, and cerebral hemispheres (frontal, temporal, parietal, and occipital lobes). From Petrovic B. Brain imaging. In: Farrell TA, ed. Radiology 101. 5th ed. Wolters Kluwer; 2020:268-292. Figure 7.1.

MANAGEMENT

Airway Management

In the setting of TBI, primary airway injury may result from concomitant craniofacial trauma or neck trauma, bleeding, or vomiting. Secondary airway compromise may be caused by loss of brainstem reflexes, or may result from agitation, hypotension, or mental status changes limiting the patient's ability to protect their airway. In the setting of existing or anticipated airway compromise, the airway should be secured early to prevent secondary injury from hypoxia or hypoventilation. A brief neurologic examination should be conducted before advanced airway management with sedation or paralysis.

Before endotracheal intubation, the patient should be preoxygenated to avoid hypoxia during the intubation attempt. Volume resuscitation is paramount to avoid hypotension during intubation, especially when giving medications that may blunt sympathetic drive and its compensatory effect on blood pressure. If there is concern that the patient might become hypotensive during or immediately after intubation, vasopressors either as a drip or in push-dose should be administered before or during the intubation attempt.

Supraglottic stimulation during airway manipulation leads to a release of systemic catecholamines, resulting in a transient increase in ICP. Lidocaine to blunt this response or a defasciculating dose of succinylcholine have shown no benefit in patient-centered outcomes and are no longer recommended. Administration of a short-acting opioid, such as fentanyl at a dose of 3 mcg/kg, may blunt the sympathetic reflex and should be considered, but any benefit must be balanced against risks of hypotension.

RSI is safe and effective in the emergent setting, decreasing the risk of aspiration and increasing the likelihood of first pass success. Although research studies have not demonstrated a clear benefit of RSI over other techniques in terms of outcomes, it remains the preferred method of airway management in the patient with TBI. Etomidate (0.3 mg/kg) is the drug of choice owing to its hemodynamic stability. Ketamine (1-2 mg/kg) is an alternative, especially in a hypotensive patient. Although the use of ketamine in TBI has historically been controversial because of a purported transient increase in ICP after ketamine administration, it is generally considered safe and effective for this indication.[15,16] Rocuronium (1.2 mg/kg) is a nondepolarizing agent and as such does not cause the fasciculations and corresponding rise in ICP seen with the depolarizing agents. However, its duration of action can exceed 1 hour, making repeat neurologic assessments challenging. As such, succinylcholine (1.5 mg/kg) is the drug of choice for paralysis in patients with TBI. Rocuronium would be a second-line agent for those with contraindications to succinylcholine.

Ventilator Management Following TBI

Following intubation, ventilation parameters should be carefully controlled and eucapnia meticulously maintained. The partial pressure of arterial carbon dioxide ($PaCO_2$) is a potent regulator of cerebral arteriolar diameter, impacting ICP and in turn CBF. (see **Figure 12.2**). Reductions in $PaCO_2$ cause reflex vasoconstriction throughout the brain, whereas hypercapnia results in vasodilatation. Although hyperventilation decreases ICP, the corresponding decrease in cerebral perfusion leads to worse patient outcomes. Unfortunately, unintentional hyperventilation during manual ventilation following intubation is common, underscoring the importance of using quantitative $ETCO_2$. Although hypocapnia may be deleterious, hypercarbia ($PaCO_2 > 45$ mm Hg) has also been associated with increased hospital mortality and should similarly be avoided.

Controlled hyperventilation can acutely reduce intracranial blood volume and thereby lower ICP, albeit at the potential cost of inducing cerebral ischemia. If acute cerebral herniation is suspected on the basis of clinical examination findings, it is reasonable to use a brief period of hyperventilation in conjunction with sedation and hyperosmolar therapy to rapidly lower ICP as a temporizing measure en route to a definitive neurosurgical procedure.

The most important priority with respect to ventilator management is maintaining adequate oxygen delivery to the injured brain tissue. Cerebral vasodilation occurs in response to arterial hypoxemia when PaO_2 falls to < 58 mm Hg, corresponding to an SpO_2 of roughly 90%. In the brain-injured patient, oxygen saturation should be maintained above 95%, although minimizing excessive fraction of inspired oxygen (FiO_2) is an important aspect of ventilator management that should not be overlooked.

$$CBF = \frac{(MAP) - (ICP)}{(CVR)}$$

Figure 12.2: Cerebral blood flow. CBF; CVR, cerebrovascular resistance; ICP, intracranial pressure; MAP, mean arterial pressures.

Blood Pressure Control and Targets

CBF is directly proportional to the perfusion pressure of the intracranial compartment (CPP), which is equal to the systemic MAP minus the ICP (Figure 12.2). Rises in ICP are related to increases in one or more of the substances inside the skull; CSF, edematous brain tissue, mass lesions including extravascular blood, and intravascular blood volume, either in the arterial or venous compartments. The optimal CPP is that which triggers maximal cerebral arteriolar vasoconstriction (decreasing intracranial arterial volume) while maintaining CBF at sufficient levels to meet the brain's metabolic demand. At higher pressures, CBF is supranormal, potentially leading to increased edema or hematoma expansion. At lower pressures, autoregulatory vasodilation increases instantaneous cerebral blood volume, although not necessarily blood *flow*, and increases the risk of intracranial hypertension.

Although the generally accepted MAP goal of 65 to 70 mm Hg may be sufficient to maintain vital organ perfusion in many disease states, the presence of an intracranial mass lesion may necessitate targeting significantly higher systemic blood pressures to ensure cerebral perfusion and prevent the counterintuitive rise in ICP that may be exacerbated by relative hypotension. Even a brief episode of hypotension with SBP < 90 mm Hg has been associated with an increase in mortality. Unfortunately, precise blood pressure targets have not been well defined. Systolic blood pressure should be maintained above 100 mm Hg, and >110 mm Hg in those older than 70 years of age.[17,18]

At the other extreme, systemic hypertension has also been associated with higher rates of mortality after TBI. Hypertension may occur as a result of pain and anxiety or may be an adaptive response to neuronal injury and increased ICP. Uncontrolled hypertension has the potential to worsen cerebral edema, cause arterial distension, or contribute to hematoma expansion. However, in the setting of elevated ICP, lowering blood pressure acutely could be detrimental by inducing reflex cerebral arteriolar vasodilation and worsening cerebral ischemia.

Hyperosmolar Therapy

Immediate medical management of patients with suspected elevations in ICP includes proper head positioning, sedation and analgesia, controlled ventilation and avoidance of hypoxia, and optimization of blood pressure. For patients with signs of increased ICP despite these measures, hyperosmolar therapy is a mainstay of treatment. Mannitol and the various available concentrations of HTS have been the most utilized drugs for the acute treatment of intracranial hypertension. Existing evidence is insufficient to support the use of either mannitol or HTS preferentially.[19]

Mannitol is administered as a 20% solution given as an infusion at a dose of 0.25 to 1 g/kg. It is a metabolically inert polysaccharide that is thought to lower ICP by exerting a dehydrating effect on brain tissue and CSF, thereby decreasing intracranial volume; but it may also work by lowering blood viscosity, leading to vasoconstriction in small cerebral arteries. Immediately after administration, mannitol expands intravascular volume, but is then rapidly excreted by the kidneys, promoting brisk diuresis. Because of the strong diuretic effect of the drug, it may worsen hypovolemia, especially in those patients with traumatic blood loss.

HTS comes in varying concentrations from 3% to as high as 30%. In the ED, a typical bolus dose of HTS is 150 to 200 cc of 3% HTS. There has been speculation that using ultraconcentrated solutions (such as 23.4%) may confer an advantage over more dilute solutions by more rapidly generating an osmolar gradient across the blood-brain barrier. However, to date there is no strong evidence for using one concentration of HTS over another. Infusion of 3% HTS is safe through a 16- to 20-g peripheral line at rates up to 50 mL/hr if central venous access is not available,[20,21] although peripheral infusion of more highly concentrated solutions have not been studied.

Anticoagulant and Antiplatelet Agent Reversal

Reversing defects in coagulation after TBI is an important therapeutic intervention to limit secondary injury related to hematoma growth. The use of oral anticoagulants and antiplatelet medications has been associated with increased rates of intracerebral hemorrhage (ICH), hematoma expansion, and mortality in patients with TBI, with warfarin and DOACs associated with a 2- to 5-fold increase in the odds of mortality.[22,23] Given the potential of these agents to contribute to expanding hemorrhage, physicians should address pharmacologic reversal as soon as possible.

Reversal of Oral Anticoagulants

Warfarin inhibits the production of vitamin K–dependent clotting factors II, VII, IX, and X. Reversal of the medication's effects traditionally includes the repletion of vitamin K and the replacement of deficient clotting factors with the transfusion of fresh frozen plasma (FFP). In the setting of life-threatening hemorrhage, anticoagulation should be accomplished as fast as possible using prothrombin complex concentrate (PCC).[24-26] Recombinant factor VIIa is not recommended for warfarin reversal if PCC is available because of higher rates of venous thromboembolism associated with its use.[27] PCC dosing is typically 25 to 50 U/kg and should be followed by a repeat check of INR 30 to 60 minutes after the infusion is completed. Repeat dosing can be considered for patients whose INR has failed to correct after the initial dose.

The DOACs include the direct thrombin inhibitor dabigatran and three anti-Xa inhibitors, apixaban, edoxaban, and rivaroxaban. Dabigatran was the first agent to have a drug-specific antidote designed for the reversal of its anticoagulant effect. Idarucizumab is a monoclonal antibody fragment that binds dabigatran with 350 times more affinity than does thrombin, its target molecule in the coagulation cascade. Thrombin time is exquisitely sensitive to dabigatran, and may be used as a reliable marker of exposure to the drug when the history is in question, provided it can be obtained quickly. Idarucizumab effectively neutralizes dabigatran within 4 hours of administration, and it is the recommended treatment for traumatic ICH associated with dabigatran use. If idarucizumab is not available, PCC should be given in the setting of life-threatening TBI.

The other three DOACs commonly encountered, apixaban, rivaroxaban, and edoxaban, exert their anticoagulant effect by inhibiting activated factor X from catalyzing the conversion of prothrombin to thrombin, the common mediator of coagulation in both the intrinsic and extrinsic clotting pathways. Andexanet alfa, a decoy factor Xa molecule, has been shown to reduce anti-factor Xa activity by 92% within 15 to 30 minutes,[28] although its effect begins to wane 4 hours after infusion. The unclear bioavailability of andexanet alfa, coupled with its high cost,[29] has led to some resistance in adopting its use. Although a direct head-to-head comparison of andexanet alfa and PCC has not been performed, four-factor PCC does provide an effective alternative for major bleeding, and, in our opinion, is a reasonable option in this setting.

Reversal of Antiplatelet Drugs and Platelet Transfusion

Platelets play an essential role in hemostasis after TBI, and deficits in platelet count or function may contribute to worsening intracranial injury. Thrombocytopenia with a platelet count $<150 \times 10^6$/L is an independent risk factor for progression of hemorrhagic injury after TBI, and platelet transfusion should be initiated to a goal of at least 50-100 $\times 10^6$/L.[30]

Preinjury aspirin and clopidogrel exposure is associated with increased mortality in patients with TBI, with dual antiplatelet regimens conferring more risk than do single antiplatelet agents.[31] However, despite the clear relationship between thrombocytopenia or platelet dysfunction and worse outcome, the benefit of platelet transfusion in patients on preinjury aspirin is unclear, and the available evidence is not sufficient to recommend for or against the use of platelet transfusion in patients taking preinjury antiplatelet agents. A single unit of platelets containing a pool of four to six whole-blood platelet concentrates will reverse the effect of aspirin, but the normalization of platelet reactivity in patients taking clopidogrel requires two platelet units in most situations.

The use of desmopressin (1-deamino-8-d-arginine vasopressin, DDAVP) may have benefit for at least the partial reversal of aspirin and clopidogrel in patients with traumatic ICH. DDAVP causes a rise in circulating von Willebrand factor (vWF) and factor VIII. In small groups of patients taking aspirin with spontaneous ICH, intravenous (IV) DDAVP (0.4 mcg/kg) improves platelet function within 30 minutes of administration.[32-34] Although the evidence for clinical benefit of using IV DDAVP to reverse antiplatelet medications is not robust, a single dose of the medication should be considered in those patients on aspirin or any of the P2Y12 inhibitors with CT evidence of intracranial hemorrhage.

Targeted Temperature Management

In the setting of cardiac arrest, induced hypothermia improves neuronal survival through a combination of inhibition of inflammatory cells and cytokine production, reducing free radical damage, suppressing epileptic electrical activity, reducing cerebral metabolism, and lowering ICP. However, the effect of targeted temperature management on outcomes following TBI is less clear.[35,36] The use of targeted temperature management or induced hypothermia for patients with TBI in the ED is not currently recommended.[17]

Seizure Prophylaxis

Post-traumatic seizures (PTSs) are classified as early when they occur within 7 days of injury or late when they occur after 7 days following injury. Up to 12% of all patients who sustain blunt head trauma and 50% of those with penetrating head trauma develop early PTS. Early seizures can theoretically worsen secondary brain injury by causing hypoxia, hypercarbia, release of excitatory neurotransmitters, and increasing ICP. Although early PTSs have not been associated with worse outcomes, antiepileptic drugs (AEDs) following severe TBI are nevertheless recommended to decrease the incidence of early PTS.[17]

In the case of active seizure, benzodiazepines should be administered as first-line agents. Lorazepam (0.05-0.1 mg/kg IV) is the preferred agent for aborting seizures because of its high effectiveness and prolonged duration of action. Diazepam (0.1-0.2 mg/kg) or midazolam (0.05-0.1 mg/kg) are effective alternatives. IM midazolam is recommended for actively seizing patients in whom IV access has not been established.[37] Owing to the rapid downregulation of gamma-aminobutyric acid (GABA) receptors, an adequate initial benzodiazepine dose is preferable to incremental dosing.

For long-term anticonvulsant activity and seizure prophylaxis in early PTS, levetiracetam (40 mg/kg IV), phenytoin, or fosphenytoin (phenytoin equivalents, 15–20 mg/kg) can be administered and are equally effective.[38-40] Fosphenytoin is preferable to phenytoin owing to its rapid administration and less potential for hypotension. However, levetiracetam is increasingly used because of its slightly favorable side effect profile and reduced incidence of drug-drug interactions.

The occurrence of late PTS has been associated with significant morbidity and decrease in quality of life.[41] The development of late PTS appears to be more common in those who have experienced early PTS, but no strategy of pharmacologic prophylaxis has been shown to modify this long-term risk. Prophylactic use of AEDs is not recommended for preventing late PTS unless the patient has had at least one seizure as a result of the insult.

Intracranial Pressure Monitoring

The Monroe-Kellie doctrine emphasizes that intracranial compliance is directly related to the combined constituent volumes of brain tissue, edema, blood, and CSF, with the reduction in the intracranial volume of any of these components resulting in a drop in ICP. Owing to the relative ease of removing CSF, using a drain to divert fluid can help control ICP and prevent downward herniation. External ventricular drain (EVD) placement requires the insertion of a flexible catheter into the lateral or third ventricle. The EVD has a dual purpose of serving as an ICP monitor when it is closed to drainage and as a therapeutic device for lowering ICP when opened. Risks of EVD insertion include intraparenchymal or intraventricular hemorrhage and ventriculitis.

Although there is no strong evidence to support the routine placement of an EVD in patients with severe TBI, it should be considered to manage elevated ICP in select patients. In patients for whom an emergent EVD is to be placed in the ED, the emergency physician's role is to manage sedation and analgesia while maintaining hemodynamic stability. Because EVD infections result in ventriculitis, which is itself a life-threatening complication, ensuring a sterile environment for the placement of the drain in the ED is essential.

Steroids

Studies have consistently failed to show benefit when steroids are used in severe TBI. In fact, administration of steroids results in an increase in adverse events including infection, gastrointestinal bleeding, and mortality.[42] In patients with severe TBI, high-dose methylprednisolone is associated with increased mortality and is contraindicated.[17]

Antibiotics

In patients with penetrating head trauma or an open skull fracture, there is concern for developing intracranial infection or meningitis. There is no evidence to support the use of antibiotic prophylaxis for the prevention of meningitis or other infection in patients with blunt basilar skull fractures. However, contamination with skin, bone, hair, and tissue may be widespread when there is cavitation caused by a missile and guidelines support the use of IV prophylactic, broad-spectrum antibiotics to cover for staphylococci, gram-negative bacilli, and anaerobes for penetrating craniocerebral trauma. We recommend a combination of vancomycin 1 g twice daily, gentamycin 80 mg 3 times daily, and metronidazole 500 mg 4 times daily.[43] Infection is also a concern for patients undergoing invasive ICP monitoring, although there is insufficient evidence to commend for or against routine use of prophylactic antibiotics. Appropriate high-quality sterile technique is paramount in reducing the risk of infection.

Progesterone

Research suggesting better cognitive outcomes following TBI for female patients has led to the hypothesis that female sex hormones may be neuroprotective. In early studies, progesterone showed promise in achieving improved neurologic outcomes following TBI. Unfortunately, the available evidence has failed to show any long-term benefit of progesterone on outcomes following TBI, and progesterone is not recommended as a management strategy.[44]

Tranexamic Acid

The antifibrinolytic agent TXA has been used to decrease bleeding in traumatic injury, with a 1.5% decrease mortality when administered within 3 hours of injury in patients with traumatic hemorrhage.[45] In the setting of TBI, TXA may likewise improve clot formation and decrease the volume of intracranial bleeding. A recent large, multinational randomized trial suggests that TXA may improve head injury–related mortality in patients with GCS <13 when patients with devastating neurologic injuries are excluded.[46] However, in this study, there was no significant difference in all-cause mortality or functional neurologic outcomes with administration of TXA. The administration of TXA 1 g load over 10 minutes followed by an additional 1 g over 8 hours is a ***reasonable option for patients*** with moderate head injury.

Surgical Decompression

The care of severe TBI almost always requires the combined efforts of emergency physicians, the trauma team, and neurosurgeons. Early surgical intervention is considered in patients with unilateral temporal or temporoparietal lesions, in those patients with initial GCS score of at least 6 with contusion volume >20 cc or evidence of midline shift or cisternal effacement, or in those patients with lesions of >50 cc regardless of midline shift or cisternal compression. The presence of altered mental status, pupillary abnormalities, abnormal motor posturing, medical comorbidities, age, and imaging findings all factor in the decision to operate.

Mortality following surgical evacuation of SDH is high, especially in older patients and in those presenting with more severe neurologic deterioration. Surgical evacuation of acute SDH should be performed if clot thickness is >10 mm or if midline shift exceeds 5 mm, regardless of presenting GCS score. Patients with EDH tend to fare much better than do similar patients requiring surgery for SDH, and surgical management of EDH is generally recommended if the clot thickness is >15 mm or if there is >5 mm of midline shift.

In contrast to SDHs and EDHs that put external pressure on the brain tissue, parenchymal contusions result from disruption of vessels within the brain tissue itself. Although the majority of contusions do not require operative management, these lesions can be associated with edema and mass effect, causing secondary brain injury that requires surgical evacuation or decompression.

TIPS AND PEARLS

- Elevating the head of the bed to 30 degrees improves venous drainage and may lower ICP.
- Hyperventilation may be useful as a means to delay impending herniation, but should be used cautiously and for as short a time as possible.
- Maintaining oxygenation and perfusion are paramount. Blood pressure goals for patients with TBI may be higher than that in patients with other traumatic injuries.
- An isolated GCS is not as predictive of outcome as a change in GCS. The GCS should be checked regularly and any changes noted.
- There is no strong evidence to support the use of either HTS or mannitol as the hyperosmolar therapy of choice. Institutional guidelines on hyperosmolar therapy should be developed to guide management.
- Effacement of the basal cisterns may be an early indicator of increasing ICP. The basal cisterns should be specifically evaluated when reviewing CT imaging of patients with TBI.

EVIDENCE

What are the key concepts in the prehospital management of the patient with suspected TBI?

The field management of patients with TBI focuses on limiting secondary injury, with specific attention to oxygenation and blood pressure. A controlled, before-after, multisystem, intention to treat statewide trial in Arizona evaluated a protocol for TBI focusing on (a) prevention/treatment of hypoxia, (b) airway interventions to optimize oxygenation and ventilation in patients with GCS <9, with endotracheal intubation when basic airway interventions were inadequate, (c) prevention of hyperventilation, and (d) avoidance and treatment of hypotension. The study enrolled 21,852 patients across 130 EMS systems over almost 8 years. Adjusted survival doubled among patients with severe TBI and tripled in patients requiring endotracheal intubation.[47]

Although permissive hypotension may be beneficial in trauma patients overall, hypotension of even short duration has been shown to increase mortality in patients with TBI. In a statewide prospective study of 13,151 patients with moderate to severe TBI, any episode of hypotension below 90 mm Hg was 28% as compared to 5.6% in those without hypotension.[48] Both magnitude of hypotension and duration also play a role. In the same statewide cohort, mortality was directly correlated to hypotension "dose," a composite measure including the depth of hypotension as well as the total duration of hypotensive episodes.[49] Although guidelines recommend maintaining a systolic blood pressure above 110 mm Hg, there is little evidence for a specific blood pressure target. One study demonstrated a nearly 19% increase in mortality for each 10 mm Hg drop in blood pressure between 40 and 120 mm Hg.[1]

Management of ventilation and oxygenation are also critical components of prehospital care. One area of particular controversy is the use of endotracheal intubation for patients with TBI managed in the field. Unfortunately, the literature involving prehospital endotracheal intubation of patients with TBI is heterogeneous, involving providers of different skill levels, a variety of treatment protocols, and different enrollment criteria. A randomized controlled trial comparing intubation in the field compared to intubation on arrival at the ED for patients with TBI demonstrated favorable neurologic outcomes at 6 months (51% compared to 39%) for patients intubated in the field.[50] However, paramedics in this study had a 97% success rate for intubation, and paramedic skill level does impact outcomes for patients with TBI undergoing endotracheal intubation in the field. A large retrospective database study demonstrated worse outcomes for patients intubated by providers with less skill in endotracheal intubation,[51] a finding supported by a meta-analysis looking at six studies with a combined 4772 patients demonstrating twice the odds of death when intubation was performed by a provider with limited experience in endotracheal intubation.[52]

Inadvertent hyperventilation, particularly in the immediate post-intubation period, can also result in adverse outcomes and must be avoided. A prospective study of 418 patients with severe TBI demonstrated a significantly higher mortality rate (56% vs 30%) in patients with inadvertent hyperventilation. The use of end-tidal CO_2 may help prevent inadvertent hyperventilation, and in this same cohort inadvertent hyperventilation with pCO_2 <25 on ED arrival was reduced from 13.4% to 5.6% when end-tidal CO_2 was used.[53] Further, hypoxia during and following field intubation is associated with increased mortality,[54] although in one small study of prehospital intubation of patients with severe TBI, 84% of desaturation events occurred in patients with a starting oxygen saturation of >90%.[55] The combination of hypoxia and hypotension is particularly devastating, with a mortality rate of 43.9% in one study and twice the odds of death for patients with both as compared to either in isolation.[48]

Is there evidence to support seizure prophylaxis following severe brain injury?

The incidence of early PTS, defined as seizures occurring within the first 30 days of injury, may be as high as 30% in patients with severe TBI. Because seizures can cause hypoxia and hypercarbia and may result in increased ICP, there is a theoretical risk that early PTS may cause worsening of secondary injury and adversely affect patient outcomes following TBI. However, the effect of AEDs on the incidence of early PTSs remains unclear. In a large meta-analysis of 10 studies with 2326 patients, early administration of AEDs resulted in an odds ratio of early PTS of 0.42 (95% CI 0.23-0.73), although the overall quality of the data was poor. No difference was found in the incidence of late seizures. Further, there were no mortality differences when AEDs were administered.[39,56] A more recent meta-analysis of 16 studies reached the same conclusions.[57]

If an AED is to be administered, levetiracetam and phenytoin are both acceptable choices. A prospective observational study of 813 patients with a GCS of <9 or CT findings of TBI receiving either levetiracetam or phenytoin demonstrated equivalent rates of early PTS. Likewise, both groups had similar rates of adverse events and similar mortality rates.[58] Although early PTSs have not been consistently associated with worse outcomes, guidelines recommend AED use to decrease the incidence of early PTS when the overall benefit is thought to outweigh the risk of complications associated with such treatment.[17] Although there is no clear outcome benefit, cost and ease of administration should be considered when determining the AED to administer.

What are the appropriate blood pressure targets in patients with a brain injury?

Blood pressure plays a critical role in TBI, with even a single episode of hypotension associated with increased mortality. Unfortunately, there is no clear, evidence-based blood pressure threshold for patients with TBI. Traditional definitions of hypotension are systolic blood pressure below 90 mm Hg. However, contemporary research suggests that the threshold may be higher. A large retrospective database study of 15,733 patients with moderate to severe TBI suggests a more appropriate blood pressure threshold of 110 mm Hg systolic. Specifically, the best fit model for blood pressure, minimizing the risk of death, was >110 mm Hg for those patients 15 to 49 years of age and >70 years of age, and >100 mm Hg for those 50 to 69 years of age.[18]

However, even this more conservative blood pressure threshold may be insufficient. In the prehospital environment, not only depth but duration of hypotension has also been shown to increase mortality.[49] Further, in a large prospective observational study of 3844 patients with moderate to severe TBI managed in the prehospital setting, an 18.8% increase in odds of death was found for each 10 mm Hg drop in systolic blood pressure below 140 mm Hg.[1] Although current guidelines recommend maintaining a systolic blood pressure of >110 mm Hg,[17] maintaining a systolic blood pressure of at least 140 mm Hg may be appropriate, although further well-controlled trials are needed.

Is there evidence to support hyperosmolar therapy in severe TBI?

In patents with suspected elevations in ICP that is refractory to sedation, analgesia, and CSF drainage, hyperosmolar fluids are used in an effort to reduce ICP. However, in the emergent setting, the evidence base for hyperosmolar fluids, and more specifically which fluid to use, is poor.

Few studies have directly compared HTS to mannitol. In one meta-analysis of 12 randomized trials, inclusive of 464 patients, no differences were found in mortality or neurologic outcome, although there was a trend in favor of HTS.[59] Further, CPP was higher with HTS, and ICP lower, at 90 to 120 minutes. Unfortunately, the limited number of patients included in these studies precludes any recommendation from the authors as to benefit of HTS over mannitol. Another meta-analysis of 11 studies likewise found no benefit to using one agent over another.[60] Finally, a Cochrane review of six trials including 287 subjects found no difference in neurologic outcomes or mortality using either agent,[19] although rebound hypotension was seen more frequently in subjects receiving mannitol. Overall, the authors found very poor-quality evidence and could make no firm conclusions or recommendations. The Brain Trauma Foundation notes that although hyperosmolar therapy may reduce ICP, there was insufficient evidence about effects on clinical outcomes to support a specific recommendation for patients with severe TBI.[17]

What is the utility of platelet administration in traumatic intracranial hemorrhage for patients on antiplatelet therapy?

Although it is clear that preinjury use of antiplatelet agents increases mortality in patients with severe TBI, especially among the elderly,[31] the impact of post-injury platelet transfusion is not clear. Although a large randomized control trial demonstrated a higher likelihood of death in patients with spontaneous ICH receiving platelet transfusion,[61] similar well-controlled studies have not been done in patients with traumatic ICH.

A systematic review of 11 observational studies of patients with severe TBI and preinjury antiplatelet agent use did not find any mortality difference in patients receiving platelet transfusion.[62] Two additional systematic reviews found similar results, although studies were of poor quality and the authors were unable to make any definitive recommendations.[63,64] On the basis of a review of five observational studies involving 635 patients, the American Association of Blood Banks (AABB) clinical practice guideline was unable to recommend for or against the use of platelet transfusion.[65] A recent small study suggests that platelet transfusion may be beneficial in those with measurable platelet dysfunction on TEG,[66] although it is insufficient to make a clear recommendation.

References

1. Spaite DW, Hu C, Bobrow BJ, et al. Mortality and prehospital blood pressure in patients with major traumatic brain injury: implications for the hypotension threshold. *JAMA Surg.* 2017;152(4):360-368.

2. Badjatia N, Carney N, Crocco TJ, et al. Guidelines for prehospital management of traumatic brain injury 2nd edition. *Prehosp Emerg Care.* 2008;12(Suppl 1):S1-S52.

3. Bulger EM, May S, Brasel KJ, et al. Out-of-hospital hypertonic resuscitation following severe traumatic brain injury: a randomized controlled trial. *JAMA.* 2010;304(13):1455-1464.

4. Cooper DJ, Myles PS, McDermott FT, et al. Prehospital hypertonic saline resuscitation of patients with hypotension and severe traumatic brain injury: a randomized controlled trial. *JAMA.* 2004;291(11):1350-1357.

5. Cole JB, Klein LR, Nystrom PC, et al. A prospective study of ketamine as primary therapy for prehospital profound agitation. *Am J Emerg Med.* 2018;36(5):789-796.

6. Green SM, Cote CJ. Ketamine and neurotoxicity: clinical perspectives and implications for emergency medicine. *Ann Emerg Med.* 2009;54(2):181-190.

7. Isbister GK, Calver LA, Page CB, Stokes B, Bryant JL, Downes MA. Randomized controlled trial of intramuscular droperidol versus midazolam for violence and acute behavioral disturbance: the DORM study. *Ann Emerg Med.* 2010;56(4):392-401.E1.

8. Isenberg DL, Jacobs D. Prehospital Agitation and Sedation Trial (PhAST): a randomized control trial of intramuscular haloperidol versus intramuscular midazolam for the sedation of the agitated or violent patient in the prehospital environment. *Prehosp Disaster Med.* 2015;30(5):491-495.

9. Chou R, Totten AM, Carney N, et al. Predictive utility of the total Glasgow Coma Scale versus the motor component of the Glasgow Coma Scale for identification of patients with serious traumatic injuries. *Ann Emerg Med.* 2017;70(2):143-157.E6.

10. Wiegele M, Schöchl H, Haushofer A, et al. Diagnostic and therapeutic approach in adult patients with traumatic brain injury receiving oral anticoagulant therapy: an Austrian interdisciplinary consensus statement. *Crit Care.* 2019;23(1):62.

11. Connon FF, Namdarian B, Ee JL, Drummond KJ, Miller JA. Do routinely repeated computed tomography scans in traumatic brain injury influence management? A prospective observational study in a level 1 trauma center. *Ann Surg*. 2011;254(6):1028-1031.

12. Naraghi L, Larentzakis A, Chang Y, et al. Is CT angiography of the head useful in the management of traumatic brain injury? *J Am Coll Surg*. 2015;220(6):1027-1031.

13. Balinger KJ, Elmously A, Hoey BA, Stehly CD, Stawicki SP, Portner ME. Selective computed tomographic angiography in traumatic subarachnoid hemorrhage: a pilot study. *J Surg Res*. 2015;199(1):183-189.

14. Koziarz A, Sne N, Kegel F, et al. Bedside optic nerve ultrasonography for diagnosing increased intracranial pressure: a systematic review and meta-analysis. *Ann Intern Med*. 2019;171(12): 896-905.

15. Cohen L, Athaide V, Wickham ME, Doyle-Waters MM, Rose NG, Hohl CM. The effect of ketamine on intracranial and cerebral perfusion pressure and health outcomes: a systematic review. *Ann Emerg Med*. 2015;65(1):43-51.E2.

16. Zeiler FA, Teitelbaum J, West M, Gillman LM. The ketamine effect on ICP in traumatic brain injury. *Neurocrit Care*. 2014;21(1):163-173.

17. Carney N, Totten AM, O'Reilly C, et al. Guidelines for the management of severe traumatic brain injury, fourth edition. *Neurosurgery*. 2017;80(1):6-15.

18. Berry C, Ley EJ, Bukur M, et al. Redefining hypotension in traumatic brain injury. *Injury*. 2012;43(11):1833-1837.

19. Chen H, Song Z, Dennis JA. Hypertonic saline versus other intracranial pressure-lowering agents for people with acute traumatic brain injury. *Cochrane Database Syst Rev*. 2020;(1):CD010904.

20. Perez CA, Figueroa SA. Complication rates of 3% hypertonic saline infusion through peripheral intravenous access. *J Neurosci Nurs*. 2017;49(3):191-195.

21. Jones GM, Bode L, Riha H, Erdman MJ. Safety of continuous peripheral infusion of 3% sodium chloride solution in neurocritical care patients. *Am J Crit Care*. 2016;26(1):37-42.

22. Collins CE, Witkowski ER, Flahive JM, Anderson FA Jr, Santry HP. Effect of preinjury warfarin use on outcomes after head trauma in Medicare beneficiaries. *Am J Surg*. 2014;208(4):544-549.E1.

23. Scotti P, Séguin C, Lo BWY, de Guise E, Troquet JM, Marcoux J. Antithrombotic agents and traumatic brain injury in the elderly population: hemorrhage patterns and outcomes. *J Neurosurg*. 2019;133(2):486-495.

24. Sarode R, Milling TJ Jr, Refaai MA, et al. Efficacy and safety of a 4-factor prothrombin complex concentrate in patients on vitamin K antagonists presenting with major bleeding: a randomized, plasma-controlled, phase IIIb study. *Circulation*. 2013;128(11):1234-1243.

25. Zeeshan M, Hamidi M, Feinstein AJ, et al. Four-factor prothrombin complex concentrate is associated with improved survival in trauma-related hemorrhage: a nationwide propensity-matched analysis. *J Trauma Acute Care Surg*. 2019;87(2):274-281.

26. Joseph B, Pandit V, Khalil M, et al. Use of prothrombin complex concentrate as an adjunct to fresh frozen plasma shortens time to craniotomy in traumatic brain injury patients. *Neurosurgery*. 2015;76(5):601-607; discussion 607.

27. Barton CA, Hom M, Johnson NB, Case J, Ran R, Schreiber M. Protocolized warfarin reversal with 4-factor prothrombin complex concentrate versus 3-factor prothrombin complex concentrate with recombinant factor VIIa. *Am J Surg*. 2018;215(5):775-779.

28. Connolly SJ, Crowther M, Eikelboom JW, et al. Full study report of andexanet alfa for bleeding associated with factor Xa inhibitors. *N Engl J Med*. 2019;380(14):1326-1335.

29. Frontera JA, Bhatt P, Lalchan R, et al. Cost comparison of andexanet versus prothrombin complex concentrates for direct factor Xa inhibitor reversal after hemorrhage. *J Thromb Thrombolysis*. 2020;49(1):121-131.

30. Picetti E, Rossi S, Abu-Zidan FM, et al. WSES consensus conference guidelines: monitoring and management of severe adult traumatic brain injury patients with polytrauma in the first 24 hours. *World J Emerg Surg*. 2019;14:53.

31. Ohm C, Mina A, Howells G, Bair H, Bendick P. Effects of antiplatelet agents on outcomes for elderly patients with traumatic intracranial hemorrhage. *J Trauma*. 2005;58(3):518-522.

32. Kapapa T, Röhrer S, Struve S, et al. Desmopressin acetate in intracranial haemorrhage. *Neurol Res Int*. 2014;2014:298767.

33. Naidech AM, Maas MB, Levasseur-Franklin KE, et al. Desmopressin improves platelet activity in acute intracerebral hemorrhage. *Stroke*. 2014; 45(8):2451-2453.

34. Barletta JF, Abdul-Rahman D, Hall ST, et al. The role of desmopressin on hematoma expansion in patients with mild traumatic brain injury prescribed pre-injury antiplatelet medications. *Neurocrit Care*. 2020;33(2):405-413.

35. Crompton EM, Lubomirova I, Cotlarciuc I, Han TS, Sharma SD, Sharma P. Meta-analysis of therapeutic hypothermia for traumatic brain injury in adult and pediatric patients. *Crit Care Med*. 2017;45(4):575-583.

36. Chen H, Wu F, Yang P, Shao J, Chen Q, Zheng R. A meta-analysis of the effects of therapeutic hypothermia in adult patients with traumatic brain injury. *Crit Care*. 2019;23(1):396.

37. Silbergleit R, Durkalski V, Lowenstein D, et al. Intramuscular versus intravenous therapy for prehospital status epilepticus. *N Engl J Med*. 2012;366(7):591-600.

38. Khan NR, VanLandingham MA, Fierst TM, et al. Should levetiracetam or phenytoin be used for posttraumatic seizure prophylaxis? A systematic review of the literature and meta-analysis. *Neurosurgery*. 2016;79(6):775-782.

39. Thompson K, Pohlmann-Eden B, Campbell LA, Abel H. Pharmacological treatments for preventing epilepsy following traumatic head injury. *Cochrane Database Syst Rev*. 2015;(8):CD009900.

40. Yang Y, Zheng F, Xu X, Wang X. Levetiracetam versus phenytoin for seizure prophylaxis following traumatic brain injury: a systematic review and meta-analysis. *CNS Drugs*. 2016;30(8):677-688.

41. Semple BD, Zamani A, Rayner G, Shultz SR, Jones NC. Affective, neurocognitive and psychosocial disorders associated with traumatic brain injury and post-traumatic epilepsy. *Neurobiol Dis*. 2019;123:27-41.

42. Edwards P, Arango M, Balica L, et al. Final results of MRC CRASH, a randomised placebo-controlled trial of intravenous corticosteroid in adults with head injury-outcomes at 6 months. *Lancet*. 2005;365(9475):1957-1959.

43. Harmon LA, Haase DJ, Kufera JA, et al. Infection after penetrating brain injury—an Eastern Association for the Surgery of Trauma multicenter study oral presentation at the 32nd annual meeting of the Eastern Association for the Surgery of Trauma, January 15-19, 2019, in Austin, Texas. *J Trauma Acute Care Surg*. 2019;87(1):61-67.

44. Ma J, Huang S, Qin S, You C, Zeng Y. Progesterone for acute traumatic brain injury. *Cochrane Database Syst Rev*. 2016;(12):CD008409.

45. CRASH-2 Trial Collaborators, Shakur H, Roberts I, et al. Effects of tranexamic acid on death, vascular occlusive events, and blood transfusion in trauma patients with significant haemorrhage (CRASH-2): a randomised, placebo-controlled trial. *Lancet*. 2010;376(9734):23-32.

46. CRASH-3 Trial Collaborators. Effects of tranexamic acid on death, disability, vascular occlusive events and other morbidities in patients with acute traumatic brain injury (CRASH-3): a randomised, placebo-controlled trial. *Lancet*. 2019;394(10210):1713-1723.

47. Spaite DW, Bobrow BJ, Keim SM, et al. Association of statewide implementation of the prehospital traumatic brain injury treatment guidelines with patient survival following traumatic brain injury: the Excellence in Prehospital Injury Care (EPIC) study. *JAMA Surg*. 2019;154(7):e191152.

48. Spaite DW, Hu C, Bobrow BJ, et al. The effect of combined out-of-hospital hypotension and hypoxia on mortality in major traumatic brain injury. *Ann Emerg Med*. 2017;69(1):62-72.

49. Spaite, DW, Hu C, Bobrow BJ, et al. Association of out-of-hospital hypotension depth and duration with traumatic brain injury mortality. *Ann Emerg Med*. 2017;70(4):522-530.E1.

50. Bernard SA, Nguyen V, Cameron P, et al. Prehospital rapid sequence intubation improves functional outcome for patients with severe traumatic brain injury: a randomized controlled trial. *Ann Surg*. 2010;252(6):959-965.

51. Haltmeier T, Benjamin E, Siboni S, Dilektasli E, Inaba K, Demetriades D. Prehospital intubation for isolated severe blunt traumatic brain injury: worse outcomes and higher mortality. *Eur J Trauma Emerg Surg*. 2017;43(6):731-739.

52. Bossers SM, Schwarte LA, Loer SA, Twisk JW, Boer C, Schober P. Experience in prehospital endotracheal intubation significantly influences mortality of patients with severe traumatic brain injury: a systematic review and meta-analysis. *PLoS One*. 2015;10(10):e0141034.

53. Davis DP, Dunford JV, Ochs M, Park K, Hoyt DB. The use of quantitative end-tidal capnometry to avoid inadvertent severe hyperventilation in patients with head injury after paramedic rapid sequence intubation. *J Trauma*. 2004;56(4):808-814.

54. Davis DP, Dunford JV, Poste JC, et al. The impact of hypoxia and hyperventilation on outcome after paramedic rapid sequence intubation of severely head-injured patients. *J Trauma*. 2004;57(1):1-8; discussion 8-10.

55. Dunford JV, Davis DP, Ochs M, Doney M, Hoyt DB. Incidence of transient hypoxia and pulse rate reactivity during paramedic rapid sequence intubation. *Ann Emerg Med*. 2003;42(6):721-728.

56. Wat R, Mammi M, Paredes J, et al. The effectiveness of antiepileptic medications as prophylaxis of early seizure in patients with traumatic brain injury compared with placebo or no treatment: a systematic review and meta-analysis. *World Neurosurg*. 2019;122:433-440.

57. Wilson CD, Burks JD, Rodgers RB, Evans RM, Bakare AA, Safavi-Abbasi S. Early and late posttraumatic epilepsy in the setting of traumatic brain injury: a meta-analysis and review of antiepileptic management. *World Neurosurg*. 2018;110:e901-e906.

58. Inaba K, Menaker J, Branco BC, et al. A prospective multicenter comparison of levetiracetam versus phenytoin for early posttraumatic seizure prophylaxis. *J Trauma Acute Care Surg*. 2013;74(3):766-771; discussion 771-773.

59. Schwimmbeck F, Voellger B, Chappell D, Eberhart L. Hypertonic saline versus mannitol for traumatic brain injury: a systematic review and meta-analysis with trial sequential analysis. *J Neurosurg Anesthesiol*. 2019;33(1):10-20.

60. Berger-Pelleiter E, Émond M, Lauzier F, Shields JF, Turgeon AF. Hypertonic saline in severe traumatic brain injury: a systematic review and meta-analysis of randomized controlled trials. *CJEM*. 2016;18(2):112-120.

61. Baharoglu MI, Cordonnier C, Al-Shahi Salman R, et al. Platelet transfusion versus standard care after acute stroke due to spontaneous cerebral haemorrhage associated with antiplatelet therapy (PATCH): a randomised, open-label, phase 3 trial. *Lancet*. 2016;387(10038):2605-2613.

62. Kumar A, Mhaskar R, Grossman BJ, et al. Platelet transfusion: a systematic review of the clinical evidence. *Transfusion*. 2015;55(5):1116-1127; quiz 1115.

63. Leong LB, David TK. Is platelet transfusion effective in patients taking antiplatelet agents who suffer an intracranial hemorrhage? *J Emerg Med*. 2015;49(4):561-572.

64. Thorn S, Güting H, Mathes T, Schäfer N, Maegele M. The effect of platelet transfusion in patients with traumatic brain injury and concomitant antiplatelet use: a systematic review and meta-analysis. *Transfusion*. 2019;59(11):3536-3544.

65. Kaufman RM, Djulbegovic B, Gernsheimer T, et al. Platelet transfusion: a clinical practice guideline from the AABB. *Ann Intern Med*. 2015;162(3):205-213.

66. Furay E, Daley M, Teixeira PG, et al. Goal-directed platelet transfusions correct platelet dysfunction and may improve survival in patients with severe traumatic brain injury. *J Trauma Acute Care Surg*. 2018; 85(5):881-887.

CHAPTER 13

Cervical Spine Trauma and Spinal Cord Emergencies

E. Megan Callan

Charles M. Andrews

THE CLINICAL CHALLENGE

The vast majority of spinal cord injuries occur from trauma, although other causes must be considered (**Table 13.1**). The mean age at the time of injury is 37 years and there is a bimodal age distribution, with the first peak between 16 and 30 years of age and the second peak older than 60 years.[1] The ratio of males to females is approximately 4:1. In descending order of prevalence, the greatest causes for acute spinal trauma are motor vehicle accidents (~40%), followed by falls (~20%), violence, and sporting injuries. The level of spinal cord injury most often occurs in cervical spine (~60%), thoracic (~32%), and lumbosacral (~9%). Injury to the spine in the setting of trauma can occur in isolation, or in polytrauma with other potential life-threatening injuries. Spinal immobilization is always an important consideration in these patients.

Spinal cord compression due to a structural abnormality is a neurosurgical emergency. Signs of injury must be recognized and urgent imaging obtained to direct treatment. About 20% of patients with a major spine injury have a second injury at a noncontiguous level; therefore, complete spine imaging with computed tomography (CT) or magnetic resonance imaging (MRI) is recommended.

PATHOPHYSIOLOGY

Trauma to the spine may involve damage to the bones, ligaments, vascular structures, and/or spinal cord. The discoligamentous complex includes the anterior longitudinal ligament, posterior longitudinal ligament, ligamentum flavum, facet capsule, and interspinous and supraspinous ligaments. The strongest component of the anterior structures is the anterior longitudinal ligament; the strongest component of the posterior structures is the facet capsule. The vertebral arteries travel through the transverse foramina of C2 to C6 and then converge to create the basilar artery.

Primary and Secondary Injury

Primary spinal cord injury encompasses the initial traumatic insult that occurs with its resulting disruption of neuronal axons. Secondary injury follows the primary insult, and can lead to ongoing progressive tissue damage for weeks after the initial injury. Secondary injury may occur because of inflammation, free radicals and oxidative stress, hypotension, hypoxia, ischemia, edema, or further mechanical disturbance of the spine. In blunt trauma, the extent of both primary and

TABLE 13.1	Differential Diagnosis of Acute Myelopathy
Pathophysiologic Cause	**Specific Cause**
Vascular	Spinal cord ischemia Vasculitis Spinal A-V malformation
Inflammatory or infectious transverse myelitis	Inflammatory: systemic lupus erythematosus, sarcoidosis, Sjögren Infectious: HIV, HTLV-1, HSV, rabies, West Nile virus, EBV, CMV, enterovirus, TB (Pott disease), Lyme disease, syphilis, mycoplasma, leptospirosis, brucellosis, schistosomiasis, filariasis Demyelinating: multiple sclerosis, neuromyelitis optica, ADEM
Structural (cord compression)	Epidural compression: metastasis, lymphoma, disk protrusion, abscess, hematoma, spondylolysis, atlantoaxial subluxation Extramedullary intradural compression: meningioma, neurofibroma Intramedullary expansion: glioma, ependymoma
Paraneoplastic	Mainly reported with lung cancer, breast cancer, and lymphoproliferative malignancies Several antibodies: CRMP-5, VGCC, amphiphysin, ganglionic AchR, VGKC, ANNA-1,2, aquaporin-4
Toxic or metabolic	Arsenic Heroin Acute B_{12} deficiency Radiation
Trauma	Motor vehicle accidents Falls Violence Sporting injuries

AchR, acetylcholine receptor; ADEM, acute disseminated encephalomyelitis; ANNA, anti-neuronal nuclear antibodies; A-V, arteriovenous; CMV, cytomegalovirus; CRMP-5, collapsing response mediator protein 5; EBV, Epstein-Barr virus; HIV, human immunodeficiency virus; HSV, herpes simplex virus; HTLV-1, human T-cell lymphotropic virus type 1; TB, tuberculosis; VGCC, voltage gated calcium channel; VGKC, voltage gated potassium channel.

Derived from Maloney PR, Jacob JT, Wijdick, EFM. Chapter 7: Acute spinal cord compression, spinal cord trauma, and peripheral nerve injury. In: Flemming K, Jones L, eds. *Mayo Clinic Neurology Board Review 2015.* Oxford University Press; 2015.

secondary injury to the cord may be directly related to the energy impact delivered at onset. A syrinx (fluid-filled cavity) may develop in some patients and lead to further neurologic deficits. Cystic cavities due to neuronal degeneration that occur ***ex vacuo*** and glial scarring from activated microglia and astrocytes can make it very difficult for damaged axons to regenerate. Even if neurites are able to regrow, oftentimes the myelin white matter surrounding them has been substantially damaged and oligodendrocyte remyelination attempts are often impaired.

Spinal shock refers to a transient loss of all neurologic function (motor, sensory, and autonomic pathways) below the level of initial spinal cord injury. Patients often have flaccid paralysis and areflexia, including loss of the bulbocavernosus reflex, from the level of the lesion down. In a select few patients, the spinal cord reflexes even above the level of injury might be depressed, known as the Schiff-Sherrington phenomenon. The duration of spinal shock most commonly dissipates within 72 hours of injury, but can persist in some patients up to 1 to 2 weeks.

Mechanism of Injury

Blunt injury is the most common mechanism for spinal trauma. Motor vehicle crashes and falls account for the majority of blunt trauma. With low-speed impacts, there may only be posterior neck muscle strain (ie, whiplash). Patients with preexisting spine disease (eg, due to degenerative spondylosis) or spine instability (eg, due to rheumatoid arthritis, Down syndrome) may develop more significant injury even at low speeds. Higher speed accidents have increased risk for spinal cord injury. Mobile parts of the spine (eg, cervical spine) and transition zones (eg, cervicothoracic and thoracolumbar) are at greatest risk for injury. Different mechanistic forces (ie, flexion, extension, distraction, compression) tend to be associated with specific injuries (**Figure 13.1**).

Penetrating traumatic spine injury is much less common than are blunt injuries, and can also be divided into low-impact (eg, knife stab) and high-impact (eg, gunshot wound) injuries. Lower impact penetration may lead to either incomplete or complete injury to the cord. High-impact penetrating spine injuries are often complete. An unstable vertebral column injury in gunshot wound patients with an intact spinal cord is very rare, and in these situations, immobilization typically offers little benefit. Gunshot wound injuries lead to damage not only by ballistic disruption of the cord but also because of blast injury forces.

The Subaxial Cervical Spine Injury Classification (SLIC) is a classification system for cervical spine injury; see **Table 13.2**.[2] Scores of 1 to 3 are typically nonsurgical, whereas scores ≥5 are surgical. A score of 4 is indeterminate.

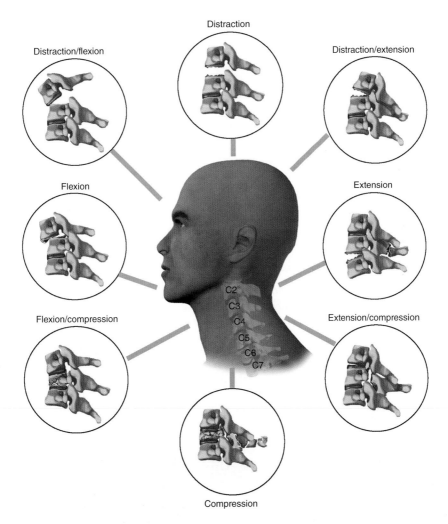

Figure 13.1: Subaxial fractures and dislocations by injury mechanism. (From Greenleaf R, Richman JD, Altman DT. General principles of verbony, ligamentous, and penetrating injuries. In: Brinker MR, ed. *Review of OrthoTrauma*. 2nd ed. Philadelphia, PA: Lippincott Williams & Wilkins; 2013:406-417. Figure 26.6)

TABLE 13.2   Subaxial Spine Injury Classification (SLIC) Severity Score

Injury Characteristics	Points
Morphology of injury	
No abnormality	0
Compression	1
Burst	2
Distraction[a]	3
Translation/rotation[b]	4
Integrity of discoligamentous complex	
Intact	0
Indeterminate[c]	1
Disrupted[d]	2
Neurologic status	
Intact	0
Nerve root injury	1
Complete	2
Incomplete	3
Persistent cord compression with neuro deficit	+1

[a]For example, facet perch, hyperextension, posterior element fracture.
[b]For example, facet dislocation, unstable teardrop, advanced stage flexion compression, bilateral pedicle fracture, floating lateral mass.
[c]For example, isolated interspinous widening, magnetic resonance imaging (MRI) T2 signal changes in ligaments only.
[d]For example, widening of the disk space, facet perch or dislocation, increased signal on T2-weighted image magnetic resonance imaging (MRI) through entire disk.

Anatomic Subclassifications and Injury

When thinking of spine injuries, there may be a predilection for specific anatomic regions, and therefore dividing the spine up into these regions can help with classification. The cervical spine can be subclassified into the occipital-cervical (O-C) junction and the subaxial cervical spine (**Table 13.3**). The cervical spinal cord is the most susceptible to injury because of its mobility, accounting for nearly half of all spinal injuries. The National Emergency X-Radiography Utilization Study Group (NEXUS) study evaluated 818 patients with cervical spine injuries, and, based on that data, the levels most commonly fractured are C2 (24%), C6 (20%), and C7 (19%).[3]

Occipital-Cervical Junction Injuries

Occipital condyle fractures typically arise from an axial loading type injury (**Figures 13.2** and **13.3**). There are three types of occipital condyle fractures: type 1—crush injury between the skull and C1 lateral mass; type 2 or Anderson Montesano—extension of a skull fracture to the condyle; and type 3—avulsion of the alar ligament pulling a fragment of bone from the condyle. These axial loading injuries are rarely unstable, except for type 3. Type 3 occipital condyle fractures often occur in the context of a severe distracting injury and should raise suspicion for atlanto-occipital dislocation.

Atlanto-occipital dislocation occurs with severe distracting injuries (significant flexion), and is most commonly due to high-speed motor vehicle collisions or car versus pedestrian accidents.

TABLE 13.3   Anatomic Subclassifications of the Spine

Region	Levels
Occipital-cervical junction	Occiput-C2
Subaxial cervical spine	C3-T1
Thoracic spine	T2-T10
Thoracolumbar junction	T11-L2
Lower lumbar spine	L3-S1
Sacrum	S2-S5

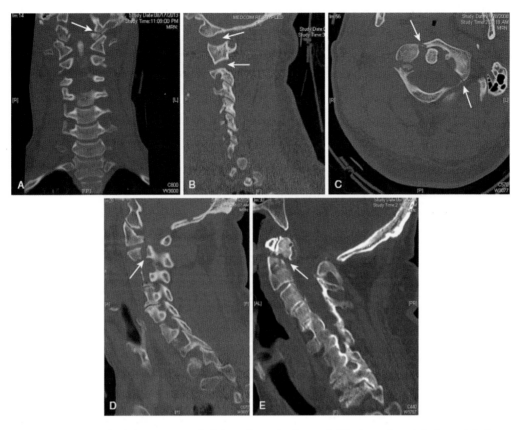

Figure 13.2: C1 and C2 fractures and dislocations. A. Coronal CT view of occipital condyle fracture. B. Sagittal CT view of atlanto-occipital dislocation. C. Axial CT view of Jefferson fracture. D. Sagittal CT view of Hangman's fracture. E. Sagittal CT view of type 2 odontoid fracture. From Schuster JM, Syre P. Chapter 30 Spine trauma and spinal cord injury. In: Kumar M, Kofke WA, Levine J, Schuster JM. *Neurocritical Care Management of the Neurosurgical Patient.* Elsevier; 2018, Figure 30.1.

This injury disrupts all the major stabilizers of the craniocervical junction: tectorial membrane, alar ligaments, apical ligament, transverse ligament, O-C1 joint, and often C1-C2 capsular ligaments. Atlanto-occipital dissociation is highly unstable, and oftentimes instantly fatal. Given the magnitude of force it takes for this dislocation to occur, there are often other associated injuries, for example, subarachnoid hemorrhage (SAH), epidural hematoma at the foramen magnum, and vertebral artery injury. Atlanto-occipital dislocation requires surgical stabilization with an O-C fusion.

C1 fractures include Jefferson fracture (or C1 burst fracture) and fractures to the C1 posterior arch. Jefferson fractures occur because of an axial loading–type injury, and there are generally two opposing fractures in the ring. About 33% of cases may have an associated C2 fracture as well. Often, there is a low incidence of neurologic injury because the C1 ring is so wide around the spinal canal. If the transverse ligament is disrupted (which may manifest as lateral displacement of the lateral masses on imaging), this is an unstable injury and surgical stabilization is indicated. Posterior C1 arch fractures occur because of extension injuries and are usually stable. However, an associated C2 fracture can occur in nearly 50% of cases, rendering this unstable.

C2 is one of the most common vertebrae fractured. There are four identified fracture types: C2 body fracture, lateral mass fracture, hangman's fracture, and fractures of the dens (or odontoid process). Both C2 body fractures and lateral mass fractures are often benign, and may be treated simply with an external brace. The hangman's fracture involves bilateral C2 pedicle and/

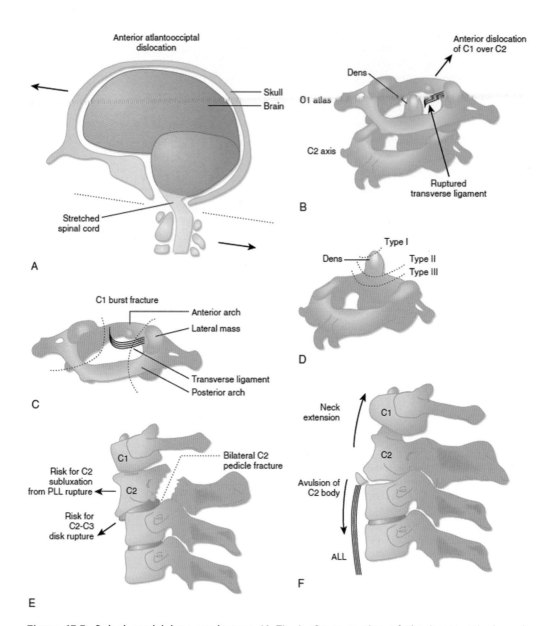

Figure 13.3: Spinal cord injury syndromes (A-F). A. Cross section of the intact spinal cord (dorsal column sensory pathway [proprioceptive pathways]: dark blue, corticospinal tract: red, spinothalamic pathway: light blue). B. Anterior cord syndrome. C. Brown-Sequard syndrome. D. Posterior cord syndrome. E. Central cord syndrome. F. Complete transection. (From Lin M, Mahadevan S. Spine Trauma and Spinal Cord Injury. In: Adams JG, Barton ED, Collings JL, DeBlieux P, Gisondi MA, Nadel ES, eds. *Emergency Medicine: Clinical Essentials.* 2nd ed. Philadelphia, PA: Elsevier; 2012. 645-660. Figure 75.3.)

or pars interarticularis fractures. This is the injury that is most classically described with judicial hangings, leading to a distraction and extension injury. However, this fracture type can often be seen with axial loading combined with flexion-type injuries. There is risk of disruption of the posterior longitudinal ligament with C2 subluxation, and C2-C3 disk rupture as well. The need for surgical stabilization may depend on the amount of angulation and displacement, but most of these fractures are unstable. There are three different fracture types of the dens. Type 1 is rare and consists of avulsion of the upper portion of the dens with an intact transverse ligament. It is often associated with a distraction-type injury. Because the ligament is intact, this injury is stable. Type 2 is the most common, and is a fracture of the dens at its base. About 10% of these patients may have rupture of the transverse ligament, which renders this injury unstable. Ligamentous injury will be seen best on MRI. Younger patients who have less displacement may be able to heal with a brace or halo; however, elderly individuals do not tolerate external bracing as well. Surgical stabilization consists typically of posterior C1-C2 fusion, but a small percentage may be amenable to stabilization anteriorly with an odontoid screw. A type 3 fracture of the dens involves extension into the C1-C2 joints bilaterally. The greater the surface area of the fractured bones, the more likely the injury is to heal with an external brace. Type 3 fractures are more stable.

Subaxial Cervical Spine Fractures (C3-T1)

Fractures that occur with mild, pure axial loading–type injuries are typically due to compression. When the axial load is more significant, burst fractures, retropulsion of bone, and traumatic disk herniation with spinal cord compression may all occur (**Figure 13.4**). If the axial load is given in combination with either a flexion and/or rotational force, there may be disruption in the posterior ligamentous complex (including interspinous, interlaminar, joint capsules, and disk capsules) and facet fractures. This may lead to subluxation of the spine and possible spinal cord injury. The classic "diving injury" consists of an axial load with hyperflexion of the neck, leading to bilateral facet joint dislocation and spinal cord injury.

The stability of these fractures in the subaxial spine depends on the degree of displacement and angulation, and whether there is associated ligamentous-disk complex injury. The following fractures are typically considered stable: articular mass fracture, burst fracture, wedge fracture, spinous process fracture, unilateral facet fracture, and transverse process fracture.

PREHOSPITAL CONCERNS

The patient with a spine injury may have injuries at multiple levels. Between 25% and 50% of patients with a spinal cord injury have also sustained a head injury, whereas spinal cord injury is seen in 10% to 30% of polytrauma patients.[4] The goal of prehospital management is to minimize secondary injury. After ensuring oxygenation and perfusion, a secondary evaluation includes enquiry about pain in the neck or back, tenderness to palpation, weakness or altered sensation, signs of incontinence, and other signs of injury. Given the mechanism of injury, prehospital providers are often tasked with removing patients from harmful situations before further evaluation and transport. Care must be taken to restrict motion of the patient's spine as much as possible during patient movement and transport. It is recommended to place the patient in a rigid cervical collar with the head stabilized in a forward-facing position. A spine log roll may be used to keep the patient in a spine-neutral position to be placed on a rigid backboard with straps. These immobilization techniques have side effects of their own, including discomfort, pressure sores, restriction of respiration, and difficulty with maintaining airway protection; see section "**Evidence**." In brief, there is only evidence to use restricted spine motion with a rigid backboard or similar device in a subset of patients: blunt trauma with altered level of consciousness, spinal pain or tenderness, neurologic disability (weakness or numbness), anatomic deformity of the spine, high-energy mechanism with either intoxication, inability to communicate, or other distracting injury.

Patients with high cervical spine injuries may have diaphragmatic weakness or respiratory accessory muscle weakness leading to respiratory failure and death. If bag mask ventilation is ineffective, an advanced airway intervention is indicated. Concomitant facial fractures or thoracic injuries (such as pneumothorax or aspiration) may confound the clinical picture. Trained emergency medical services personnel may use an advanced airway with in-line immobilization of the cervical spine. Hypotension may occur either due to hypovolemic/hemorrhagic shock or autonomic dysfunction (neurogenic shock). Crystalloid or colloid intravenous (IV) fluid volume resuscitation with at least two large-bore IVs can help maintain blood pressure until arrival at the hospital. The desired mean arterial pressure (MAP) is 90 mm Hg, and episodes of hypotension with systolic blood pressure below 90 mm Hg should be avoided because this can exacerbate neurologic injury.

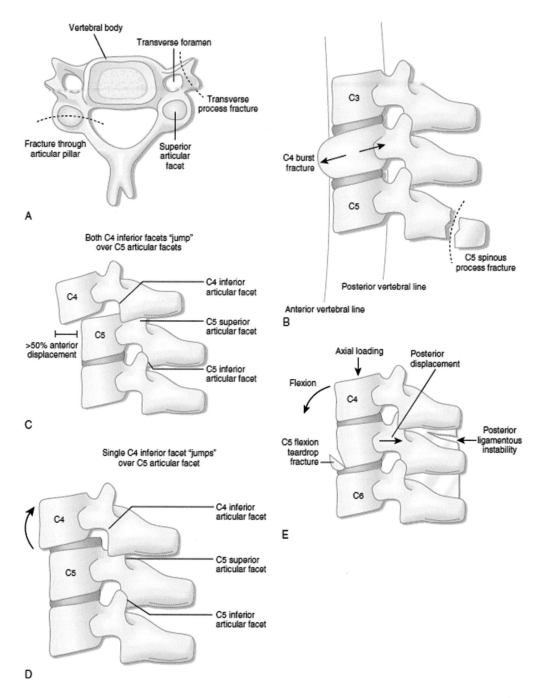

Figure 13.4: C3-T1 fractures and subluxations. A. Superior axial view of an articular pillar fracture and transverse process fracture. B. Sagittal view of a C4 burst fracture and C5 clay shoveler's (spinus process) fracture. C. Sagittal view of bilateral C4 facet dislocation. D. Sagittal view of unilateral C4 facet dislocation. E. Sagittal view of a C5 teardrop fracture.

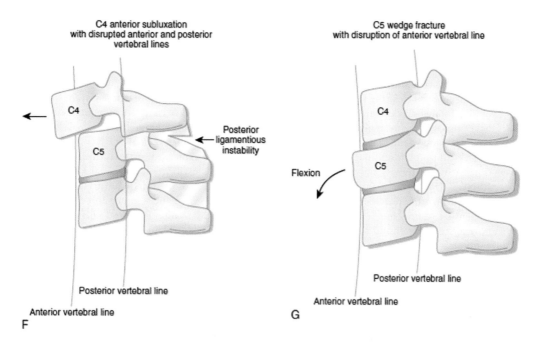

Figure 13.4: (*continued*) F. Sagittal view of C4 anterior subluxation. G. Sagittal view of a C5 wedge fracture. (From Lin M, Mahadevan S. Spine Trauma and Spinal Cord Injury. In: Adams JG, Barton ED, Collings JL, DeBlieux P, Gisondi MA, Nadel ES, eds. *Emergency Medicine: Clinical Essentials.* 2nd ed. Philadelphia, PA: Elsevier; 2012. 645-660. Figure 75.8.)

APPROACH/THE FOCUSED EXAMINATION

Trauma protocols underscore the importance of a systematic approach to spine trauma, that is, "the ABCs," neurologic disability, and potential exposures. Patients should initially have total spine precautions, with immobilization of the cervical spine in a hard collar and the use of log rolling on a rigid board to protect thoracic and lumbar spine. Major causes of death in patients with acute spinal cord injury are aspiration, respiratory failure, and shock. Labored breathing or paradoxic breathing because of weak diaphragmatic and chest wall musculature with or without autonomic instability may indicate a cervical spine lesion.

Spinal shock and neurogenic shock are two separate processes that are at times incorrectly used interchangeably. Spinal shock refers to a temporary loss or depression of all neurologic function and spinal-mediated reflexes below the level of the injury. This is especially seen as reduced motor tone or flaccidity and loss of sensation, but may include loss of the normal mediated autonomic spinal cord reflexes. Therefore, patients with spinal shock may have concomitant neurogenic shock. Neurogenic shock can persist 1 to 6 weeks after injury.

Both motor and sensory levels need to be assessed. Weak limbs are often flaccid initially, progressively becoming more spastic in days to weeks. Deep tendon reflexes are often initially reduced or absent immediately following an injury to the spinal cord, and will become more brisk in a matter of days to weeks. The patient needs to be checked for urinary retention or incontinence, and for bowel incontinence and reduced rectal tone. When log rolling the patient or loosening the collar to examine the cervical spine, a sudden "step-off" of a spinous process felt with palpation may indicate the location of injury.

Classification of Spinal Cord Injuries

Spinal cord injuries are described as complete or incomplete. By definition, a patient with an incomplete lesion has residual motor or sensory function more than three segments below the level of the injury. This can include "sacral sparing," meaning that the sensation is preserved around the anus/perineum, there is still voluntary rectal sphincter tone, and possibly voluntary toe flexion. The incomplete spinal cord syndromes are described subsequently: central cord syndrome, anterior cord syndrome, posterior cord syndrome, and Brown-Séquard syndrome (or cord hemisection) (**Figure 13.5**).

With a complete lesion, there is no preservation of any motor or sensory function more than three segments below the level of injury. A complete lesion can only be diagnosed in the absence of initial spinal shock. Some patients may end up appearing to have complete spine injury, only to have improvement to an incomplete injury within 24 to 48 hours. It is unlikely that spinal shock, or temporary loss of function below the spinal level, will continue after 72 hours.

A thorough examination of the patient using the American Spinal Injury Association (ASIA) International Standards for Neurological Classification of Spinal Cord Injury (ISNCSCI) is the best way to document the patient's degree of neurologic injury and to communicate to other providers (**Figure 13.6A**). The examination includes motor and dual-modality sensory testing, and a rectal examination for tone and sensation (**Figure 13.6B**) delineates how to score motor and sensory grades. ASIA has also developed an impairment scale that is commonly used in evaluation of patients with spinal cord injury, which categorizes patients into different classes, A to E (**Figure 13.6B**), based on function and whether the injury is complete or incomplete.

Central Cord Syndrome

Central cord syndrome most commonly occurs in the cervical spine because of the mobility of that region. It most often results from a hyperextension injury, and patients with underlying stenosis are at higher risk. Therefore, this injury pattern is fairly common in older patients with underlying degenerative disease and a higher incidence of falls. Central cord syndrome can occur without any bony fractures, and an enlarging syrinx of the central canal can also lead to symptoms. The spinothalamic pain fibers of the upper extremities are affected first, leading to a bilateral loss of pain and temperature sensation in a "cape-like" distribution. Corticospinal motor tracts may be affected, leading to weakness. The arrangement of the corticospinal fibers has upper extremity tracts more medial, leading to greater arm weakness than to leg weakness. Patients with central cord syndrome may be more susceptible to further hypotension-induced spinal cord injury, and blood pressure augmentation may help improve symptoms. In patients who require surgical stabilization and have concomitant central cord syndrome, there has been a debate about the timing of the surgery; however, most studies show these operations can be carried out early, safely, and without further injury.

Anterior Cord Syndrome

Anterior cord syndrome most commonly occurs from an infarct of the anterior spinal artery due to vascular injury or occlusion of the vessel. In trauma patients, bone fragments or retropulsed disks may also impede flow by direct compression. There may be direct injury to the anterior portion of the spinal cord as well. The anterior horn motor cells are the most affected, leading to loss of motor function below the level of the injury. Spinothalamic tracts are also impaired, and there is loss of pain and temperature sensation. The dorsal columns are spared; and, therefore, light touch, vibratory, and joint position senses are intact.

Posterior Cord Syndrome

Posterior cord syndrome is typically not a common injury seen in trauma patients unless the posterior aspect of the cord is compressed by bony elements. Posterior compression of the spinal cord may more likely result from hematoma, abscess, or tumors. An infarct of one of the posterior spinal arteries may lead to unilateral damage to the dorsal column. Subacute combined degeneration due to B_{12} or copper deficiency, and syphilis (tabes dorsalis) and human immunodeficiency virus (HIV; vacuolar myelopathy) will lead to involvement of the dorsal columns. Damage to the dorsal columns will lead to a loss of sensation—light touch, vibratory sense, and proprioception—and patients can present with a sensory ataxia.

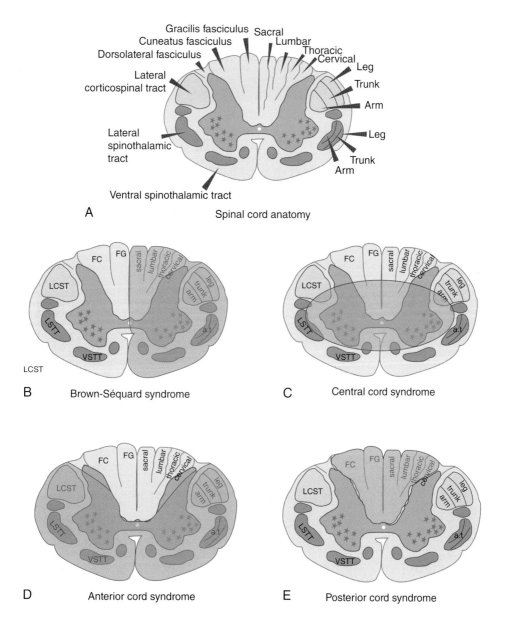

Figure 13.5: Illustrations depict cross sections of the cervical spinal cord. A. Cross-sectional anatomy of the normal cervical spinal cord shows the ascending and descending tracts and their topographic organization. B. Brown-Séquard syndrome, with hemisection of the cord. C. Central cord syndrome, with injuries to the central portion of the spinal cord affecting the arms more than the legs. D. Anterior cord syndrome, with sparing of only the posterior columns of the spinal cord. E. Posterior cord syndrome, affecting only the posterior columns. FC = fasciculus cuneatus, FG = fasciculus gracilis, LCST = lateral corticospinal tract, LSTT = lateral spinothalamic tracts, VSTT = vertical spinothalamic tracts. (From Malik AT, Yu E, Yu WD, Khan SN. Spinal Trauma. In: Liberman JR, ed. *AAOS Comprehensive Orthopaedic Review.* 3rd ed. Philadelphia, PA: Wolters Kluwer; 2019: 141-159. Originally published in: Tay BKB , Eismont F : Cervical spine fractures and dislocations. In: Fardon DF , Garfin SR , Abitbol ii , Boden SD , Herkowitz HN , Mayer TG, eds. *Orthopaedic Knowledge Update: Spine.* 2nd ed. Rosemont, IL: American Academy of Orthopaedic Surgeons; 2002: 247-262.)

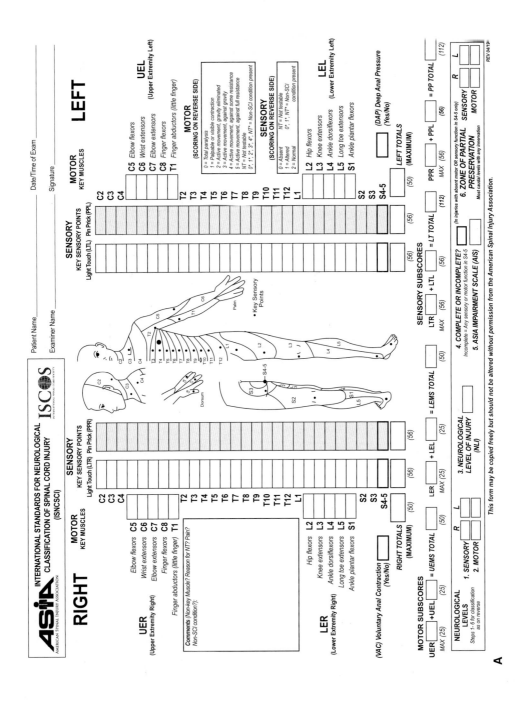

Figure 13.6: International Standards for Neurological Classification of SCI (ISNCSCI). A. ISNCSCI worksheet.

Muscle Function Grading

0 = Total paralysis

1 = Palpable or visible contraction

2 = Active movement, full range of motion (ROM) with gravity eliminated

3 = Active movement, full ROM against gravity

4 = Active movement, full ROM against gravity and moderate resistance in a muscle specific position

5 = (Normal) active movement, full ROM against gravity and full resistance in a functional muscle position expected from an otherwise unimpaired person

NT = Not testable (ie, due to immobilization, severe pain such that the patient cannot be graded, amputation of limb, or contracture of >50% of the normal ROM)

0*, 1*, 2*, 3*, 4*, NT* = Non-SCI condition present[a]

Sensory Grading

0 = Absent   1 = Altered, either decreased/impaired sensation or hypersensitivity

2 = Normal   NT = Not testable

0*, 1*, NT* = Non-SCI condition present [a]

[a]Note: Abnormal motor and sensory scores should be tagged with a "*" to indicate an impairment due to a non-SCI condition. The non-SCI condition should be explained in the comments box together with information about how the score is rated for classification purposes (at least normal / not normal for classification).

When to Test Non-key Muscles:

In a patient with an apparent AIS B classification, non-key muscle functions more than three levels below the motor level on each side should be tested to most accurately classify the injury (differentiate between AIS B and C).

Movement	Root level
Shoulder: Flexion, extension, abduction, adduction, internal and external rotation **Elbow:** Supination	C5
Elbow: Pronation **Wrist:** Flexion	C6
Finger: Flexion at proximal joint, extension **Thumb:** Flexion, extension and abduction in plane of thumb	C7
Finger: Flexion at MCP joint **Thumb:** Opposition, adduction and abduction perpendicular to palm	C8
Finger: Abduction of the index finger	T1
Hip: Adduction	L2
Hip: External rotation	L3
Hip: Extension, abduction, internal rotation **Knee:** Flexion **Ankle:** Inversion and eversion **Toe:** MP and IP extension	L4
Hallux and Toe: DIP and PIP flexion and abduction	L5
Hallux: Adduction	S1

ASIA Impairment Scale (AIS)

A = Complete. No sensory or motor function is preserved in the sacral segments S4-5.

B = Sensory Incomplete. Sensory but not motor function is preserved below the neurological level and includes the sacral segments S4-5 (light touch or pin prick at S4-5 or deep anal pressure) AND no motor function is preserved more than three levels below the motor level on either side of the body.

C = Motor Incomplete. Motor function is preserved at the most caudal sacral segments for voluntary anal contraction (VAC) OR the patient meets the criteria for sensory incomplete status (sensory function preserved at the most caudal sacral segments S4-5 by LT, PP or DAP), and has some sparing of motor function more than three levels below the ipsilateral motor level on either side of the body. (This includes key or non-key muscle functions to determine motor incomplete status.) For AIS C—less than half of key muscle functions below the single NLI have a muscle grade ≥ 3.

D = Motor Incomplete. Motor incomplete status as defined above, with at least half (half or more) of key muscle functions below the single NLI having a muscle grade ≥ 3.

E = Normal. If sensation and motor function as tested with the ISNCSCI are graded as normal in all segments, and the patient had prior deficits, then the AIS grade is E. Someone without an initial SCI does not receive an AIS grade.

Using ND: To document the sensory, motor and NLI levels, the ASIA Impairment Scale grade, and/or the zone of partial preservation (ZPP) when they are unable to be determined based on the examination results.

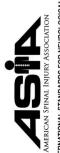
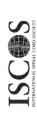

AMERICAN SPINAL INJURY ASSOCIATION

ISCOS
INTERNATIONAL SPINAL CORD SOCIETY

INTERNATIONAL STANDARDS FOR NEUROLOGICAL CLASSIFICATION OF SPINAL CORD INJURY

Steps in Classification

The following order is recommended for determining the classification of individuals with SCI.

1. Determine sensory levels for right and left sides.
The sensory level is the most caudal, intact dermatome for both pin prick and light touch sensation.

2. Determine motor levels for right and left sides.
Defined by the lowest key muscle function that has a grade of at least 3 (on supine testing), providing the key muscle functions represented by segments above that level are judged to be intact (graded as a 5).
Note: in regions where there is no myotome to test, the motor level is presumed to be the same as the sensory level, if testable motor function above that level is also normal.

3. Determine the neurological level of injury (NLI).
This refers to the most caudal segment of the cord with intact sensation and antigravity (3 or more) muscle function strength, provided that there is normal (intact) sensory and motor function rostrally respectively.
The NLI is the most cephalad of the sensory and motor levels determined in steps 1 and 2.

4. Determine whether the injury is Complete or Incomplete.
(ie, absence or presence of sacral sparing)
If voluntary anal contraction = No AND all S4-5 sensory scores = 0 AND deep anal pressure = No, then injury is Complete.
Otherwise, injury is Incomplete.

5. Determine ASIA Impairment Scale (AIS) Grade.

Is injury Complete?   If YES, AIS = A

NO ↓

Is injury Motor Complete? If YES, AIS = B

NO ↓   (No = voluntary anal contraction OR motor function more than three levels below the motor level on a given side, if the patient has sensory incomplete classification)

Are at least half (half or more) of the key muscles below the neurological level of injury graded 3 or better?

NO ↓   YES ↓

AIS = C   AIS = D

If sensation and motor function is normal in all segments, AIS=E
Note: AIS E is used in follow-up testing when an individual with a documented SCI has recovered normal function. If at initial testing no deficits are found, the individual is neurologically intact and the ASIA Impairment Scale does not apply.

6. Determine the zone of partial preservation (ZPP).
The ZPP is used only in injuries with absent motor (no VAC) OR sensory function (no DAP, no LT and no PP sensation) in the lowest sacral segments S4-5, and refers to those dermatomes and myotomes caudal to the sensory and motor levels that remain partially innervated. With sacral sparing of sensory function, the sensory ZPP is not applicable and therefore "NA" is recorded in the block of the worksheet. Accordingly, if VAC is present, the motor ZPP is not applicable and is noted as "NA."

B

Figure 13.6: (*continued*) B. Muscle function, sensory, and impairment grading. (American Spinal Injury Association: International Standards for Neurological Classification of Spinal Cord Injury, revised 2019; Richmond, VA.)

Brown-Séquard Syndrome

Brown-Séquard syndrome is most commonly due to penetrating trauma to the spine, such as a stabbing or gunshot wound. Although well described, it is rarely seen clinically. A unilateral facet fracture dislocation may also lead to a similar injury. Nontraumatic causes may include compression by a neoplasm or abscess. This syndrome consists of transection of only one half of the spinal cord, leading to damage of both ascending and descending fibers on one side of the cord. Therefore, patients will have ipsilateral loss of motor function, light touch, vibration, and proprioception, as well as contralateral loss of pain and temperature sensation below the level of the injury.

Cervical Spine Clearance and Imaging

Trained providers can safely clear the cervical spine without imaging if the patient is awake, alert, cooperative, not intoxicated, and does not have any obvious neurologic deficit or distracting injuries (**Figure 13.7**).[3,5] The patient must not have bony point tenderness and be able to complete a functional range of motion (ROM) test without pain. If the patient cannot do these things, then some

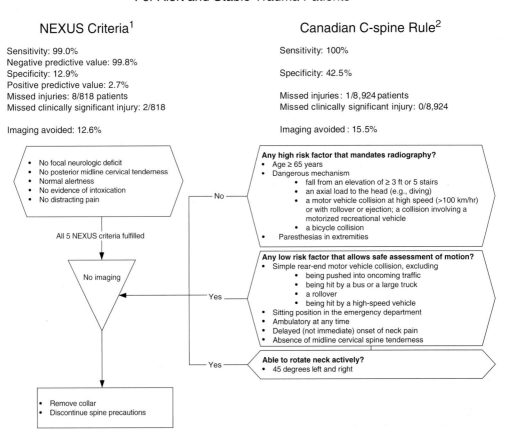

For Alert and Stable Trauma Patients

NEXUS Criteria[1]

Sensitivity: 99.0%
Negative predictive value: 99.8%
Specificity: 12.9%
Positive predictive value: 2.7%
Missed injuries: 8/818 patients
Missed clinically significant injury: 2/818

Imaging avoided: 12.6%

- No focal neurologic deficit
- No posterior midline cervical tenderness
- Normal alertness
- No evidence of intoxication
- No distracting pain

All 5 NEXUS criteria fulfilled

No imaging

- Remove collar
- Discontinue spine precautions

Canadian C-spine Rule[2]

Sensitivity: 100%

Specificity: 42.5%

Missed injuries: 1/8,924 patients
Missed clinically significant injury: 0/8,924

Imaging avoided: 15.5%

Any high risk factor that mandates radiography?
- Age ≥ 65 years
- Dangerous mechanism
  - fall from an elevation of ≥ 3 ft or 5 stairs
  - an axial load to the head (e.g., diving)
  - a motor vehicle collision at high speed (>100 km/hr) or with rollover or ejection; a collision involving a motorized recreational vehicle
  - a bicycle collision
- Paresthesias in extremities

Any low risk factor that allows safe assessment of motion?
- Simple rear-end motor vehicle collision, excluding
  - being pushed into oncoming traffic
  - being hit by a bus or a large truck
  - a rollover
  - being hit by a high-speed vehicle
- Sitting position in the emergency department
- Ambulatory at any time
- Delayed (not immediate) onset of neck pain
- Absence of midline cervical spine tenderness

Able to rotate neck actively?
- 45 degrees left and right

[1]Hoffman JR et al. Validity of a set of clinical criteria to rule out injury to the cervical spine in patients with blunt trauma. National Emergency X-Radiography Utilization Study Group. N Engl J Med 2000;343.

[2]Stiell IG et al. The Canadian C-spine rule for radiography in alert and stable trauma patients. JAMA 2001;286:1841.

Figure 13.7: Comparison of NEXUS Criteria and Canadian C-spine Rule for avoiding imaging in alert, examinable trauma patients. NEXUS, National Emergency X-ray Utilization Study. (From Adeniran AO, Pearson AM, Mirza SK. Principles of Spine Trauma Care. In: Court-Brown C, Heckman JD, McKee M, McQueen MM, Ricci W, Tornetta P, eds. *Rockwood and Green's Fractures in Adults.* 8th ed. Philadelphia, PA: Wolters Kluwer; 2015:1645-1676. Figure 43.5.)

type of imaging is recommended. In young alert patients without underlying spine disease and a low suspicion for spine/spinal cord injury, a three-view (anteroposterior [AP], lateral, and open mouth) cervical x-ray series may be sufficient. This has become less utilized given the inadequacy of x-rays and availability of CT (**Figure 13.8**).

In older patients with potential degenerative changes, in any patient in whom there is a concern for spinal cord injury (ie, a neurologic deficit), or in patients with encephalopathy, high-resolution CT with thin cuts (1.5-3 mm) is recommended. If there is a neurologic injury that cannot be explained by CT scan, an MRI can be obtained to look for soft-tissue/ligamentous injury, spinal cord edema, hemorrhage, and demyelination. In patients who have a contraindication to MRI, CT myelogram can be considered; however, it is advised to use caution when performing a lumbar puncture to introduce contrast because changes in the pressure of the spinal column may exacerbate the neurologic injury.

In the comatose patient, it is more difficult to clear the C-spine. If the patient cannot be cleared clinically, it is safest to keep the patient stabilized in a cervical collar, especially if there are other traumatic injuries that need to be tended to first, or if the patient is likely to wake up and become examinable in the near future. It is not recommended to use flexion and extension radiographs for spine clearance in a patient who cannot be clinically examined and cleared. MRI of the cervical spine is an option; however, it may overestimate the degree of soft-tissue injury. There can be nonspecific signal changes in the paraspinal muscles without any significant disruption of discoligamentous structures. MRI can also be useful in patients with degenerative changes seen on CT.

Given the course the vertebral arteries take through the cervical spine, any patient with a C-spine injury should be screened for vertebral artery injury. Carotid vessels can be injured as well, depending on the mechanism and force of injury. Screening is typically done with a CT angiogram of the neck, and in many cases, it is just as good as a digital subtraction angiogram as well as being less invasive.[6] The Denver Screening Criteria for Vascular Injury can be used as a guide to help determine who needs a screening angiogram (**Table 13.4**). In patients who are found to have carotid or vertebral artery injury, treatment often consists of antiplatelet medication or anticoagulation

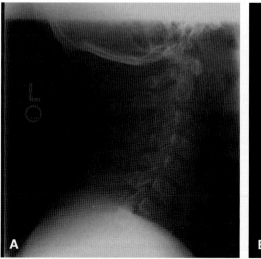
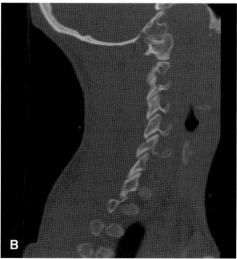

Figure 13.8: A nondiagnostic plain film in a symptomatic patient who had a C6 fracture seen on computed tomography (CT). A. Seemingly normal lateral x-ray of the cervical spine. B. CT reveals a nondisplaced fracture at C6. (Courtesy of Dr William Krantz, West Virginia University, Department of Radiology and from Tadros A. Cervical spine imaging in trauma. In: Tews M, eds. Clerkship Directors in Emergency Medicine (CDEM). Accessed March 5, 2021. https://www.saem .org/cdem/education/online-education/m3-curriculum/group-traumatic-and-orthopedic-injuries/cervical-spine-imaging-in-trauma)

TABLE 13.4	Denver Screening Criteria for Blunt Vascular Injury
Risk Factors for Vascular Injury	
Infarct on head CT	
Cervical hematoma	
Massive epistaxis	
Anisocoria or Horner syndrome	
Severe TBI with GCS < 8	
Cervical bruit or thrill	
Focal neurologic deficit	
Severe facial fractures (LaForte II or III, mandible fracture)	
Cervical spine fracture	
Fracture of the skull base or occipital condyles	
Thoracic vascular injury	
Blunt cardiac rupture	
Upper rib fracture	
Hanging injury	

CT, computed tomography; GCS, Glasgow Coma Scale; TBI, traumatic brain injury.

pending no contraindications. Endovascular intervention may be warranted for patients who have pseudoaneurysms or fistulas, and in some cases of dissection. In rare cases, occlusive embolization of the vessel may need to be done.

MANAGEMENT

Cervical Spine Bracing

Various types of collars and bracing devices exist (**Figure 13.9**). Soft sponge collars do not immobilize the cervical spine or stabilize it to any significant degree. The function of soft collars is mostly to remind the patient to reduce their own neck movements. Rigid cervical collars are better for spine stabilization, but may not be adequate for upper and mid-cervical spine injury or prevention of rotation. Rigid collars include Miami J, Aspen, and Philadelphia. Both the Miami J and Aspen collars have removable pads, whereas the Philadelphia collar's pads are not removable.

Cervicothoracic orthoses (**Figure 13.10**) include the two-poster brace, Minerva brace, sternal occipital mandibular immobilizer (SOMI) brace, and the Yale brace. These orthoses consist of a neck collar that incorporates some form of a body vest to immobilize the cervical spine. The cervicothoracic orthoses do a better job limiting flexion-extension and rotation as compared to hard cervical collars alone.[7,8] They are not as good in prevention of lateral bending in comparison to a halo-vest.

The halo-vest brace can help immobilize the upper or lower cervical spine, but is not quite as good for mid-cervical lesions. Overall, the halo-vest reduces flexion, extension, and lateral bending and rotation more than do other nonsurgical external stabilizing devices. This device consists of a halo with pins that screw into the skull for fixation, and the ring is then connected to a vest by four rods. Newer versions have more of a half halo with an opening posteriorly.

Cervical Traction

In some patients, cervical traction can be used initially before surgical stabilization for closed reduction in cases of fracture dislocation. Traction can rapidly decompress neural elements, but should only be performed by an experienced clinician; it also requires having an awake and cooperative patient to closely monitor the neurologic examination. Gardner Wells tongs

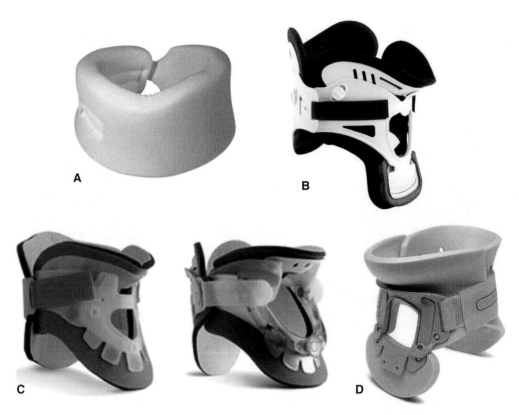

Figure 13.9: Different types of collars. A. Soft foam collar. B. Miami J cervical collar. C. Aspen cervical collar. D. Philadelphia cervical collar.

(**Figure 13.11**) are generally used with weights progressively suspended from the head. With each increment of weight, the patient is reexamined neurologically and radiologically to visualize the dislocation. This process is continued until one of the following: reduction is obtained, two-third patient body weight is reached, there is a neurologic change, or if excessive distraction is seen on x-ray. Following initial reduction, the alignment of the cervical spine can often be maintained with less weight than what was needed to reduce the dislocation. A disadvantage of using cervical traction is that the patient must remain supine, which may lead to difficulty with airway protection. Beds that can move into reverse Trendelenburg may help to some degree. Traction is contraindicated if a patient has atlanto-occipital dislocation, traumatic disk herniation, or other additional rostral injuries.

Early Decompression and Stabilization

It is advised that decompression of neural elements and stabilization of a mechanically unstable spine be done in a timely manner. The definition of spinal instability may be debated, but, in general, it can be described as a loss of structural integrity that poses a risk of the following: neurologic decline, progressive deformity, or persistent pain under normal physiologic loads and ROM. As noted previously, some fractures are more stable than are others and can be treated with external brace stabilization, whereas other injuries with significant bony and ligamentous disruption require internal surgical stabilization. In patients who have a neurologic deficit, early decompression and stabilization of the spine may improve outcomes, especially if the patient has an incomplete injury. The sooner a patient goes in for surgical stabilization, the sooner they may be mobilized and have decreased risk of venous thromboembolism (VTE) and pulmonary complications. In patients with a neurologic deficit, there are data to suggest that the earlier the surgical decompression, the outcome in that ongoing compression may contribute to secondary injury.[9-11] Depending on the study, "early" decompression could mean within 8 to 12 hours of

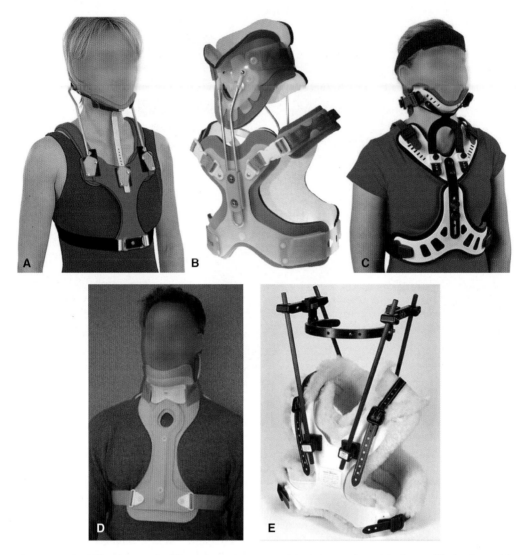

Figure 13.10: Different cervicothoracic orthoses. A. SOMI (sternal occipital mandibular immobilizer) brace. B. Aspen CTO brace. C. Minerva CTO halo brace. D. Yale brace. E. Halo vest with cervical traction.

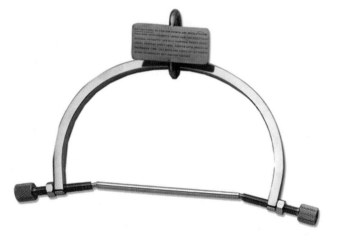

Figure 13.11: Gardner Wells traction tongs.

the injury or within 24 hours. Although earlier surgical stabilization is the ideal, in the poly-trauma patient before consideration for spine surgery, it is important to make sure there is adequate resuscitation and there are no other potentially life-threatening injuries that might take precedence.

Autonomic Derangements and Neurogenic Shock

Immediate attention should be given to blood pressure management in a patient presenting with acute spinal cord injury. Hypotension and bradycardia occur fairly often in cervical or high thoracic spinal cord injuries (T6 level or above) because of damage of the sympathetic chain fibers; hypoperfusion to the injured spinal cord leading to further damage may result from hypotension.

Neurogenic shock is a distributive shock state that is caused by loss of sympathetic tone leading to profound hypotension, bradycardia, and peripheral vasodilation. It is estimated to occur in up to 20% of patients with cervical injury.[1] Patients may require vasopressors after volume resuscitation to maintain a normal MAP that allows for adequate tissue perfusion. Hemorrhagic shock, tension pneumothorax, and cardiac tamponade must be considered in these patients. Bradycardia and hypotension in patients with neurogenic shock may be exacerbated by anything that increases vagal tone (ie, suctioning, defecating) as well as turning, and hypoxia.

Acute-Phase Blood Pressure Recommendations

Current guidelines suggest blood pressure augmentation may be helpful in the acute phase post the injury. The suggested MAP target is 85 to 90 mm Hg, and goal systolic blood pressure >90 mm Hg. The length of blood pressure augmentation is up to 1 week. MAP augmentation can be done with both fluids and vasopressors, with caution advised so as not to volume overload the patient. The Consortium for Spinal Cord Medicine suggests that a vasopressor with inotropic, chronotropic, and vasoconstrictive properties be used: see section "Evidence."[11,12]

The risks and benefits of blood pressure augmentation obviously must be assessed for each individual patient because prolonged use of vasopressors and keeping patients in bed connected to IV poles also have their negative side effects. In our opinion, it is acceptable to reevaluate the patient's ability to tolerate lower MAP goals following decompression/stabilization and demonstrating clinical stability of their neurologic examination.

Subacute—Chronic Orthostatic Hypotension, Other Autonomic Derangements, and Autonomic Dysreflexia

Symptomatic orthostatic hypotension may continue even past the acute phase of injury that impedes patient mobilization and rehabilitation. Abdominal binders and thigh-high compression stockings can be used to help with venous dilatation and return to the heart. Pharmacologic agents can be started to help treat hypotension and include midodrine or ephedrine.

Aside from cardiovascular autonomic changes such as hypotension and bradyarrhythmias, patients can have other autonomic concerns. Temperature regulation becomes more problematic in patients with spinal cord injury. Hypothermia is a common problem because of the inability of blood vessels to vasoconstrict, and loss of shivering response. Heat dissipation when patients have elevated body temperatures is impaired because of the inability of the body to redistribute blood to surfaces and impaired sweating. Bladder and bowel dysfunction is common. There may be incontinence and retention, with an inability to void or defecate.

Autonomic dysreflexia may emerge and consists of acute hypertension, bradycardia, flushing, diaphoresis, blurred vision, and headache. Of note, systolic blood pressure elevations in adults > 20 mm Hg above baseline may suggest autonomic dysreflexia. The most common cause of autonomic dysreflexia is distended viscus, such as overdistended bladder or bowel with retention. This stimulus then leads to a massive sympathetic outflow. The Consortium for Spinal Cord Medicine guidelines recommend some easy things to check first: if the blood pressure is high, sit the patient upright if they are laying supine, loosen any tight clothing or other constrictive devices, survey the patient for instigating urinary causes (check indwelling catheter if there is one, bladder scan, in and out catheterization, etc.), and evaluate the patient for fecal impaction. If none of these are the inciting problem, the patient may need further evaluation and temporary treatment with an antihypertensive that has both a rapid onset of action and short duration while other etiologies are explored.

Pulmonary and Airway Issues

Both pulmonary function and airway mechanics need to be assessed and managed in a patient with cervical spinal cord injury. Lesions above C5 impair diaphragmatic function. Even with C5 injury or below, accessory muscles of respiration can be affected, leading to paradoxic breathing, reduced tidal volumes, atelectasis, and respiratory failure. Patients have reduced ability to cough and clear their airway, leading to aspiration events. Dysphagia and bulbar dysfunction can complicate matters, leading to even more difficulty managing secretions.

Patients with cervical spine injury are considered to have a difficult airway because spinal alignment must remain stable during intubation. There is decreased ROM of the neck to align a patient in the "sniffing" position needed for direct laryngoscopy. In patients with trauma to the head or face, fractures or bleeding in the naso- or oropharynx increase the complexity, making the provider potentially unable to bag mask ventilate or visualize structures in the airway.

Fiberoptic intubation or video laryngoscopy is the recommended technique for intubating the patient with a C-spine injury because they are performed with the patient's neck in a neutral position. Jaw thrust maneuvers are generally safe, but it is not recommended to tilt the patient's head or perform a chin lift. Manual in-line stabilization of the neck by a second provider with the anterior portion of the collar off may be performed to assist more emergent intubation; however, this technique is known to affect the grade view during laryngoscopy, and rescue airway equipment should be available. In trauma patients with injuries to the face and bleeding obstructing the airway, a surgical airway may be preferred.

Higher tidal volumes can be considered in patients with respiratory failure due to cervical spinal cord injury and difficulty weaning from the ventilator. The Consortium for Spinal Cord Medicine recommends a tidal volume of approximately 15 to 20 cc/kg ideal body weight, because higher tidal volumes may help promote recruitment, prevent atelectasis, and be better tolerated in patients with healthy lung physiology.[13,14] The risks and benefits of using higher tidal volumes leading to possible volutrauma and barotrauma must be considered in patients with polytrauma acutely at risk for acute respiratory distress syndrome; alternative to higher volumes, more external positive end-expiratory pressure (PEEP) can help patient comfort and synchrony. Up to half of patients with cervical spinal cord injury may require a tracheostomy for chronic respiratory failure. Patients with a complete spinal cord injury have higher rates of tracheostomy than do those with incomplete lesions.

Prevention of Venous Thromboembolism

Patients with spinal cord injury are at high risk for VTE, especially those patients with neurologic motor deficits. Mechanical pneumatic compression devices should be placed early after injury. Low-molecular-weight heparin (LMWH) or unfractionated heparin (UFH) are recommended for pharmacologic prophylaxis and should be initiated within 72 hours. In some instances, pharmacologic prophylaxis may need to be temporarily held before surgical stabilization and decompression; however, it should be resumed as soon as possible, typically within 24 hours postoperatively.

Steroids

There is controversy over the use of corticosteroids to improve outcomes in patients with spinal cord injury. At present, there is no clear evidence to demonstrate that steroids improve outcomes, especially if they are administered > 8 hours post injury, see section "**Evidence**."

PEDIATRIC ISSUES

Spinal cord injury is fairly uncommon in the pediatric population. The ratio of head injury to spinal cord injury in pediatric patients is about 30:1, and of all spinal cord injuries only about 5% occur in children. As in adults, the cervical spine is the region most commonly injured in pediatric patients. In children who are younger than or equal to age 9 years, about two-third of the injuries occur at the OC junction, but with increasing age, subaxial cervical spine involvement may be seen. Children have larger heads in relation to their body size as compared to adults, which changes the fulcrum. The vertebral bodies are not completely ossified, making the spine more flexible. Ligaments are firmly attached to articular bone surfaces. In the pediatric population, ligamentous injury of the spine is more common than are bony fractures. This is because the ligaments have more laxity and the paraspinal muscles are underdeveloped. It is also possible that neural damage may occur even without significant musculoskeletal injury in young children because of immaturity and flexibility of the bony ligamentous structures. In comparison to adult patients with neurologic injury, children have a better prognosis for recovery.

Spinal cord injury without radiographic abnormality (SCIWORA) was originally described in the 1980s in children who presented with either ongoing or transient neurologic deficits following an injury, but had no acute signs of injury on imaging. With the increasing availability of MRI, many of these patients with presumed "SCIWORA" actually have demonstrable injury to the spinal cord and/or soft-tissue components of the spinal column.[15] The spine in children is more mobile and malleable, which may be why patients may present with neurologic deficits and no obviously bony injuries on plain films or CT scan. There is a small percentage of patients who still do not have defined injuries seen on MRI, and these individuals without signal change to the spinal cord typically have excellent neurologic recovery. SCIWORA can occur in adults and in pediatric patients, but is less common.

TIPS AND PEARLS

- The primary injury refers to the initial compression, contusion, stretching, and/or laceration of the spinal cord. Secondary injury occurs at the cellular level following initial injury.
- The ASIA impairment scale helps document a patient's initial neurologic status following a spinal cord injury.
- Cervical spine bracing and immobilization on a rigid board with straps is typically implemented prehospitalization to help protect the spine from further mechanical injury and prevent further neurologic dysfunction.
- Decision rules help determine who needs radiographs.
- Early surgical decompression and stabilization of a mechanically unstable spine may lead to better outcomes.
- Airway and pulmonary issues are common in patients with cervical spinal cord injury and may lead to aspiration, paradoxic breathing, and respiratory failure.
- Patients with cervical spine injury/trauma are considered difficult intubations because of the need for in-line immobilization and stabilization of the neck and inability to perform head tilt and chin lift maneuvers. The use of video laryngoscopes or flexible fiberoptic scopes can ease placement of endotracheal airways.
- Autonomic dysfunction can frequently occur with cervical spinal cord injuries and commonly consists of hypotension, bradycardia, urinary retention, slow transit bowel constipation, and changes in temperature regulation.
- In the acute trauma patient, hemorrhagic/hypovolemic shock needs to be ruled out before considering neurogenic shock. After volume resuscitation, vasopressors can be considered for treatment of neurogenic shock.
- Neurogenic shock is a distributive type of shock resulting from cervical spine or high thoracic injury, and is due to loss of sympathetic vascular tone and bradycardia. Spinal shock is an initial acute depression or loss of all neurologic function below the level of a spinal cord injury that has improvement over time. Neurogenic shock may occur acutely during spinal shock.
- In spinal cord injury, blood pressure augmentation to help increase spinal cord perfusion with fluids and vasopressors may be considered with a target pressure of > 85 to 90 mm Hg.
- In patients with cervical spine fractures, screening for arterial injury with a CT angiogram is recommended based on the Denver Screening Criteria.
- At this time, there is no strong evidence to support the use of corticosteroids or hypothermia for neuroprotection in patients with acute spinal cord injury

EVIDENCE

What is the best way to immobilize the spine?

Historically, complete spinal immobilization was used for emergency transport of patients with blunt injury trauma with the use of a long backboard, cervical collar, and head immobilization device. The thought process being that complete immobilization would reduce the risk of neurologic deterioration due to forces that may exacerbate the initial injury. Studies have been performed to evaluate the benefit of long board immobilization, and the potential risks.[16,17] The use of hard backboards may lead to increased pain and discomfort (boards are not padded and do not align with the natural curvature of the spine, this clearly being most pronounced in patients with baseline kyphotic or lordotic spine deformities), can cause pressure ulcers (patients are on the board much longer than intended), delay in resuscitation (delays in intubation have arisen out of fear for movement of the spine), and increases in intracranial pressure (due to head of bed flat positioning and cervical collars that were perhaps placed too tightly). On the basis of spine biomechanics, some have noted that the amount of force required to create bony and ligamentous injury to the spine is rather significant, and therefore for further injury to occur, forces would need to be directed to the injured site exceeding the normal ROM.[16]

In 2013, the National Association of EMS Physicians made a statement calling for decreased use of long spine boards, noting that it may still have use in a subset of patients: blunt trauma with altered consciousness, spinal pain or tenderness, neurologic disability (weakness or numbness), anatomic deformity of the spine, high-energy mechanism with intoxication, inability to communicate, or other distracting injury.[17] There is a shift toward "spinal motion restriction" over "spinal immobilization."[18] Patients with blunt trauma can be transported with a hard cervical collar in a scoop stretcher, padded litter, vacuum splint, ambulance cot, or a longboard—but immobilization should be removed as quickly as possible after arrival at the hospital.[17,18] There is no role for spinal motion restriction in patients with penetrating traumas.[18]

Can the C-spine be safely cleared using clinical criteria?

Both the NEXUS criteria[3] and the Canadian C-spine Rule[5] can be used to identify trauma patients who require imaging. Before the development of these guidelines, there was a seemingly excessive amount of C-spine imaging being performed in part due to the high morbidity of missing an injury and the medicolegal risks. The NEXUS criteria validation study used three-view x-ray imaging of the neck, unless a CT or an MRI was also performed. While developing the Canadian C-spine Rule, patients underwent plain x-ray films or CT of the neck based on physician discretion. Both of these guidelines have high sensitivity to detect injury, 99% and 100%, respectively; the NEXUS criteria have a negative predictive value of 99.8%, whereas the Canadian C-spine Rule has a negative predictive value of 100%.[3,5]

What is the best vasopressor for managing neurogenic shock?

A common first choice is norepinephrine; however, dopamine or epinephrine might also be considered, and vasopressin may be added in refractory cases. Phenylephrine can be used, but has a risk for worsening bradycardia because it is a pure alpha agonist. In patients with profound bradycardia, inotropic vasopressors can be used, but other treatments to consider are atropine, glycopyrrolate, aminophylline, or theophylline, and in refractory cases a cardiac pacer.[11,12]

Do steroids improve outcomes in patients with acute spinal cord injury?

Corticosteroids were once thought to offer some degree of neuroprotection through modulation of the immune/inflammatory process, inhibition of cytokine production, and reduction of lipid peroxidation/development of free radicals.[19] The National Acute Spinal Cord Injury Study I (NASCIS I), NASCIS II, and NASCIS III trials all looked at the use of methylprednisolone as a neuroprotective agent post injury. The primary analyses in these studies did not demonstrate any significant difference in either motor or sensory recovery between groups. Posthoc analyses of NASCIS II, which compared placebo to methylprednisolone, revealed an improvement in neurologic function only in those patients who received methylprednisolone within 8 hours of injury. Those receiving steroids after 8 hours actually had worse neurologic outcomes than did those on placebo. The NASCIS III trial did not have a placebo arm, but instead compared duration of steroid treatment for either 24 or 48 hours. The difference between groups was not statistically significant; however, in posthoc analyses, greater improvement was demonstrated in those patients who received the methylprednisolone for a period of 48 hours if started between 3 and 8 hours after injury. That being said, the longer duration of treatment portended an increased risk of infection. These studies have had criticisms over biases and the use of posthoc analyses following initial negative primary findings. A Cochrane review performed by the same investigator completing NASCIS trials suggested that in clinical practice, methylprednisolone, if given within 8 hours of injury, can lead to improved outcomes, and further improvement may occur if the duration of therapy is extended to 48 hours.[20]

The Consortium for Spinal Cord Medicine guidelines note there is no definitive evidence to recommend the use of any neuroprotective agents, including steroids, at this time. The efficacy is questionable, and there is a possibility for severe side effects with the use. Other authors have suggested that repeat randomized controlled trials need to be done looking at treating patients specifically within 8 hours of injury to see if there is, in fact, reliable improvements in neurologic function.[21]

Does therapeutic hypothermia improve outcomes in patients with acute spinal injury?

There is not enough high-quality data at this time to support the use of therapeutic hypothermia in spinal cord injury. A few small trials and case reports of the use of hypothermia for high-grade spinal cord injuries that suggest potential benefit have been published, but more research is needed.[22] Induced hypothermia has its own host of risks and complications, including infections, coagulopathy, and electrolyte derangements. There is evidence that fever in patients with spinal cord injury can be detrimental, and utilizing devices such as intravascular catheters or cooling pads to keep patients normothermic and prevent hyperthermic injury to cells can be considered if other measures to treat elevated temperatures fail.[23]

References

1. Ahuja CS, Wilson JR, Nori S, et al. Traumatic spinal cord injury. *Nat Rev Dis Primers*. 2017;3(17018):1-21.

2. Vaccaro AR, Hulbert RJ, Patel AA, et al. The subaxial cervical spine injury classification system: a novel approach to recognize the importance of morphology, neurology, and integrity of the disco-ligamentous complex. *Spine*. 2007;32(21):2365-2374.

3. Hoffman JR, Mower WR, Wolfson AB, Todd KH, Zucker MI. Validity of a set of clinical criteria to rule out injury to the cervical spine in patients with blunt trauma. *N Engl J Med*. 2000;343(2):94-99.

4. Bernhard M, Gries A, Kremer P, Böttiger BW. Spinal cord injury – prehospital management. *Resuscitation*. 2005;66:127-139.

5. Stiell IG, Wells GA, Vandemheen KL, et al. The Canadian C-spine rule for radiography in alert and stable trauma patients. *JAMA*. 2001;286(15):1841-1848.

6. Brommeland T, Helseth E, Aarhus M, et al. Best practice guidelines for blunt cerebrovascular injury (BCVI). *Scand J Trauma Resusc Emerg Med*. 2018;26:90.

7. Holla M, Huisman JMR, Verdonschot N, Goosen J, Hosman AJF, Hannink G. The ability of external immobilizers to restrict movement of the cervical spine: a systematic review. *Eur Spine J*. 2016;25:2023-2036.

8. Ivanic PC. Do cervical collars and cervicothoracic orthoses effectively stabilize the injured cervical spine? *Spine*. 2013;38(13):E767-E774.

9. Furlan JC, Noonan V, Cadotte DW, Fehlings MG. Timing of decompressive surgery of spinal cord after traumatic spinal cord injury: an evidence based examination of preclinical and clinical studies. *J Neurotrauma*. 2011;28:1371-1399.

10. Wilson JR, Tetreault LA, Kwon BK, et al. Timing of decompression in patients with acute spinal cord injury: a systematic review. *Global Spine J*. 2017;7(3S):95S-115S.

11. Witiw CD, Fehlings MG. Acute spinal cord injury. *J Spinal Disord Tech*. 2015;28(6):202-210.

12. Consortium for Spinal Cord Medicine. Clinical practice guidelines: early acute management in adults with spinal cord injury. *J Spinal Cord Med*. 2008;31(4):403-479.

13. Consortium for Spinal Cord Medicine. Clinical practice guidelines: respiratory management following spinal cord injury. *J Spinal Cord Med*. 2005;28(3):259-293.

14. Vázquez RG, Sedes PR, Fariña MM, Marqués AM, Ferreiro Velasco ME. Respiratory management in the patient with spinal cord injury. *Biomed Res Int*. 2013;2013:168757.

15. Pang D. Spinal cord injury without radiographic abnormality in children, 2 decades later. *Neurosurgery*. 2004;55(6):1325-1343.

16. Hauswald M. A re-conceptualization of acute spinal care. *Emerg Med J*. 2013;30:720-723.

17. Feld FX. Removal of the long spine board from clinical practice: a historical perspective. *J Athl Train*. 2018;53(8):752-755.

18. Fischer PE, Perina DG, Delbridge TR, Fallat ME, et al. Spinal motion restriction in the trauma patient – a joint position statement. *Prehosp Emer Care*. 2018;22(6):659-661.

19. Kwon BK, Tetzlaff W, Grauer JN, Beiner J, Vaccaro AR. Pathophysiology and pharmacologic treatment of acute spinal cord injury. *Spine J*. 2004;4:451-464.

20. Bracken MB. Cochrane library review: steroids for acute spinal cord injury. *Cochrane Database Syst Rev*. 2012;1:CD001046.

21. Nesathurai S. Steroids and spinal cord injury: revisiting the NASCIS II and NASCIS III trials. *J Trauma*. 1998;45(6):1088-1093.

22. Dietrich WD, Cappuccino A, Cappuccino H. Systemic hypothermia for the treatment of acute cervical spine injury in sports. *Curr Sports Med Rep*. 2011;10(1):50-54.

23. Guadalupe Castillo-Abrego. Update on therapeutic temperature management: hypothermia in spinal cord injury. *Crit Care*. 2012;16(Suppl 2):15-17.

Thoracic and Lumbar Spine

Lauren M. Post

Angela Hua

CLINICAL CHALLENGE

In the emergency department (ED), low back pain is one of the most common musculoskeletal chief complaints and affects approximately 80% of adults at some point in their lives.[1] The complaint of low back pain was responsible for approximately 4% of ED visits from 2000 to 2016.[2] "Spinal conditions," which include neck and back pain, comprise the third largest portion of total national health spending in the United States, behind diabetes and heart disease.[3] The majority of patients presenting to the ED will complain of neck or lower back pain rather than thoracic-level pain. Thoracic back pain has been documented less frequently, with < 20% of people reporting symptoms within their lifetime.[4] Many will have benign etiologies that will resolve with conservative management, but the small percentage that requires immediate intervention must be quickly identified. In addition, patients with nonemergent conditions require a well-thought out strategic plan to manage their condition and maximize function.

A broad differential diagnosis and an evaluation that is systematic without bias is fundamental to managing low back pain; see **Table 14.1**. In addition to primary spinal pathology, processes that may refer pain to the back must be considered. Failure to address these alternative diagnoses in the face of localized pain is a common oversight in many case reviews.[5] Because of the lower frequency of thoracic back pain, vascular emergencies and other causes of referred pain must remain high on the differential for patients with this complaint.

PATHOPHYSIOLOGY

Musculoskeletal strain, arthritic degeneration, spinal stenosis, and stable fractures may be painful and contribute to overall morbidity, but are not usually associated with acute neurologic deficits. Many of the more serious causes of back pain can be categorized as being "compressive," with the inciting pathology filling the limited amount of space within the spinal canal. **Figure 14.1** shows the relative location of the potential spaces in and around the spinal column.

The spinal cord tapers to the conus medullaris around the L1 level; the cauda equina is the bundle of nerve roots that continues to innervate the lower extremities, perineum, and bladder. Compressive lesions, including herniated disks, tumors, hematomas, and abscesses, can fill these spaces and exert pressure on the cord and nerve roots. This pressure may reduce blood flow, inducing ischemia of neural tissue and may cause transient, acute dysfunction as well as permanent infarction if not decompressed. Some of the more benign pathologies may develop a compressive component as well and may progress to requiring surgical intervention.

TABLE 14.1	Differential Diagnosis of Adult Patients Presenting with Back Pain
Primary Benign	**Primary Serious**

Stable fracture
Sprains and strains
Degeneration
Spinal stenosis
Posterolateral disk herniation
	Unstable fracture
	Malignancy
	  • Epidural metastatic disease
	  • Intradural metastatic disease
	  • Intramedullary tumor
	Infection
	  • Osteomyelitis
	  • Epidural abscess
	  • Infectious diskitis
	Hematoma
	  • Epidural
	  • Subarachnoid
	  • *Central disk herniation*

Secondary[a]	

Vascular
  • Aneurysm
  • Dissection
  • Thromboembolism
Gastrointestinal
  • Malignancy
  • Pancreatitis
  • Gallbladder disease
  • Peptic ulcer
Cardiac ischemia
  • *Pulmonary*
  • Malignancy
  • Infection
Retroperitoneal
  • Malignancy
  • Renal colic
  • Infection
  • Hemorrhage
  • Localized abscess	

[a]May still be considered serious.

Radiculopathy, the pain and weakness associated with nerve root impingement, results from one of the compressive mechanisms of injury. Spinal disk disease is usually benign and self-limited, with approximately 80% to 90% of cases getting symptomatic relief with medical management. Lumbar disk disease results from changes in disk alignment and integrity, resulting in abnormal bony movement and pain. Compression of microvasculature feeding the spinal cord and nerve roots produces ischemia within these structures. The resulting inflammation and degradation cause an increase in inflammatory mediators, that is, cytokines, tumor necrosis factor alpha (TNF-α), and macrophages. This process causes loss of disk and foraminal height, the inability to cushion the spinal column, and neuropathic pain. Increased mechanical stress also causes bony distortion at the facets, and osteophyte formation. A combination of these factors leads to the clinical presentation of lumbar radiculopathy, pain, and weakness as a result of nerve root impingement. Epidural compression may occur at the levels of the spinal cord, conus medullaris, or cauda equina. This compression occurs most commonly from disk herniation, followed by tumor and infection, with a small percentage caused by hemorrhage.[6,7] Conus medullaris syndrome occurs when there is a compressive force from T12 to L2, and cauda equina syndrome from compression of the nerve roots from L3 to L5. Both of these syndromes may present as back pain with neurologic deficits including urinary retention and lower extremity weakness.

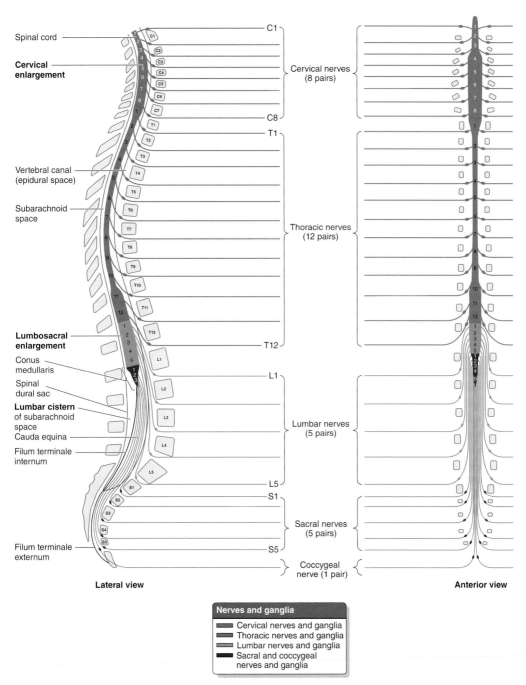

Figure 14.1: Anatomy of the spinal column.

PREHOSPITAL CONSIDERATIONS

When the emergency medical system is activated, the prehospital provider becomes the first point of triage, with the mechanism of injury determining the initial resources and the transport destination. Traumatic injuries require a rapid primary survey, with an evaluation for the presence of additional injuries and mechanical stabilization of potential fractures. These patients may require immobilization and log-roll precautions to prevent any further complications. Patients with concomitant head injuries or meeting trauma activation criteria should be transported to a facility with appropriate specialty coverage. Because the etiology of atraumatic back pain is varied, a more comprehensive secondary survey may be needed to determine stability. Abnormal vital signs or motor deficits can provide important information before arrival at the receiving ED, and also guiding further evaluation. It is also critical that the prehospital provider attempt to obtain additional medical history, medications, and alcohol or substance use.

PEDIATRIC ISSUES

The pediatric population adds another level of complexity to the evaluation of back pain. **Table 14.2** lists some of the more common causes of back pain in this group. Musculoskeletal causes of thoracic back pain tend to be more frequent in the adolescent population than in other pediatric age groups.[4] Overuse injuries are frequent, and the rapid growth of adolescence can cause pain as well as potentially worsening scoliosis. Interestingly, the use of school backpacks and their increasing weight has been suggested as contributing to the preponderance of musculoskeletal back pain in older children and adolescents.[4] Younger patients tend not to have the degenerative changes present in adults, making acute disk herniation a less likely process. The pediatric spine is more flexible than in adulthood, leading to spinal cord injuries without radiographic abnormality (SCIWORA) in cases of trauma.

As in adults, infection and malignancy should be considered in a patient presenting with acute back pain. Primary pediatric malignancies such as lymphomas and leukemias frequently cause back pain. Unlike many adult malignancies, cancers affecting children appear less likely to metastasize to the bony spine. Infectious diskitis and infectious spondylodiskitis are rare but potentially devastating infections of the intervertebral disk and surrounding vertebral bodies. Most cases are due to hematogenous spread of *Staphylococcus aureus*; however, in endemic areas, *Mycobacterium tuberculosis* is also a frequent cause. The clinical presentation of these infections is usually nonspecific, with low-grade fever associated with lower back pain and stiffness. Neurologic deficits are not usually present until later stages, when nerve compression occurs or the infection breaks into

TABLE 14.2	Causes of Back Pain in Children and Adolescents
Mechanical	• Fracture • Overuse • Herniated disk • Scoliosis
Tumors	• Osteoid osteoma • Bone cyst • Ewing tumor • Osteogenic sarcoma • Neuroblastoma • Wilms tumor • Lymphoma • Leukemia
Infection/Inflammation	• Diskitis/spondylodiskitis • Osteomyelitis • Collagen vascular diseases • Ankylosing spondylitis
Referred pain	• SCFE • Hip/knee abnormalities • Gait abnormalities causing strain • Additional causes of secondary pain as noted in Table 14.1

Slipped capital femoral epiphysis SCFE.

the spinal canal. Most cases are mild and treated with rest and symptomatic pain relief, but if left untreated, these infections can lead to permanent deformities, spinal instability, or extension into the spinal canal.

Conditions referring pain into the back are similar to those in adults. In addition, children with genetic conditions affecting the connective tissue such as Marfan and Ehlers-Danlos syndromes may also present with back pain due to spinal instability or mechanical stress.

APPROACH/THE FOCUSED EXAMINATION

The history in patients with back pain should include a review of systems, prior medical problems, time course, modifying factors, associated symptoms, and prior episodes. Specifically asking about neurologic changes, reviewing medications, and previous records will help narrow the differential diagnosis. **Figure 14.2** provides a framework for evaluating the patient presenting with acute back pain. The use of "red flags" to suggest serious underlying pathology in back pain is a useful tool (**Table 14.3**). These factors help identify patients at risk for more serious etiologies of back pain, including malignancy, infection, and hemorrhage.

A comprehensive physical examination including, but not limited to, neurologic and musculoskeletal systems is required. General observation of patients complaining of back pain can contribute to a differential diagnosis and subsequent workup. Watching during common movements such as walking, sitting, and standing can provide insight into the degree of discomfort and limitation of function. Many patients with mechanical low back pain will find certain positions or postures more comfortable. Observing for guarding or avoidance of specific movements may also be helpful, because this may suggest a referred or intra-abdominal cause of the pain. In addition, looking for general changes in physical appearance such as muscle wasting or the stigmata of substance abuse can aid in stratifying these patients.

Vital signs are a critical component of the evaluation of back pain, and may provide important clues to the cause of pain that may otherwise be overlooked. Elevated temperature or recent history of fevers highly suggests an infectious process. In combination with the complaint of back pain, a fever may be the only other evidence of infection, especially within the deeper structures. Although uncommon, some patients may report a recent fever but present as afebrile. The measurement of blood pressure helps in screening for intra-abdominal catastrophes that can present as back pain. Hypertension is a risk factor for both aortic dissection and abdominal aortic aneurysm, and blood pressure control may precipitate or worsen a developing process. In the initial stages of these conditions, a patient may present with an elevated blood pressure, but as the dissection extends or the aneurysm ruptures, hypotension will likely be found. Although these conditions often are associated with changes in blood pressure, a normal reading does not eliminate the need for a high level of suspicion.

Abdominal pain is often difficult for patients to describe completely, and when back pain accompanies it or is more prominent, the back pain may become the focus of the complaint. In addition, some intrathoracic and intra-abdominal processes, such as myocardial infarctions and aortic dissections, may not present with their classic symptoms, but rather referring pain into the back. Uncovering upper quadrant tenderness may suggest gall bladder or peptic ulcer disease, pancreatitis, or bowel obstruction. A pulsatile abdominal mass would necessitate an investigation for abdominal aneurysm. Lower quadrant tenderness may suggest appendicitis or diverticulitis with pain referred to the back. In addition, suprapubic tenderness or the presence of a palpable bladder could suggest urinary retention, increasing concern for spinal cord compression or cauda equina syndrome. Patients with urinary retention should be examined for rectal tone and perineal numbness.

An examination of the back should include inspection of the skin, palpation of bony areas, palpation of paraspinal musculature, and an assessment of the patient's range of motion. Skin examination should look for changes or erythema that would suggest herpes zoster or other infectious processes as well as ecchymosis that would indicate trauma. Bony point tenderness, misalignment or step offs may localize traumatic injuries or infection. The spine should also be examined for abnormal curvature because scoliosis and subsequent degenerative changes produce pain. This is especially relevant in the pediatric population where back pain may be the earliest indication of scoliosis. Palpation of the paraspinal musculature may reveal muscle spasm.

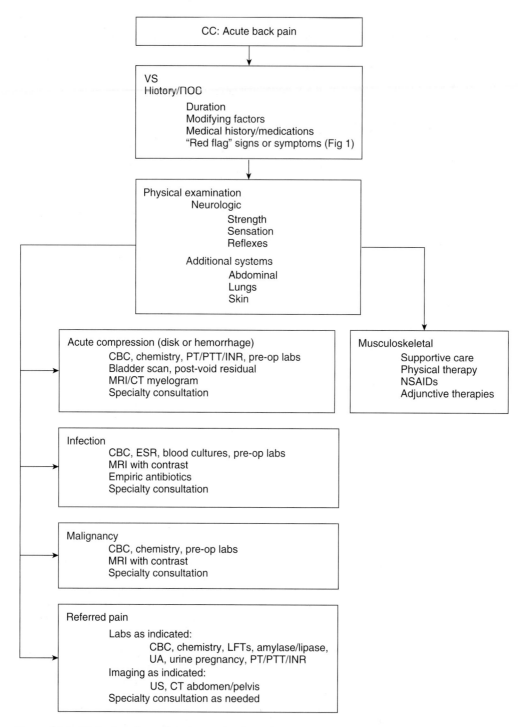

Figure 14.2: Clinical pathway for the evaluation of acute back pain. CBC, complete blood count; CC, chief complaint; CT, computed tomography; ESR, erythrocyte sedimentation rate; LFT, liver function test; MRI, magnetic resonance imaging; NSAIDs, nonsteroidal anti-inflammatory drugs; PT/PTT/INR, prothrombin time/partial prothrombin time/international normalized ratio; ROS, review of systems; UA, urine analysis; US, ultrasound; VS, vital signs.

TABLE 14.3	Red Flag History and Physical Examination Findings
Finding	**Increased Concern**
Age < 20 yr	Infection, malignancy
Age > 50 yr	Malignancy, vascular disease
Sudden severe pain, especially thoracic	Vascular catastrophe, infection
Unexplained weight loss	Infection, malignancy
Night sweats or unexplained fever	Infection, malignancy
Immunocompromised state (HIV, steroids, immunosuppressing drugs)	Infection
Prior medical history (malignancy, IV drug abuse, infection, AAA)	Metastatic disease, infection/abscess, retroperitoneal hemorrhage
Urinary retention, incontinence, saddle anesthesia	Cauda equina
Motor deficit	Cord or nerve root compression
Pain at rest or at night	Infection, malignancy
Osteoporosis, trauma, steroid use	Fracture
Anticoagulant/antiplatelet use (especially with recent spinal injection)	Hemorrhage, hematoma

AAA, abdominal aortic aneurysm; HIV, human immunodeficiency virus; IV, intravenous.

The neurologic examination should always include an evaluation of sensation, strength, and reflexes in the lower extremities. This allows the examiner to document neurologic deficits, to localize the lesion, and provides a baseline for repeated evaluations. Examination techniques, including the straight leg raise, may suggest increased dural tension as a cause of radiculopathy. The musculoskeletal evaluation should include an assessment of the lower extremity joints. Primary pathology or altered mechanics of the hip, knee, or ankle joints may cause secondary back pain. The pain of lumbar radiculopathy is often described as sharp or burning and follows the area of sensory innervation. Nerve dysfunction can present as motor weakness, sensory loss, or a combination of both. Pairing examination findings with known levels of innervation will lead the physician to a possible location of the lesion (**Table 14.4**).

Physical examination findings may vary depending on the degree of compression over one or more spinal levels. Owing to the overlap in anatomy, the clinical presentation of cauda equina and conus medullaris syndromes can be similar. Both syndromes are due to compression of the spinal cord and nerves exiting at the L1 to L5 levels. Symptoms of conus medullaris compression may include upper motor neuron signs, producing increased tone and reflexes in the lower extremities.

TABLE 14.4	Localizing the Lesion	
Disk Level	**Location of Pain**	**Motor Deficit**
T12-L1	Inguinal region, medial thigh	Usually none
L1-2	Anterior and medial thigh	Mild quadricep weakness Mildly diminished patellar reflex
L2-3	Anterolateral thigh	Quadricep weakness Diminished patellar reflex
L3-4	Posterolateral thigh Anterior tibia	Quadricep weakness Diminished patellar reflex
L4-5	Dorsal foot	Extensor weakness of ankle and great toe
L5-S1	Lateral foot	Diminished Achilles reflex

Compression of the cauda produces lower motor neuron signs in the lower limbs and can cause neurogenic bladder, loss of rectal tone, and saddle anesthesia. The most common finding is that of urinary retention with or without overflow incontinence.[8,9] Other clinical features seen may include back pain, sensory loss, incontinence, or bilateral sciatica.[6,8,9] **Table 14.5** summarizes the differences in these two syndromes. If a compression syndrome is suspected, urinary retention should be evaluated by bladder scan, postvoid residual, or Foley catheter placement. Emergent computed tomography (CT) myelogram, or magnetic resonance imaging (MRI) is indicated to confirm the diagnosis. Owing to the incidence of metastatic disease and skip lesions, imaging of the entire spinal column is preferred, if possible, especially in the pediatric population.[10]

LABORATORY AND DIAGNOSTIC STUDIES

Laboratory testing, in cases of low back pain, is usually not helpful in most patients. Urine pregnancy testing should be considered in all appropriate patients both to facilitate any imaging and to evaluate for an intra-abdominal cause of the pain. Urinalysis can be used to support a clinical decision of renal colic or pyelonephritis as a source of referred pain. If infection or malignancy is suspected, a complete blood count (CBC), erythrocyte sedimentation rate (ESR), and blood cultures may be indicated. Anticoagulated patients and those in whom intervention may be necessary should have a coagulation profile and blood bank typing performed. See the **Evidence** section for further discussion of the utility of laboratory tests.

Emergency department ultrasound (EDUS) may be used to evaluate for intra-abdominal causes of back pain, including gall bladder disease, ectopic pregnancy, and abdominal aortic aneurysm. In addition, EDUS may be used to evaluate for urinary retention and postvoid residual volumes in patients with urinary retention due to cauda equina syndrome.

In the absence of any "red flags" (Table 14.3) or abnormal neurologic findings, imaging in atraumatic back pain is rarely necessary. The increasing frequency of imaging in patients with low back pain contributes to the overall costs of treating back pain. In evaluating the financial burden of imaging, the costs of follow-up testing, physician consultation, and potential interventions must be considered in addition to the lifetime dose of radiation that patients are being subjected to. The increased use of spinal imaging has led to a higher rate of spinal surgery, with a questionable decrease in morbidity.[11] In addition, many imaging modalities demonstrate incidental findings that prompt additional investigation both within the ED and outpatient settings.

TABLE 14.5	**Distinguishing Conus Medullaris from Cauda Equina Syndrome**	
	Conus Medullaris	**Cauda Equina**
Anatomy	Terminal end of spinal cord	Nerves and nerve roots extending from conus
Vertebral Level	T12-L2	L1-L5
Spinal Nerve Level	Sacral plexus	Lumbar plexus Sacral plexus
Clinical Presentation	Sudden, bilateral pain	Gradual, unilateral pain
Radiculopathy	Uncommon	Common
Low Back Pain	Common	Uncommon
Motor/Sensory Impairment Reflexes	Bilateral and symmetric weakness Loss of ankle reflex UMN signs may be present: spasticity, hyperreflexia	Unilateral and asymmetric weakness Loss of **both** knee and ankle reflexes
Sphincter Dysfunction Sexual Dysfunction	Early incontinence Impotence common	Late incontinence Impotence uncommon

UMN, upper motor nerve.

Plain film x-rays can detect underlying structural conditions such as fractures, subluxations, and lytic lesions. Imaging in patients with back pain after body motion without precipitating trauma is rarely helpful in the initial ED evaluation. The incidence of nonclinically suspected, intervenable lesions found on x-rays is approximately 1:2500 patients.[12] Documented trauma with bony tenderness is the most appropriate indication for x-rays; however, many clinicians will consider plain film x-rays in patients in whom back pain has been present consistently for >1 month, or in the presence of other "red flags" suggesting malignancy or infection. Other modalities such as CT or MRI may be able to better define the causative lesion, but plain film x-rays may help direct future imaging.

CT scanning provides increased resolution for the evaluation of osseous structures and moderate detail for the evaluation of disk herniation. This modality is not sensitive for compression syndromes, ligamentous instability, or lesions within the spinal canal. The addition of contrast, especially with myelography, facilitates identification of these lesions. The sensitivity of CT scan remains lower than that of MRI, yet despite this limitation, it does provide an option for those patients who are unable to undergo MRI testing.

MRI has become the study of choice in the evaluation of disk herniation and radiculopathy; however, emergent imaging may be reserved for those patients where the results will guide immediate intervention. This is also the preferred modality for evaluation of epidural abscess; therefore, emergent MRI is indicated in situations of progressive neurologic deficits with the suggestion of malignancy, infection, inflammation, or acute disk herniation. Contrast is indicated when there is suspicion of infection, tumor, or vascular anomaly. **Figure 14.3** demonstrates differences in x-ray, CT, CT myelograph, and MRI images.

MANAGEMENT

Spinal Subarachnoid/Epidural Hemorrhage

Hemorrhages within subarachnoid, subdural, and epidural spaces are usually associated with an underlying cause, with < 1% determined to be idiopathic.[13] The most common causes are direct trauma, vascular abnormalities, spinal tumors, hypertension, and anticoagulation/thrombolysis. Patients present clinically with acute pain and symptoms consistent with compression of the cord segments affected. Intracranial subarachnoid blood may migrate to the lower subarachnoid spaces, producing pain in these areas. A careful review of medical history, medications, and "red flag"

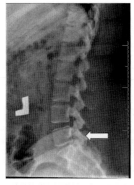 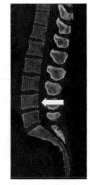 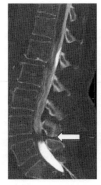 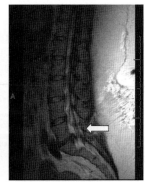

A. X-ray   B. Non-contrast CT   C. CT myelogram   D. T2 MRI

Figure 14.3: Examples of x-ray (A), computed tomography (CT) (B), CT myelogram (C), and magnetic resonance imaging (MRI) (D) images of a compressive lesion in the lumbar spine. Courtesy of Alexander Post, MD FAANS, Department of Neurosurgery, Augusta University Medical Center.

symptoms may be the only information that can move a physician closer to this diagnosis because the clinical presentation may be very similar to other causes of compressive syndromes.

When suspecting a spinal hemorrhage, MRI with magnetic resonance (MR) angiography is the preferred modality of choice because this can further define the anatomy involved. Laboratory studies should include CBC, prothrombin time/partial prothrombin time/international normalized ratio (PT/PTT/INR), and blood bank testing to determine whether reversal of coagulopathy is needed. Urgent specialty consultation is also recommended because catheter angiography may be necessary for better delineation of the lesion, endovascular treatment, or preoperative planning.

Lumbar Radiculopathy

The natural history of lumbar disk disease is that almost 90% of patients will improve within 6 weeks and resolve within 3 months, with or without treatment.[14] Approximately 20% of patients will report a recurrence within 6 months.[15] The initial treatment for lumbar disk disease is usually nonoperative and should involve nonopiate pain medications, exercise, and physical therapy.[14]

Literature demonstrates that an expeditious return to ordinary activity leads to faster and better outcomes than does bedrest.[16] If the patient has relief from bed rest, then a short duration (2 days) is associated with faster recovery than do longer courses.[16] Exercise is not acutely recommended.[16] Pharmacologically, expert opinion and guidelines recommend nonnarcotic analgesics.[16-18] However, in practice, emergency clinicians commonly use opioids; one large national sample showed a rate of approximately 61%.[16] Nonsteroidal anti-inflammatory drugs (NSAIDs) and acetaminophen should be considered first-line medications for back pain.[16-18] Muscle relaxants have often been added to the regimen, although the evidence is somewhat mixed. One randomized controlled trial compared functional outcomes and pain control among patients receiving a 10-day treatment of (a) naproxen and placebo, (b) naproxen and cyclobenzaprine, and (c) naproxen and oxycodone/acetaminophen.[19] The study found no improvement in outcome with the addition of either muscle relaxant or opiate in the short-term management of back pain at the patients' 1-week follow-up.[19] A Cochrane review of 30 randomized controlled trials found evidence that muscle relaxants are more effective than is placebo for patients with acute low back pain.[20] Evidence for the use of oral steroids is mixed and largely negative, but there are some studies showing a possible benefit in patients with a radiculopathy component to their back pain.[16,18]

One of the most important aspects of treating patients with acute back pain is adequate counseling and careful instructions on return precautions (ie, red flags). Physical therapy is often used in conjunction with medication for management of back pain. Physical therapy focusing on strengthening of core muscle groups (abdominal wall and lumbar musculature) has demonstrated positive effects.[14] Patients who present with acute neurologic findings—sensory alterations, weakness, incontinence—have a higher rate of functional recovery if decompressed within 24 to 48 hours of the time of onset.[21,22]

Cauda Equina/Conus Medullaris Syndrome

Acute compression syndromes are a surgical emergency, necessitating timely consultation and intervention. There is increasing evidence that physiologic deterioration in compressive syndromes occurs as a cascade rather than in a stepwise manner. Because of this, there is still a large amount of uncertainty in the literature regarding the timing of surgical intervention. The general recommendation in the literature has been to support a 48-hour window from time of admission for surgical decompression. An earlier review of both animal and human subjects notes that the level of neurologic dysfunction at the time of surgery (incomplete cauda equina syndrome versus cauda equina syndrome with retention) is the most significant determinant of overall prognosis. They note that it is likely that the earlier the intervention, the more beneficial the effects on the compressed nerve, but did not discuss the optimal timing of intervention.[23] Two more recent reviews of 4066 and 20,924 patients support the recommendation of decompression within 48 hours of hospital admission. Both reviews note that decompression after 48 hours is associated with increased inpatient mortality, total complications, prolonged length of stay, increased cost of hospitalization, and nonfavorable discharges.[13,24]

TABLE 14.6 Antibiotics for Epidural Abscess	
Empiric Therapy	**Alternative Therapies**
Vancomycin IV q8-12h *Target serum trough concentration 15-20 mcg/mL* Ceftriaxone 2 mg IV q12h	Vancomycin allergy
	Linezolid 600 mg IV BID Daptomycin 6-10 mg/kg once daily Trimethoprim-sulfamethoxazole (5 mg/kg of trimethoprim q8-12h)
	Beta-lactam/carbapenem allergy
	Moxifloxacin 400 mg daily

BID, twice a day; IV, intravenous.

Epidural Abscess

Spinal epidural abscesses are rare, but potentially devastating infections, and data suggests that their incidence has been increasing over the past few decades.[25,26] This process is more common in the older adult population, with common risk factors including diabetes, alcoholism, cancer, immunocompromised states, and prior instrumentation. Intravenous (IV) drug abuse is also a contributory factor in younger populations.

Abscesses develop in the epidural space between the dura and the spinal canal wall, causing compression of the cord or vascular thrombosis. The resulting injury may lead to paraplegia, quadriplegia, and death. The most common organism cultured is *Staphylococcus aureus,* usually as a result of bacteremia. Direct extension from neighboring infection or instrumentation has also been documented.[26,27]

The initial clinical presentation may be nonspecific, including fever and malaise, with approximately half of the cases being initially misdiagnosed.[28] The classic triad of fever, back pain, and neurologic deficit is present in only a small proportion of patients.[23,25-28] Laboratory testing may show leukocytosis and elevation of ESR. The preferred imaging is MRI with gadolinium, again with imaging of the entire column if possible. CT with contrast or CT myelogram may also be an acceptable alternative to MRI.

The goal of management is to reduce and eliminate the infectious mass, decompress the spinal cord, and eradicate the causative organism. Treatment is usually a combination of surgical decompression and IV antibiotics; however, there has been discussion suggesting guided aspiration versus open decompression in smaller abscesses.[23] Recommended antibiotics include vancomycin with cefotaxime, ceftriaxone, cefepime, ceftazidime, or meropenem depending on the clinical situation.[27] See **Tables 14.6** and **14.7** for suggested antibiotic regimens.

TABLE 14.7 Targeted Antibiotics for Organisms Identified in Epidural Abscess		
Microorganism	**Recommended Therapy**	**Alternative Therapies**
Streptococcus pneumoniae	Vancomycin IV q8-12h Serum trough 15-20 mcg/mL Ceftriaxone 2 g IV q12h	Moxifloxacin 400 mg daily
Pseudomonas aeruginosa	Cefepime 2 g q8h **or** Ceftazidime 2 g q8h	Aztreonam 2 g q6-8h Meropenem 2 g q8h Ciprofloxacin 400 mg q8-12h

Staphylococcus aureus
  Methicillin susceptible
  Methicillin resistant
	Nafcillin 2 g q4h
	Oxacillin 2 g q4h
	Vancomycin 15-20 mg/kg q8-12h
		Meropenem 2q q8h
		Linezolid 600 mg q12h
		Linezolid 600 mg q12h
		Daptomycin 6-10 mg/kg daily
		Trimethoprim-sulfamethoxazole (5 mg/kg of trimethoprim q8-12h)

(continued)

TABLE 14.7	Targeted Antibiotics for Organisms Identified in Epidural Abscess (*continued*)	
Microorganism	**Recommended Therapy**	**Alternative Therapies**
Escherichia coli and other *Enterobacteriaceae*	Ceftriaxone 2 g q12h	Aztreonam 2 g q6-8h Meropenem 2 g q8h Moxifloxacin 400 mg daily Ampicillin 2 g q4h Trimethoprim-sulfamethoxazole (5 mg/kg of trimethoprim q8-12h)
Neisseria meningitidis	Ceftriaxone 2 g q12h	Aztreonam 2 g q6-8h Moxifloxacin 400 mg daily Chloramphenicol 1-1.5g q6h
Listeria monocytogenes	Ampicillin 2 g q4h	Trimethoprim-sulfamethoxazole (5 mg/kg of trimethoprim q8-12h)

IV, intravenous.

TIPS AND PEARLS

- *Review the patient's chart and medications:* Although patient-reported "red flags" are important to consider, they have low sensitivity and specificity for the identification of serious pathologies. Red flags from the patient's medical record are slightly more accurate, but there is poor agreement between patient-reported red flags and those obtained from the medical record.[29]
- *Remember to consider referred pain when evaluating for the cause of back pain:* Pain from intrathoracic and intra-abdominal pathology can cause pain that is felt in the back and these processes should be considered early in the evaluation to avoid a catastrophic miss. As mentioned, failure to include pathology outside the spine and spinal musculature has been noted to be one of the key findings in many legal case reviews.[5]
- *Choose imaging wisely:* Because back pain is a common complaint and frequently becomes a lifelong medical problem, the use of radiation-based imaging should be limited to minimize total lifetime dose exposure. Plain films may demonstrate fractures, bony misalignment, and grossly lytic lesions, but provide little information about the ligaments, disks, and potential spaces of the spinal column. CT and MRI provide more information in these areas, and can be reformatted for surgical planning.
- *Be specific when documenting the physical examination:* Often, the decision to intervene emergently can depend on the progression of a neurologic deficit. Be as specific as possible when documenting sensation and strength, as well as any perceived change. An isolated examination provides less information to subsequent physicians than do serial examinations noting any changes.

SUMMARY

In conclusion, back pain is a very common presenting complaint, and the critical step in ED management is the rapid recognition of the infrequent causes that will benefit from immediate intervention. Although many of these problems present with similar characteristics, a careful review of medical history, medications, and red flags can focus the additional workup. Referred pain may prompt an ED visit for "back pain," and the more serious causes must be considered. Acute pain with demonstrable neurologic findings suggests one of the more serious causes of pain, which often fall into the compressive category. Imaging and laboratory studies should be guided by the most likely serious causes of back pain, as well as the potential for surgical intervention. Specialty consultation from Spine Surgery, Radiology, Oncology, and Infectious Diseases should be initiated as early as possible to help prevent further neurologic injury.

EVIDENCE

Are "the red flags" sensitive indicators of underlying emergent causes of back pain?

Much of the literature associated with the diagnosis and management of lower back pain is based on primary care or specialty clinic settings. The prevalence of presenting complaints requiring urgent intervention was 2.5% to 5.1% in prospective studies and 0.7% to 7.4% in retrospective studies. These conditions included unstable vertebral fractures, malignancies, infections, cord compression, and vascular anomalies.[5] However, the prevalence of serious pathology presenting to the ED has been demonstrated to be higher than in the primary care population.[6] Many of the algorithms addressing back pain were developed from this literature and support the use of these common red flags, but there has been little prospective evaluation, especially within Emergency Medicine.[7, 12, 30,34]

Therefore, the difficulty lies in developing an efficient, cost-conscious, and effective plan for the evaluation of back pain in the ED.[34] These red flags can help guide the workup, but a serious pathology should not be excluded on the basis of this information.

Unfortunately, the severity of pain and the presence of neurologic abnormalities are not definitive in their ability to risk stratify a patient in the ED with back pain. Many of the benign causes present with debilitating pain and occasional neurologic findings, whereas some of the serious causes may be more indolent. As mentioned, the commonly discussed "red flags" provide some guidance in the evaluation of back pain, but have not been prospectively validated. Patient reports of this information have been demonstrated to be less predictive than those found in the medical record.[12]

Are ESR and C-reactive protein (CRP) necessary in the evaluation of back pain?

In the cases of suspected infection or malignancy as the etiology of back pain, laboratory testing, consisting of CBC, ESR, CRP, and urinalysis may be of some use. Urinalysis may be useful for diagnosing pyelonephritis. For spinal infections, the laboratory sensitivities are as follows: increased white blood count (WBC), 35% to 61%; increased ESR, 76% to 95%; and increased CRP, 82% to 98%.[8, 10] An increased ESR also has a sensitivity of 78% and specificity of 67% in the diagnostic evaluation of occult malignancy.[8, 10] As evidenced by these numbers, an elevated WBC is not a sensitive evaluation for spinal infections. Similarly, the percentage of neutrophils and the presence of immature forms (bands) are not adequately sensitive.[8]

Inflammatory markers, such as ESR and CRP, may be highly sensitive but nonspecific. Of note, the timing differs between these two markers: CRP levels rise at the onset of inflammation and return more quickly to normal than do ESR levels.[8] One single-center study of patients with suspected spinal epidural abscess compared clinical outcomes before and after the implementation of a diagnostic guideline using ESR (cutoff of 20 mm) and CRP. The study found a decrease in diagnostic delays from 84% to 10%, and the proportion of patients with motor abnormalities at the time of diagnosis dropped from 82% to 19%. However, keep in mind that the lower the threshold definition of a positive/elevated ESR, the higher the sensitivity but the poorer the specificity. Using an ESR cutoff of > 20 mm has a sensitivity approaching 100% for epidural abscess, but with poor specificity.[8] Given the poor specificity of ESR and CRP, these laboratory tests are not routinely recommended in patients with back pain without suspicion of infection or malignancy.

Are muscle relaxants beneficial in the treatment of back pain?

If a musculoskeletal etiology is the suspected cause of back pain, an important treatment goal is to provide adequate analgesia. First-line pharmacologic agents are considered to be nonopioid analgesic agents, including acetaminophen and NSAIDs.[9, 14] Muscle relaxants are frequently added on for patients with back pain in the ED. A Cochrane review of 51 trials with 6057 patients found NSAIDs to be effective for short-term symptomatic relief in patients with acute back pain.[19] There were no notable differences in the efficacy of various NSAIDs.[19] Another Cochrane review of 30 randomized controlled trials found evidence that muscle relaxants are more effective than is placebo for patients with acute low back pain.[26] With the exception of one trial finding superiority of carisoprodol to diazepam, no one muscle relaxant was found superior to another in this review, including benzodiazepines (diazepam and tetrazepam), nonbenzodiazepine antispasmodics (cyclobenzaprine, carisoprodol, chlorzoxazone, meprobamate, methocarbamol, metaxalone, orphenadrine, tizanidine, and flupirtine), and antispasticity drugs (baclofen and dantrolene sodium).[20] The review suggests that muscle relaxants could be of benefit to patients with acute low back pain, reducing the duration of their discomfort and accelerating recovery, but at the cost of potentially greater adverse events. In particular, results indicate that muscle relaxants are associated with more prevalent central nervous system events, most commonly drowsiness and dizziness, and the medications must be used with caution.[20]

Are NSAIDs as effective as opioids in managing back pain?

Opioid analgesics may be considered as a third-line alternative, and are best reserved for those experiencing severe acute back pain that is inadequately controlled with nonnarcotic agents.[9] Data from studies on opioid superiority compared with NSAIDs or acetaminophen are inconclusive: Opioids have not been shown to be more effective for initial treatment of acute lower back pain, nor do they increase the likelihood to return to work.[17] When prescribing opioids, ensure that patients are cautioned on their side effects, including constipation, confusion, and sedation. There is no role for starting any long-acting chronic pain medications (eg, methadone, fentanyl patches) in the ED.

Do steroids promote recovery in patients with acute back pain? Chronic back pain?

Oral glucocorticoids do not confer a clear benefit in patients with lower back pain, with or without sciatica.[9] Many practitioners continue to prescribe glucocorticoids for patients with radiculopathy, but any benefit is modest and probably transient.[8,9,14] Epidural glucocorticoid injections seem to be most effective for patients with radiculopathy caused by a herniated disk, but do not confer a benefit beyond 4 to 6 weeks, and do not delay surgery in those who are already surgical candidates.[9] Generally, this procedure is part of outpatient pain management. Other alternative methods include acupuncture and massage therapy. Evidence is overall poor. A few systematic reviews of trials found inconclusive results for the management of acute back pain, but possibly a benefit in chronic pain.[35-37] Ultimately, one of the most important aspects of treating acute musculoskeletal back pain in patients is adequate counseling.

Is there a role for adjunctive pain management modalities in treating back pain?

There have been few high-quality studies investigating the use of acupuncture in the treatment of nonspecific back pain. Several articles reviewed the evidence for the use of acupuncture, but noted that the clinical trials were limited in patient number and technique, making specific recommendations difficult. On the basis of these, acupuncture may provide a clinically meaningful reduction in the degree of self-reported symptoms and degree of disability compared to no treatment. The results are inconsistent when compared to the medication regimens as discussed previously, because there is a statistical difference, but no obvious clinical benefit.[25,38,39] With the relative low incidence of side effects, acupuncture may provide an alternative therapy for pain relief when contraindications exist to systemic medications.

References

1.   Maher C, Underwood M, Buchbinder R. Non-specific low back pain. *Lancet*. 2017;389:736-747.

2.   Edwards J, Hayden J, Asbridge M, Gregoire B, Magee K. Prevalence of low back pain in emergency settings: a systematic review and meta-analysis. *BMC Musculoskelet Disord*. 2017;18:143.

3.   Dieleman JL, Baral R, Birger M, et al. US spending on personal health care and public health, 1996–2013. *JAMA*. 2016;316:2627-2646.

4.   Briggs AM, Smith AJ, Straker LM, et al. Thoracic spine pain in the general population: prevalence, incidence and associated factors in children, adolescents and adults: a systematic review. *BMC Musculoskelet Disord*. 2009;2910:77.

5.   Pope JV, Edlow JA. Avoiding misdiagnosis in patients with neurological emergencies. *Emerg Med Int*. 2012;2012:949275.

6.   Fraser S, Roberts L, Murphy E. Cauda equina syndrome: a literature review of its definition and clinical presentation. *Arch Phys Med Rehabil*. 2009;90:1964-1968.

7.   Korse NS, Pijpers JA, van Zwet E, Elzevier HW, Vleggeert-Lankamp CLA. Cauda Equina Syndrome: presentation, outcome, and predictors with focus on micturition, defecation, and sexual dysfunction. *Eur Spine J*. 2017;26(3):894-904.

8. Singleton J, Edlow JA. Acute nontraumatic back pain. *Emerg Med Clin North Am*. 2016;34(4):743-757.

9. Corwell BN. The emergency department evaluation, management, and treatment of back pain. *Emerg Med Clin North Am*. 2010;28(4):811-839.

10. Deyo RA, Weinstein JN. Low back pain. *N Engl J Med*. 2001;344:363-370.

11. Balasubramanian K, Kalsi P, Greenough CG, Kuskoor Seetharam MP. Reliability of clinical assessment in diagnosing cauda equina syndrome. *Br J Neurosurg*. 2010;24:383-386.

12. Verhagen AP, Downie A, Popal N, Maher C, Koes BW. Red flags presented in current low back pain guidelines: a review. *Eur Spine J*. 2016;25:2788-2802.

13. Hogan WB, Kuris EO, Durand WM, et al. Timing of surgical decompression for cauda equina syndrome. *World Neurosurg*. 2019;132:e732-e738.

14. Deyo RA. Cascade effects of medical technology. *Annu Rev Public Health*. 2002;23:23-44.

15. Kim YH, Cho KT, Chung CK, Kim HJ. Idiopathic spontaneous spinal subarachnoid hemorrhage. *Spinal Cord*. 2004;42:545-547.

16. Vakili M, Crum-Cianflone NF. Spinal epidural abscess: a series of 101 cases. *Am J Med*. 2017;130: 1458-1463.

17. Darouiche RO. Spinal epidural abscess. *N Engl J Med*. 2006;355:2012-2020.

18. Patel AR, Alton TB, Bransford RJ, Lee MJ, Bellabarba CB, Chapman JR. Spinal epidural abscesses: risk factors, medical versus surgical management, a retrospective review of 128 cases. *Spine J*. 2014;14:326-330.

19. Van Tulder MW, Scholten RJPM, Koes BW, Deyo RA. Nonsteroidal anti-inflammatory drugs for low back pain: a systematic review within the framework of the cochrane collaboration back review group. *Spine*. 2000;25(19):2501-2513.

20. Reihsaus E, Waldbaur H, Seeling W. Spinal epidural abscess: a meta-analysis of 915 patients. *Neurosurg Rev*. 2000;23:175-204; discussion 205.

21. Madigan L, Vaccaro AR, Spector LR, Milam RA. Management of symptomatic lumbar degenerative disk disease. *J Am Acad Orthop Surg*. 2009;17:102-111.

22. Cassidy JD, Cote P, Carroll LJ, Kristman V. Incidence and course of low back pain episodes in the general population. *Spine (Phila Pa 1976)*. 2005;30:2817-2823.

23. Chau AM, Xu LL, Pelzer NR, Gragnaniello C. Timing of surgical intervention in cauda equina syndrome: a systematic critical review. *World Neurosurg*. 2014;81(3-4):640-650.

24. Thakur JD, Storey C, Kalakoti P, et al. Early intervention in cauda equina syndrome associated with better outcomes: a myth or reality? Insights from the nationwide inpatient sample database (2005–2011). *Spine J*. 2017;17(10):1435-1448.

25. Friedman BW, Dym AA, DAvitt M, et al. Naproxen with cyclobenzaprine, oxycodone/acetaminophen, or placebo for treating acute low back pain: a randomized clinical trial. *JAMA*. 2015;314:1572-1580.

26. Van Tulder MW, Touray T, Furlan AD, Solway S, Bouter L. Muscle relaxants for nonspecific low back pain: a systematic review within the framework of the Cochrane collaboration. *Spine*. 2003;28(17):1978-1992.

27. Ahn UM, Ahn NU, Buchowski JM, Garrett ES, Sieber AN, Kostuik JP. Cauda equina syndrome secondary to lumbar disc herniation: a meta-analysis of surgical outcomes. *Spine (Phila Pa 1976)*. 2000;25:1515-1522.

28. Albert R, Lange M, Brawanski A, Schebesch KM. Urgent discectomy: clinical features and neurological outcome. *Surg Neurol Int*. 2016;7:17.

29. Ropper AE, Ropper AH. Acute spinal cord compression. *N Engl J Med*. 2017;376:1358-1369.

30. Domen PM, Hofman PA, van Santbrink H, Weber WE. Predictive value of clinical characteristics in patients with suspected cauda equina syndrome. *Eur J Neurol*. 2009;16:416-419.

31. Davis DP, Wold RM, Patel RJ, et al. The clinical presentation and impact of diagnostic delays on emergency department patients with spinal epidural abscess. *J Emerg Med*. 2004;26:285-291.

32. Arko Lt, Quach E, Nguyen V, Chang D, Sukul V, Kim BS. Medical and surgical management of spinal epidural abscess: a systematic review. *Neurosurg Focus*. 2014;37:E4.

33. Tsiang JT, Kinzy TG, Thompson N, et al. Sensitivity and specificity of patient-entered red flags for lower back pain. *Spine J*. 2019;19:293-300.

34. Galliker G, Scherer DF, Trippolini MA, Rasmussen-Barr E, LoMartire R, Wertli MM. Low back pain in the emergency department: prevalence of serious spinal pathologies and diagnostic accuracy of red flags. *Am J Med*. 2020;133:60-72.e14.

35. van Tulder MW, Cherkin DC, Bermn B. The effectiveness of acupuncture in the management of acute and chronic low back pain: a systematic review within the framework of the Cochrane Collaboration Back Review Group. *Spine*. 1999;24(11):1113-1123.

36. Furlan AD, van Tulder MW, Cherkin D, et al. Acupuncture and dry-needling for low back pain. *Cochrane Database Syst Rev* 2005;(1): CD001351.

37. Cherkin DC, Sherman KJ, Deyo RA, et al. A review of the evidence for the effectiveness, safety, and cost of acupuncture, massage therapy, and spinal manipulation for back pain. *Ann Intern Med*. 2003;138(11):898-906.

38. Lee JH, Choi TY, Lee MS, et al. Acupuncture for acute low back pain: a systematic review. *Clin J Pain*. 2013;29(2):172-185.

39. Lam M, Glavin R, Curry P. Effectiveness of acupuncture for nonspecific chronic low back pain: a systematic review and meta-analysis. *Spine*. 2013;38(24):2124-2138.

Acute Stroke

Christopher A. Lewandowski
Edward P. Sloan

THE CLINICAL CHALLENGE

Stroke is characterized as a neurologic deficit attributed to an acute focal injury of the central nervous system (CNS) from a vascular cause.[1,2] The definition includes cerebral infarction or acute ischemic stroke (AIS), intracerebral hemorrhage (ICH), and subarachnoid hemorrhage (SAH). AIS is caused by vascular occlusion with interruption of cerebral blood flow (CBF) leading to infarction. Transient ischemic attacks (TIAs) were defined as a brief episode of neurologic dysfunction caused by focal brain or retinal ischemia, with clinical symptoms typically lasting <1 hour, and without evidence of acute infarction.[1,3] Nontraumatic spontaneous ICH is caused by bleeding into the cerebral and cerebellar cortices as well as the into CNS or ventricular system. This chapter discusses AIS, TIAs, and ICH. SAHs and cerebral venous thrombosis (CVT) are discussed in **Chapter 16: Headache**.

The clinical challenge for emergency clinicians is to diagnose an acute stroke, TIA, or hemorrhage accurately and quickly, separating it from other conditions that mimic stroke (false positives) as well as diagnosing masquerading strokes that are called chameleons (false negatives), which initially suggest another diagnosis. Patients with ICH may have focal neurologic symptoms similar to AIS, but frequently present with altered mental status, and may have an unstable airway, extreme hypertension (HTN), new-onset seizures, or elevated intracranial pressure (ICP). All patients with acute stroke require emergent diagnosis, stabilization, and proper therapy. This all needs to happen in a brief period to save the dying brain from infarction or limit harm from an ICH or prevent its expansion. As many of the current therapies are highly time sensitive, including access to interventional radiology or neurosurgical intervention, successful management requires streamlined systems of care to promote optimal patient outcomes.

EPIDEMIOLOGY

There are nearly 800,000 strokes that occur per year in the United States, 1 every 40 seconds; 87% are ischemic, 10% are ICHs, and 3% are SAHs. Approximately 600,000 are first strokes and 200,000 are recurrent strokes. The prevalence of stroke in the United States is 2.7%; but varies from 1.3% to 4.7% depending on the state.[4] Despite the incidence falling by 32% per 10-year period from 1987 to 2017, it is projected that the prevalence in adults will rise to 4% by 2030 as the population ages[4,5] (**Figure 15.1**).

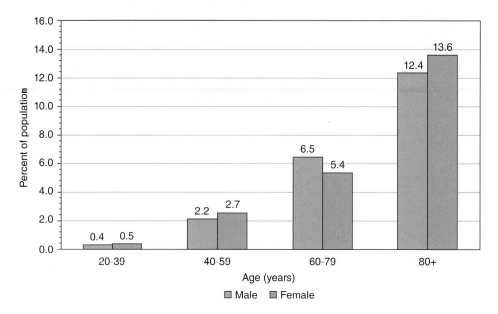

Figure 15.1: Stroke prevalence by age and sex (NHANES, 2015-2018). From Virani SS, Alonso A, Aparicio HJ, et al. Heart disease and stroke statistics—2021 update: a report from the American Heart Association. *Circulation*. 2021;143(8):e254-e743. Data from unpublished National Heart, Lung, and Blood Institute tabulation using NHANES, 2015 to 2018.

In 2018, there were almost 150,000 deaths from stroke, a rate of about 37.1/100,000 people, making it the fifth leading cause of death in the United States. The all-cause mortality rate after stroke is 10.5% at 30 days, 21.2% at 1 year, and 40% at 5 years. The mortality for ICH is especially high, at 44% at 30 days. Two-thirds of stroke deaths were thought to be outside of the hospital setting. Death rates vary significantly based on sex, race/ethnicity, and region of the country (**Figure 15.2**), especially in the southeastern United States known as the "Stroke Belt" (**Figure 15.3**).

Most importantly, stroke is the leading cause of adult disability in the United States. There are over 7 million stroke survivors, many of whom require many years of support and care and live with chronic disabilities. The direct and indirect cost of stroke is approximately $50 billion annually, and is projected to increase to nearly $95 billion by 2030.[4] The quality adjusted life years (QALYs) lost is about 5 years for the first-ever AIS and 6.2 years for an ICH.[6] As a result, stroke trials most often focus on decreasing disability rather than on preventing death.

Globally, stroke is the second leading cause of death and a major cause of disability with a prevalence of over 100 million. The worldwide incidence of stroke is 11.6 million for AIS and 5.3 million for ICHs per year.[7,8] The global lifetime risk of stroke is 24.9% for those older than 25 years.

Transient Ischemic Attacks

TIAs have an incidence of 5 million per year. About 2.3% of Americans have experienced a TIA. As with AIS, there is an increasing incidence with age, for males, and for Blacks and Mexican Americans. TIA features associated with subsequent disabling stroke include age older than 60, diabetes, focal symptoms (motor weakness, abnormal speech), and symptom duration over 10 minutes. Up to 30% to 40% of patients with these high-risk features will have a lesion on magnetic resonance imaging (MRI) that amplifies their risk of subsequent disabling stroke.

Recent improvement in the care of patients with TIA has resulted in an overall risk of subsequent disabling stroke of 1.2% at 2 days and 7.4% at 90 days. Currently, the 1-year risk of stroke is 5%, and the 5-year risk is 9.5%.

TIAs are also a marker of cardiovascular disease and carry a 6.2% 1-year and a 12% 5-year risk of stroke, acute coronary syndrome, or death. The 10-year risk for stroke, myocardial infarction, or death is 43%.[9] For these reasons, patients with TIAs need to have a rapid follow-up or admission to ensure timely evaluation and treatment.[4]

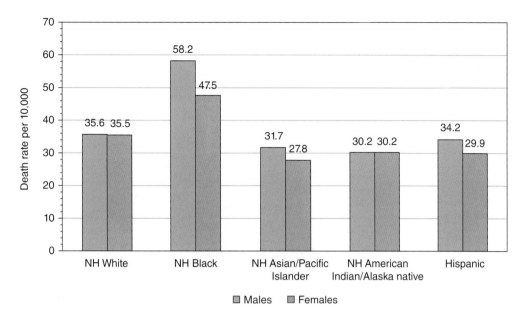

Figure 15.2: **Death rates by race and sex.** Death rates for the American Indian or Alaska Native and Asian or Pacific Islander populations are known to be underestimated. Stroke includes *International Classification of Diseases, 10th Revision* codes I60 through I69 (cerebrovascular disease). Mortality for NH Asian people includes Pacific Islander people. NH indicates non-Hispanic. From Virani SS, Alonso A, Aparicio HJ, et al. Heart disease and stroke statistics—2021 update: a report from the American Heart Association. *Circulation.* 2021;143(8):e254-e743. Data from unpublished National Heart, Lung, and Blood Institute tabulation using Centers for Disease Control Prevention Wide-Ranging Online Data for Epidemiological Research.

Risk Factors for Stroke

The risk factors for stroke include both modifiable and nonmodifiable factors. Eighty-seven percent of strokes are due to modifiable risk factors, and 47% are thought to be due to behavioral factors such as smoking, sedentary lifestyle, and diet. Black Americans, Mexican Americans, and American Indians have a higher risk of stroke compared to White Americans. Women have a higher risk of stroke and fatal strokes not only because they live longer but also due to such factors as pregnancy-associated complications, oral contraception, and hormonal therapy.[4] The major modifiable risk factors include HTN, atrial fibrillation (AF), smoking, diabetes, obesity, sedentary lifestyle, and hyperlipidemia. The nonmodifiable risks include age, sex race/ethnicity, prior stroke or TIA, family history, and air pollution.[10,11] Management of the major modifiable risk factors decreases not only stroke risk but also cardiovascular risk, all-cause mortality, and cancer risk.[12]

PATHOPHYSIOLOGY OF ACUTE ISCHEMIC STROKE

The brain receives 20% of the cardiac output, but is only 2% of the total body weight. It has minimal energy reserves, and is highly dependent on continuous supply of oxygen and glucose.[13] When CBF is interrupted to a portion of the brain, an AIS occurs and causes brain injury with focal neurologic dysfunction characteristic of the vascular distribution involved. In the case of TIAs, blood flow returns spontaneously, and the symptoms resolve.[14]

Blood flow can be interrupted by multiple different mechanisms. The most common classification of stroke mechanisms uses the "TOAST" criteria, and includes small vessel occlusions, large artery atherosclerosis, cardioembolism, cryptogenic stroke, and other pathologies.[15] The degree of brain injury from a stroke depends on the severity of ischemia (degree of flow restriction) and on the duration of ischemia. As the CBF falls, the brain tissue becomes electrically silent and then suffers membrane failure. The time required to produce irreversible damage is related to the severity

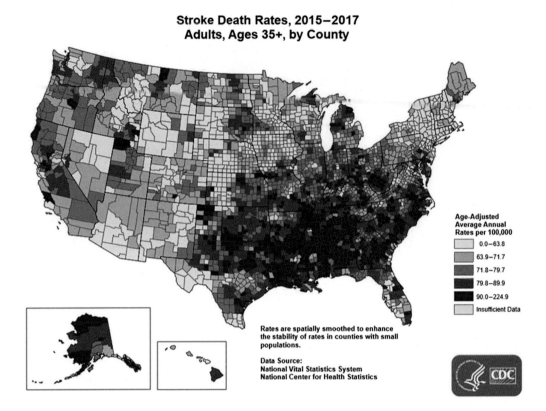

**Stroke Death Rates, 2015–2017
Adults, Ages 35+, by County**

Age-Adjusted
Average Annual
Rates per 100,000

	0.0–63.8
	63.9–71.7
	71.8–79.7
	79.8–89.9
	90.0–224.9
	Insufficient Data

Rates are spatially smoothed to enhance
the stability of rates in counties with small
populations.

Data Source:
National Vital Statistics System
National Center for Health Statistics

Figure 15.3: The Stroke Belt. Rates are spatially smoothed to enhance the stability of rates in counties with small populations. *International Classification of Diseases, 10th Revision* codes for stroke: I60 through I69. From National Center for Health Statistics, National Vital Statistics System. Stroke death rates. Accessed April 6, 2020. https://www.cdc.gov/dhdsp/maps/pdfs/stroke_all.pdf

of the ischemia over minutes to hours[16,17] (**Figure 15.4**). The areas with the most severe ischemia, the core, are irreversibly damaged and die relatively quickly. The surrounding areas with less severe ischemia, the penumbra, are alive, electrically silent, detected on examination, and can be salvaged if reperfusion is rapidly established[18] (**Figure 15.5**). Surrounding the penumbra is a zone of benign oligemia that eventually survives. Without reperfusion, the core infarct eventually extends to involve the penumbra, which results in a larger final stroke volume.

Secondary injury from ischemia is caused by an acute "excitotoxic" response triggered by membrane failure with release of excitatory amino acids, aspartate and glutamate, from the presynaptic membrane (**Figure 15.6**). These excitatory amino acids open calcium channels via N-methyl-D-aspartate (NMDA) receptors, causing calcium/sodium influx, activation of proteolytic enzymes, further membrane and blood-brain barrier failure, and repetition of the cycle. Neuroprotective agents are aimed at interrupting this cycle.

For every minute with a large vessel stroke, the average patient loses 1.9 million neurons, 14 billion synapses, and 7.5 miles of axonal fibers,[19] leading to the axiom "Time is brain." Clock time, as measured by the last known normal, is an unreliable surrogate marker for the underlying progression of these pathophysiologic processes. Variability from patient to patient from ischemic injury is explained by the amount of collateral blood flow and other individual factors. Some patients are fast progressors, whereas others progress to infarction at a slower rate.[20] With the development of computed tomography perfusion (CTP) imaging and magnetic resonance (MR) perfusion imaging, obtaining an understanding of the size of the core and penumbra for an individual patient is feasible, especially those with large vessel occlusions (LVOs).[21]

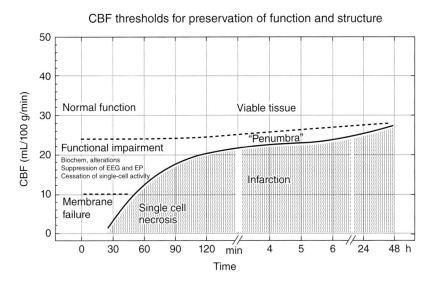

Figure 15.4: Thresholds of focal cerebral ischemia in awake monkeys. From Jones TH, Morawetz RB, Crowell RM, et al. Thresholds of focal cerebral ischemia in awake monkeys. *J Neurosurg.* 1981;54(6):773-782.

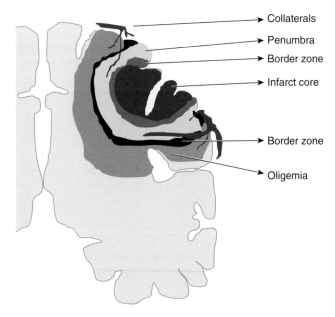

Figure 15.5: The ischemic penumbra. Schematic demonstration of the infarct core, penumbra, benign oligemia, and associated border zones. Dynamic changes in size over time occur depending on the status of the leptomeningeal collaterals and hemodynamic, physiologic, or metabolic factors. The infarct core is nonviable tissue. Penumbra is the ischemic but dysfunctional zone, and remains viable if blood flow is restored. Benign oligemia is underperfused, but functional tissue that remains viable. The threshold level for neuronal dysfunction is a cerebral blood flow (CBF) of approximately 20 mL/100 g/min, and the benign ischemia zone is above this threshold. From Liu CSJ, Dobre MC. Brain MR perfusion imaging: cerebral ischemia. In: Saremi F, ed. *Perfusion Imaging in Clinical Practice.* Wolters Kluwer; 2016:217-223. Figure 12.1.

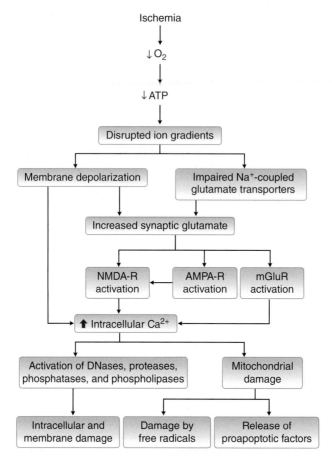

Figure 15.6: Excitotoxicity. Role of glutamate receptors in excitotoxicity. Although a multiplicity of damaging cellular processes occur as a consequence of the decreased ATP levels that result from impaired oxidative metabolism or from the superoxidative damage from activated neutrophils that invade an ischemic region, only glutamate-mediated processes are depicted here. ATP, adenosine triphosphate; AMPA-R, AMPA receptor; mGluR, NMDA-R, N-methyl-D-aspartate receptor. From Forman SA, Chou J, Strichartz GR, Lo EH. Pharmacology of GABAergic and glutamatergic neurotransmission. In: Golan DE, Tashjian AH, Armstrong EJ, Armstrong AW, eds. *Principles of Pharmacology.* 3rd ed. Wolters Kluwer; 2012:164-185. Figure 12.10.

PREHOSPITAL CONCERNS

The public is encouraged to activate emergency medical services (EMS) if there is concern for an acute stroke because it is the fastest way to get to the emergency department (ED).[22] A stroke screening tool is advised for both the dispatchers and the EMS personnel. Stroke screens are based on a brief history or examination checking for common stroke symptoms such as sensorimotor deficits and speech problems. The Los Angeles Prehospital Stroke (LAPSS) and the Cincinnati Prehospital Stroke Screen (CPSS) are reasonable validated stroke screens.[23] A Cochrane Review recommended the CPSS.[24]

With the advent of intra-arterial therapy (IAT) for stroke, EMS personnel are being asked to also perform a prehospital stroke severity scale used to detect an LVO and reroute patients to a thrombectomy-capable center (**Figure 15.7**).[25] Stroke severity scales focus on motor deficits and cortical findings such as aphasia or neglect. Most LVO scales have good accuracy, high sensitivity, and low specificity: The Rapid Arterial Occlusion Evaluation (RACE) scale and the Los Angeles Motor Scale (LAMS) are the most accurate, and the Prehospital Acute Stroke Severity (PASS)

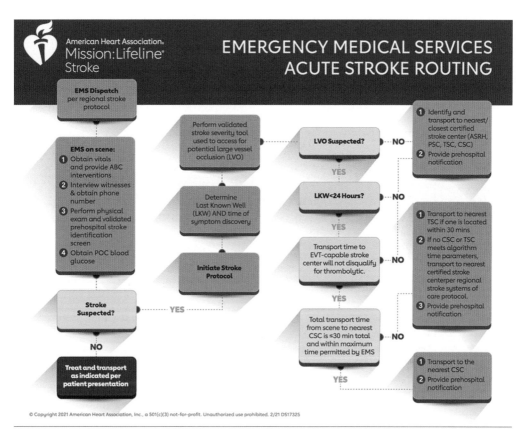

Figure 15.7: Acute stroke routing protocol. From Jauch EC, Schwamm LH, Panagos PD, et al. Recommendations for regional stroke destination plans in rural, suburban, and urban communities from the prehospital stroke system of care consensus conference: a consensus statement from the American Academy of Neurology, American Heart Association/American Stroke Association, American Society of Neuroradiology, National Association of EMS Physicians, National Association of State EMS Officials, Society of NeuroInterventional Surgery, and Society of Vascular and Interventional Neurology: Endorsed by the Neurocritical Care Society. *Stroke*. 2021;52(5):e133-e152.

scale was the most easily reconstructed from standard data collection (**Table 15.1**).[26] Alterations in mental status associated with ICH are more common than with AIS, and should be assessed using the Glasgow Coma Scale (GCS) score.

Before evaluating the patient for signs and symptoms of stroke, EMS personnel must evaluate the patient for the "ABCs" (airway, breathing, circulation), address any life-threatening issues, and provide supportive care per their local protocols. Supportive care includes evaluation of the airway, preventing aspiration, and ensuring that the oxygen saturation is over 94%. The blood pressure (BP) should be measured and treated with isotonic fluids if the patient is hypotensive. Extreme elevations in systolic blood pressure (SBP) with ICH and are independently associated with ICH volume, but it is not known if prehospital BP control attenuates ICH expansion. No specific guidelines exist for prehospital treatment of HTN. The patient should also be placed on a monitor and examined for trauma, especially the C-spine if there is a history of associated fall or syncope. A point-of-care glucose measurement is mandatory because hypoglycemia is an easily addressed stroke mimic. Seizures should be managed with benzodiazepines per the EMS protocol in a manner similar to that of any other seizure.

Rapid EMS stroke identification and transport to a thrombolytic-capable center not only improves care for patients with ischemic stroke but also shortens the time to emergency interventions.[27] If a patient is clearly outside the 4.5-hour window or has a severe stroke, transportation to a

TABLE 15.1	Prehospital Evaluation of Stroke			
Stroke Screens	Items Tested	Sensitivity for Stroke	Specificity for Stroke	Comments
CPSS	Facial droop Arm drift Abnormal speech	80%	88%	1 of 3 new findings: 72% probability AIS All 3 findings: probability AIS >85%
LAPSS	Facial smile Grip Arm strength	91%	97%	86% PPV, 98% NPV 96% overall accuracy
Stroke Severity Scales	Items Tested	Sensitivity for LVO	Specificity for LVO	
LAMS	Facial droop Arm rift Grip strength	81%	85%	For LAMS ≥4 85% accuracy for LVO LR(+) 7.36 LR(−) 0.21
RACE	Facial palsy Arm weakness Leg weakness Head, gaze deviation Neglect/aphasia	85% Score ≥ 5	68%	PPV 0.70 NPV 0.79 LR(+) 4.17 LR(−) 0.48
PASS scale	LOC Gaze deviation Arm weakness	Score ≥ 2 66%	83%	Accuracy 76% PPV 0.67 NPV 0.81

AIS, acute ischemic stroke; CPSS, Cincinnati Prehospital Stroke Screen; LAPSS, Los Angeles Prehospital Stroke Screen; LOC, level of consciousness; LR, likelihood ratio; LVO, large vessel occlusion; NPV, negative predictive value; PASS, Prehospital Acute Stroke Severity scale; PPV, positive predictive value.[1]
Prospective validation in LA, data from *The Stroke Interventionalist 2001* and Hastrup S, Damgaard D, Johnsen SP, Andersen G. Prehospital acute stroke severity scale to predict large artery occlusion: design and comparison with other scales. *Stroke.* 2016;47(7):1772-1776.

facility that can provide intra-arterial thrombectomy is reasonable if the delay is not greater than 15 to 20 minutes.[28] EMS prenotification of the patient's arrival is recommended, and bringing a family member, if possible, allows the ED physicians and stroke team to make necessary preparations.

ACUTE ISCHEMIC STROKE

APPROACH

When a patient with an acute stroke symptom presents, multiple simultaneous processes need to occur to minimize time from door to treatment. A team approach within the context of an established system of care including a stroke team is advised. The exact order of the evaluation may vary among institutions. These systems should also prepare for rapid management of adverse events.

Diagnosis of Acute Ischemic Stroke

The diagnosis of AIS is dependent on the history, physical findings, and appropriate imaging. Classically, an acute stroke has a sudden onset of symptoms with focal neurologic findings attributed to a vascular distribution. Standard neurologic examination is reviewed in **Chapter 2: The Neurologic Examination**. There are five syndromes that the emergency physician should become very familiar with[29] (**Table 15.2**).

The National Institute of Health Stroke Scale (NIHSS) is a highly reproducible stroke severity scale that was developed and validated for research purposes,[30] but was found to be highly useful in clinical care. It does not represent a complete neurologic examination. The stroke scale evaluates

TABLE 15.2	Common Stroke Syndromes		
Artery	**Symptoms**	**Comments**	
Left MCA (left dominant, right-handed person)	Aphasia[a] L gaze preference R visual field deficit R hemiparesis R hemisensory loss	The dominant cerebral hemisphere is the side that controls language function, generally the left hemisphere	L-M2 superior division L-M2 inferior division
Right MCA	Left neglect/hemi-inattention[a] R gaze preference L visual field deficit L hemiparesis L hemisensory loss		R-M2 superior division R-M2 inferior division
Lacunar syndromes	Pure motor (internal capsule) Pure sensory (thalamus) Clumsy hand/dysarthria (pons or genu of internal capsule) Ataxic hemiparesis (pons) Multi-infarct dementia	Caused by occlusion of small penetrating arteries into the basal ganglia, thalamus, brainstem	
Brainstem; vertebral and basilar arteries	Cranial nerve findings such as dizziness, diplopia, dysarthria, dysphagia, ataxia with crossed findings. The cranial nerve deficits are ipsilateral, the motor and sensory deficits are contralateral	Posterior circulation strokes range from asymptomatic to comatose in basilar artery occlusion that has a 95% mortality	
Cerebellar syndromes; vertebral and basilar arteries	Truncal/gait ataxia, limb ataxia, and skew deviation		

MCA, middle cerebral artery.
[a]Indicates cortical findings.

the 11 domains with a standard scoring system. It correlates to the size of the stroke, the risk of post lytic hemorrhage, the likelihood of an LVO, and allows for patient monitoring over time (see **Table 15.3**). In general, a stroke scale of 0 to 5 is considered mild, 6 to 15 moderate, 16 to 20 severe, and over 20 very severe strokes. The NIHSS gives higher scores to dominant hemispheric strokes compared to same-size strokes on nondominant hemispheres, and it is less sensitive for posterior circulation stroke.

Stroke outcomes are frequently measured by the modified Rankin Score (mRS), which reflects a patient's functional status (see **Table 15.4**). The mRS is also used to estimate the patient's baseline functional status before the stroke. Most thrombectomy trials only included patients with a baseline mRS of 0 to 2. Both scales require brief training and certification to ensure reliability and reproducibility.

Non-contrast computed tomography (NCCT) or MRI is the first step in imaging the patient with acute stroke.[22] The NCCT is most frequently used because it is readily available and is highly reliable in demonstrating an acute ICH. A negative NCCT finding with symptoms of an AIS makes the diagnosis. The ability of the NCCT to detect an AIS is limited in the early hours; it is about 50% sensitive and 80% specific. Diffusion-weighted imaging (DWI) on MRI is highly sensitive for AIS, and can detect the cytotoxic edema of infarcted tissue within 20 minutes of the first symptoms. The NCCT can be followed by a computed tomography angiogram (CTA) of the head and neck to diagnose an LVO and a CTP to determine the size of the penumbra. The CTA is nearly 100% sensitive and 80% to 100% specific for LVO. The CTP is now aided by postprocessing software that can identify tissue destined to infarct (the core) with a 100% sensitivity and a 91%

TABLE 15.3	**NIH Stroke Scale (abbreviated)**
1a. Level of Consciousness:	0 = Alert; keenly responsive 1 = Not alert, but arousable by minor stimulation 2 = Not alert, obtunded, requires repeated stimulation, or painful stimulation 3 = Responds only with reflex effects or totally unresponsive, flaccid, areflexic
1b. LOC Questions: What is the month? What is your age?	0 = Answers both questions correctly 1 = Answers one question correctly 2 = Answers neither question correctly
1c. LOC Commands: Open and close eyes grip and release hand	0 = Performs both tasks correctly 1 = Performs one task correctly 2 = Performs neither task correctly
2. Best Gaze: Only horizontal eye movements	0 = Normal 1 = Partial gaze palsy, but where forced deviation or total gaze paresis are not present 2 = Forced deviation, or total gaze paresis
3. Visual: Visual fields (upper and lower quadrants)	0 = No visual loss 1 = Partial hemianopia 2 = Complete hemianopia 3 = Bilateral hemianopia (blind including cortical blindness)
4. Facial Palsy:	0 = Normal symmetrical movement 1 = Minor paralysis (flattened nasolabial fold, asymmetry on smiling) 2 = Partial paralysis 3 = Complete paralysis of one or both sides

5 and 6. Motor Arm and Leg:
   5a. Left Arm
   5b. Right Arm
   6a. Left Leg
   6b. Right Leg
	Arm—10 second hold, Leg—5 second hold
	0 = No drift
	1 = Drift, limb drifts down before full 5 or 10 s; does not hit bed
	2 = Limb down to bed before 10 s, but has some effort against gravity
	3 = No effort against gravity, limb falls
	4 = No movement

7. Limb Ataxia: Finger-to-nose and heel-to-shin tests are scored only if present	0 = Absent 1 = Present in one limb 2 = Present in two limbs
8. Sensory: Pinprick and light touch on multiple body areas	0 = Normal; no sensory loss 1 = Mild to moderate sensory loss 2 = Severe to total sensory loss; patient is not aware of being touched in the face, arm, and leg
9. Best Language: Use picture or naming card	0 = No aphasia, normal 1 = Mild to moderate aphasia 2 = Severe aphasia; listener carries burden of communication 3 = Mute, global aphasia; no usable speech or auditory comprehension
10. Dysarthria:	0 = Normal 1 = Mild to moderate; patient slurs at least some words, but can be understood 2 = Severe; patient's speech unintelligible or is mute/anarthric x = Intubated or other physical barrier

TABLE 15.3 NIH Stroke Scale (abbreviated) (*Continued*)

11. Extinction, Inattention, Neglect: Visual, sensory or spatial, personal score only if present	0 = No abnormality 1 = Extinction to bilateral simultaneous stimulation in one of the sensory modalities 2 = Profound hemi-inattention or hemi-inattention to more than one modality

NIH, National Institutes of Health.

TABLE 15.4 Modified Rankin Scale

0	No symptoms at all
1	No significant disability despite symptoms; able to carry out all usual duties and activities
2	Slight disability: unable to carry out all previous activities, but able to look after own affairs without assistance
3	Moderate disability: requiring some help, but able to walk without assistance
4	Moderately severe disability: unable to walk and attend to bodily needs without assistance
5	Severe disability: bedridden, incontinent, and requiring constant nursing care and attention
6	Dead

specificity, and can identify the volume of the ischemic tissue.[31] The difference between these is the mismatch volume, and is considered to be the penumbra.

Transient Ischemic Attacks

The initial evaluation of a TIA is identical to that of an acute stroke. Seventy-five percent of TIAs resolve within 1 hour. When the patient returns to normal, the time of last known well also resets for purposes of acute treatment. The differential diagnosis of sudden focal neurologic deficits is quite large (**Table 15.5**). It is important to ensure a complete workup for the cause of the TIA as soon as possible, preferably within 24 to 48 hours. The ABCD2 score[32] is commonly used for risk stratification after a TIA to prioritize patients in need of an urgent evaluation (**Table 15.6**). This score may be skewed toward classic, clear-cut TIAs and away from TIAs with more atypical or isolated symptoms, that is, nonconsensus TIAs. In a 16-year study, the 90-day stroke risk after a TIA was 11.6% for classic TIAs and 10.6% for nonconsensus TIAs, with a 10-year risk of any major vascular of 27.1% and 31%, respectively. The nonconsensus group was more likely to have posterior circulation stenosis (odds ratio [OR] = 2.21; 95% CI: 1.59-3.1) and was less likely to follow up with a doctor.[33]

AIS Management

The ED approach is to first stabilize the patient and address any immediate life threats. Airway and ventilation need to be secured if the patient is unconscious or has significant bulbar impairment. Oxygen levels should be maintained above 94% O_2 saturation, but higher levels have not been shown to be beneficial; 100% O_2 or a non-rebreather mask should not be used unless specifically indicated. Low BP is much more detrimental than is high BP, and needs immediate attention and treatment. High BPs are common in the acute phase and typically decline during the initial evaluation and with IV fluids. An evaluation of the C-spine and for signs of major trauma is also indicated. This should be followed by a focused examination to determine the severity of the stroke. The NIHSS can be performed in 5 to 7 minutes. Simultaneously, team members should be placing intravenous (IV) lines and obtaining blood samples. Blood tests should include glucose (point of care), troponin, complete blood count (CBC), platelets, international normalized ratio (INR), prothrombin time (PT), partial thromboplastin time (PTT), and electrolytes. An electrocardiogram (ECG) and chest x-ray should be deferred until imaging is completed to avoid delays in treatment. The initial history should be focused and concentrate on the time last known normal, as compared to the time symptoms were discovered, and exclusion criteria for thrombolysis. All patients with acute stroke should start with an NCCT. Patients with AIS having an NIHSS score of 6 or more

TABLE 15.5	Differential Diagnosis of Sudden-Onset Transient Focal Deficit
Ischemic stroke	
Intracerebral hemorrhage	
Transient ischemic attack	
Hypoglycemia	
Seizure with postictal (Todd) paralysis	
Partial seizure	
Migraine with aura	
Abscess with seizure	
Tumor with bleed or seizure	
Toxic-metabolic or infectious insult with old cerebral lesion	
Subdural hematoma (acute)	
Multiple sclerosis	
Cerebritis	

TABLE 15.6	ABCD2 Score	
Feature	**Variable**	**Score**
A—age	≥60 years	1 point
B—blood pressure	≥140/90 mm Hg	1
C—clinical features	Unilateral weakness Speech impairment, no weakness	2 1
D—duration	≥60 minutes 10-59	2 1
D—diabetes	Present	1

Risk Level (Points)	**Percentage of Patients (%)**	**Stroke Risk at 2 Days (%)**	**Stroke Risk at 7 Days (%)**
High (6-7)	21	8.1	11.7
Moderate (4-5)	45	4.1	5.9
Low (0-3)	34	1.0	1.2

should undergo a CTA of the head and neck. If the onset of symptoms is over 6 hours, then CTP should be added. MRI with DWI and a magnetic resonance angiogram (MRA) can also be used for the initial imaging as long as the time to treatment is not delayed.

There are multiple proven treatments for AIS that include thrombolysis within 4.5 hours of onset of symptoms, IAT, also called mechanical thrombectomy (MT), aspirin within 24 to 48 hours, and acute stroke units (ASUs).

Thrombolysis for AIS

The National Institute for Neurological Disorders and Stroke (NINDS) recombinant tissue plasminogen activator (rt-PA) stroke trial was two consecutive randomized placebo-controlled trials that established the efficacy and safety of t-PA for the treatment of AIS in the 0- to 3-hour window and led to U.S. Food and Drug Administration (FDA) approval in June of 1996. The inclusion criteria include age 18 or older, an acute stroke with a measurable neurologic deficit, and an NCCT that excludes any hemorrhage. The exclusion criteria are designed for patient safety and have been become less restrictive over time (**Table 15.7**). The dose: 0.9 mg/kg, a maximum of 90 mg, 10% given as bolus

TABLE 15.7	Inclusion/Exclusion Criteria for Intravenous T-PA for Acute Ischemic Stroke

Inclusion Criteria

Clinical diagnosis of stroke with measurable deficit

Symptom onset ≤4.5 hours

Age 18 years or older

Absolute Exclusion Criteria

Evidence of ICH or intra-axial tumor on pretreatment CT-head

Clinical presentation suggestive of SAH

Any history of intracranial hemorrhage

Uncontrolled hypertension at time of treatment
    Blood pressure >185/110 mm Hg on two readings 5 minutes apart

Active internal bleeding or known aortic dissection

Any intracranial or spinal surgery, severe head trauma within the past 3 months

Acute bleeding diathesis:
a. INR >1.7 with current use of warfarin (Coumadin)
b. Patients taking oral direct thrombin inhibitors and oral direct factor Xa inhibitors within the past 48 hours
c. Elevated PTT with administration of unfractionated heparin or anti-Xa
d. Low-molecular-weight heparin within 24 hours (therapeutic dose)
e. Platelet count <100,000/mm^3

CT demonstrates extensive regions of clear hypodensity suggestive of acute irreversible ischemia

For patients with acute ischemic stroke and symptoms consistent with (untreated) infective endocarditis, treatment with IV t-PA is not recommended

Cautions/Warnings

Minor nondisabling symptoms, ie, sensory only

Rapidly improving stroke symptoms
    Treatment should not be delayed to monitor for further improvement

Ischemic stroke within 3 months

Blood glucose concentration <50 mg/dL and >400 mg/dL:

Pregnancy and early postpartum period (<14 days after delivery)

Seizure at onset of stroke symptoms

Recent anterior ST-elevation myocardial infarction in previous 3 months (not current) or acute pericarditis

Major surgery or serious trauma (excluding head trauma) within last 14 days

Arterial puncture, noncompressible site 7 days

Lumbar puncture within 7 days

History of frank GI or GU hemorrhage within 21 days

Known, untreated, extra-axial intracranial neoplasm

Known, untreated, and unsecured intracranial aneurysm (especially if >10 mm)

Known, untreated, intracranial vascular malformation

CT demonstrates extensive regions of clear hypodensity suggestive of acute irreversible ischemia

(continued)

TABLE 15.7	Inclusion/Exclusion Criteria for Intravenous T-PA for Acute Ischemic Stroke *(Continued)*

3-4.5 Hours from Symptom Onset-Additional Exclusions

National Institutes of Health Stroke Scale (NIHSS) score >25

Age >80—Relative exclusion

Use of warfarin regardless of INR—Relative exclusion

Diabetic patients with previous stroke—Relative exclusion

CT, computed tomography; GI, gastrointestinal; GU, genitourinary; ICH, intracerebral hemorrhage; INR, international normalized ratio; IV, intravenous; PTT, partial thromboplastin time; SAH, subarachnoid hemorrhage; t-PA, tissue plasminogen activator.

and the remainder given over 1 hour, was established in a prior dose escalation study with a focus on safety as well. The NINDS trial demonstrated that patients who receive t-PA have a greater chance of returning to normal or near normal at 90 days with an adjusted OR of 2.0 (95% CI: 1.3-3.1) for benefit that represented an absolute benefit 11% to 13%, and a relative increase in favorable outcome of 30% to 50%. There were more symptomatic ICHs (sxICHs) in the rt-PA group, 6.4% versus 0.6%, but no increase in mortality, 17% versus 21%. The sxICH rate for patients with a baseline NIHSS over 20 is 17%; this group also has the highest mortality and severe disability rate (**Table 15.8**).

IV t-PA is also recommended in the 3- to 4.5-hour window based on the Third European Cooperative Acute Stroke Study (ECASS III) trial, pooled analyses of multiple trials, and a prospective database. t-PA is not currently FDA approved in this time window, but is a IB recommendation by the American Heart Association/American Stroke Association (AHA/ASA).[22] ECASS III excluded those older than age 80, or with a combination of both previous stroke and diabetes, or with an NIHSS over 25 or early ischemic changes of more than one-third of middle cerebral artery (MCA) territory to limit the risk of sxICH. These exclusion criteria might not be warranted depending on more recent analysis. The OR for improvement (90-day mRS 0,1) was 1.34 (95% CI: 1.00-1.65) and 1.47 (95% CI: 1.10-1.97) in the per protocol population. The sxICH rate was 2.4% versus 0.2% based on the ECASS ICH criteria, which were not as strict but more relevant than was the NINDS criteria.

Special cases such as mild but disabling strokes, strokes that stabilize after rapid early improvement, and sickle cell disease (SCD)–associated stroke should also be treated. Patients who wake up with stroke symptoms or have an uncertain onset of symptoms can be treated in the 0- to 4.5-hour window after an MRI. The MR DWI will demonstrate the stroke; however, the MR FLAIR image does not show a stroke for the initial 4.5 to 5 hours. If there is a positive DWI and a negative FLAIR image (a mismatch), the stroke is still early and can be treated with IV t-PA. Rapid treatment is also preferred over delays to treatment for additional studies for patients who present with stroke symptoms that might mimic an AIS because this group has a very low risk of sxICH.

The current recommendation for the door-to-needle time for IV t-PA is 45 minutes. Treatment can proceed before the availability of laboratory results unless there is a high suspicion of

TABLE 15.8	sxICH Rate by Baseline NIHSS Score[a]
NIHSS Score	**sxICH Rate**
0-5	2%
6-10	3%
11-15	5%
16-20	4%
>20	17%

sxICH was defined as any blood on CT within 36 hours of treatment associated with a 4-point increase in NIHSS score.
NIHSS, National Institute of Health Stroke Scale; sxICH, symptomatic intracerebral hemorrhage.
[a]0- to 3-hour window.

coagulopathy or thrombocytopenia. The infusion can be stopped if abnormal results return. The half-life of IV t-PA is 7 minutes. The ECG and chest x-ray should not delay treatment either and can be completed after the NCCT. The importance of reducing onset to treatment time in the 0- to 4.5-hour window was demonstrated in an analysis by Lansberg that evaluated the number needed to treat (NNT) for benefit and harm based on shifts across the mRS[34] (**Figure 15.8**). This data is very useful in patient and family discussions of thrombolytic treatment.

Post lytic care should start as soon as the t-PA bolus has been completed. This includes adherence to the monitoring protocol regarding vital signs and neuro checks, maintaining the BP below 180/105, and being prepared to deal with any complications such as angioedema or ICH.

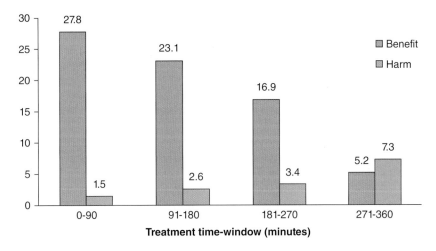

Figure 15.8: The number needed to treat (NNT) for benefit/harm by time. Number of patients who benefit and are harmed per 100 patients treated in each time window. From Lansberg MG, Schrooten M, Bluhmki E, Thijs VN, Saver JL. Treatment time-specific number needed to treat estimates for tissue plasminogen activator therapy in acute stroke based on shifts over the entire range of the modified Rankin Scale. *Stroke.* 2009;40(6):2079-2084.

Intra-arterial Therapy for Stroke

The ability of IV t-PA to recanalize arteries is proportional to the clot burden, the size of the artery, and the size of the stroke[35,36] (**Figure 15.9**). In the NINDS trial, only 10% of patients with a baseline stroke scale over 20 returned to normal and had a nearly 70% chance of being severely disabled

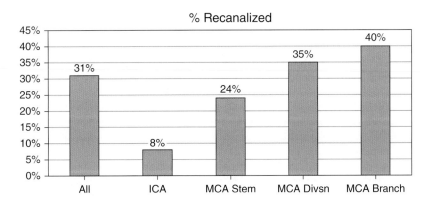

Figure 15.9: Recanalization by size of the artery. ICA, internal carotid artery; MCA, middle cerebral artery. Data from del Zoppo, GJ. *Ann Neurol* 1992 Jul;32(1):78-86.

or dead at 3 months with IV therapy alone. An NIHSS of 10 or greater is associated with an 80% chance of having an LVO. Patients with LVOs are candidates for IAT and MT.

Technical advances have produced stent retrievers and aspiration catheters that are now the mainstay of IAT. The benefit of IAT in the 6-hour window was demonstrated in five trials in 2015.[37] Between 68% and 100% of the patients were also treated with IV t-PA. These trials used the NCCT, CTA, and the ASPECTS to select patients for IAT as well as the criteria for IV t-PA. The ASPECTS score looks at 10 specified areas of the NCCT and assigns 1 point for every normal area or 0 points for every area with early ischemic changes or hypodensity that indicates infarcted tissue; a score of 6 or more was used. The NNT was 2.6 to return one patient to functional independence (mRS = 0-2) at 90 days. In the 0- to 6-hour window, a CTP was not required.

The IAT window was extended to 24 hours based on two trials: DEFUSE 3[38] and DAWN[39] using CTP or MRI for patient selection. Artificial intelligence software was used to postprocess the CTP scans in real time. The commonly used criteria for CTP now used include a core infarct of <70 mL, with a ratio of ischemia to infarct of 1.8 or more and a penumbra (mismatch) volume of over 15 mL. The NNT was approximately 2 for return to independent function, with no difference in mortality. It is recommended that all patients with an NIHSS score of 6 or more undergo CTA (or MRA) and those who present beyond 6 hours also have a CTP completed. Any patient who is also eligible for IV t-PA should receive it even if going for IAT.

Aspirin

Two large studies have demonstrated the benefit of aspirin (325 mg) as a treatment for AIS in the first 24 to 48 hours. If a patient receives IV t-PA, the aspirin is usually held for the first 24 hours. Aspirin should not be given within 90 minutes of IV t-PA because it may increase the chance of sxICH. Oral aspirin should not be given until a swallow screen is completed to prevent aspiration.

Supportive Care for All Patients with Acute Stroke

The majority of patients with AIS (70%-85%) are not eligible for acute therapy. Only 10% to 12% of these patients have an LVO, and only about 20% of the patients receive IV t-PA. Therefore, all patients should receive supportive care consistent with the type of care provided in an ASU. ASUs have been shown to provide protocolized care that decreases disability and mortality and improves the quality of life. They pay close attention to supportive care to minimize complications; this should be started in the ED. These "stroke vital signs" include attention to oxygenation, circulation, BP, glucose, temperature, and seizures.

Oxygen levels should be maintained above 94%. There is no evidence to support the use of 100% O_2 or hyperbaric oxygen. The airway must be kept patent, so intubation would be indicated if the patient is unconscious or is unable to manage their secretions. All patients, including those with TIA, should be kept NPO (nothing by mouth) to prevent aspiration until a swallow screen is performed. If the patient fails the swallow screen, a formal swallow study is indicated.

Circulation must be ensured to maintain optimal cerebral perfusion. This includes optimizing cardiovascular status. Many patients with acute stroke are volume depleted despite being hypertensive. Systolic dysfunction and myocardial suppression can occur in 13% to 28% of stroke cases, arrhythmias can occur in 5% to 30% of cases, and acute myocardial infarction can occur in 2% of the cases. All patients should be placed on a cardiac monitor, and testing for acute myocardial infarction with ECGs and troponin levels should be done. If there is an acute ST-elevation myocardial infarction (STEMI) in association with an AIS, and the patient is eligible for IV t-PA, it should be administered at the AIS dose.

Cerebral autoregulation is the brain's ability to maintain a constant CBF across a broad range of mean arterial pressures (MAPs). In the area of ischemia, autoregulation is lost and the CBF depends on the MAP. Patients with chronic HTN have a shift to higher MAPs to maintain CBF. In patients who do not receive IV t-PA, the BP should be allowed to run high. Those with chronic HTN should not be "normalized" because this will expand the area of ischemia and infarction. The recommendations are not to treat the BP until it is over 220/120. The use of short-acting, titratable medications is encouraged. BP in the IV t-PA candidate should be below 185/110 before treatment. If the BP is above this level on two readings 5 minutes apart, titratable medications such as labetalol, nicardipine, or nitroglycerine may be used to bring the BP into range.

Overall, hypotension is much more detrimental than HTN. One should seek the cause and treat the hypotension aggressively. The use of 0.9 NS (normal saline) first to ensure adequate preload is a reasonable start.

Hypoglycemia can cause hemiplegia and mimic a stroke; therefore, a point-of-care glucose should be done during the initial encounter, and levels at or below 60 mg/dL should be corrected. Routine use of D50 for "mental status changes" should be discouraged until the glucose is measured.

Glucose elevations at the time of an AIS portend a worse outcome than is normoglycemia for the same-size stroke, possibly due to lactate-related injury. Insulin is a neuroprotective, but aggressive lowering (using IV insulin with tight control) of blood glucose does not improve outcome. It is recommended to keep the glucose level between 140 and 180 mg/dL with a regular insulin sliding scale. Severe hyperglycemia should be treated more aggressively,

Temperature is very important because a fever worsens outcome especially in the first 24 hours after an AIS. Brain temperature is generally higher than is core temperature by approximately 1 °C. Elevations above 38 °C should be treated aggressively with acetaminophen or ibuprofen, and the source of the fever investigated and addressed. At this time, there is no evidence that hypothermia in AIS improves outcome, and is not recommended.

Seizures occur in approximately 5% of acute strokes and are usually generalized tonic-clonic in nature. The possible causes include severe strokes with cortical involvement, unstable tissue at risk for infarction, spreading depolarizations from the excitotoxic response, or a history of a seizure disorder. The patients should be protected from injury during the ictus, and treated in the standard manner starting with a benzodiazepine. There is no need for prophylactic seizure treatment.

Management of TIA

The management of the patient with TIA is identical to that for AIS in regard to supportive care, including a swallow screen. Therapy is based on the cause of the TIA. The urgency of the evaluation for a cause is based on risk stratification for subsequent disabling stroke using the ABCD2 score. The evaluation should be completed within a 24- to 48-hour period for high-risk patients who have a significant 2-day risk of disabling stroke. Frequently, these patients are admitted to the hospital. The evaluation begins with brain imaging, usually an NCCT, although an MRI with DWI is preferable and should be completed as early as possible. Other studies include vascular imaging of the head and neck with either a CTA or an MRA; Doppler ultrasound and transcranial Dopplers are acceptable; echocardiography (preferably transesophageal); an ECG and cardiac monitoring; routine blood tests; as well as a blood test for hypercoagulability, if indicated. The frequency of uncovering AF or paroxysmal AF is related to the duration of cardiac monitoring.[9]

The various treatments for a TIA include dual antiplatelet therapy (DAPT), generally with clopidogrel and aspirin,[40] carotid endarterectomy or stent, oral anticoagulation, possible patent foramen ovale (PFO) closure, and risk factor modification. The benefit of these therapies begins in the first 12 to 48 hours, and in the case of carotid endarterectomy or stent, it is in the first 1 to 2 weeks after the TIA. Institutional systems that facilitate rapid evaluation and treatment of the patient with TIA result in optimal outcomes.

INTRACEREBRAL HEMORRHAGE

EPIDEMIOLOGY

ICH accounts for up to 20% of all strokes, with a higher prevalence in Japan and Korea (18%-24%) as compared to the United States, United Kingdom, and Australia (8%-15%).[41] ICH prevalence is two times higher in lower income countries as compared to those with higher incomes (22 vs. 10 per 100,000 person-years). Asians have an ICH rate twice as high as other ethnic groups (51.8 per 100,000 person-years vs. 19.6-24.2 in Whites, Black, and Hispanics), and Blacks have an ICH rate nearly 2 times higher than do Whites (48.9 vs. 26.6 per 100,000). ICH incidence increases with age, with rates as high as 176 per 100,000 person-years in those 75 to 94 years old. Males have a slightly greater ICH rate as compared to females.

Modifiable behavioral risk factors for ICH include smoking, excessive alcohol use, and sympathomimetic drug abuse. Modifiable medical risk factors for ICH include HTN, anticoagulation and antiplatelet use, and low low-density lipoprotein (LDL) cholesterol and triglyceride levels. Nonmodifiable risk factors in addition to age, race, and sex, include chronic kidney disease, the presence of cerebral microbleeds, and, possibly, multiparity.

In high-income countries, the age-adjusted ICH rate has remained stable at 10 per 100,000 between 1980 and 2008, even though it has increased in low-income countries. Although ICH due to poorly controlled HTN has declined, ICH incidence has remained stable possibly due to the presence of amyloid angiopathy in a growing population of older patients.

Following ICH, up to 40% of patients can achieve long-term functional independence. The ICH case fatality rate is 40% at 1 month and 54% at 1 year. Less than one-third of patients with ICH survive to 5 years. Prognostic factors that predict a poorer outcome following ICH include age 80 or older, low body weight, chronic kidney disease, admission hyperglycemia, advanced white matter lesions, and lower GCS scores. Hemorrhage-specific poor prognostic factors include ICH volume ≥30 mL, intraventricular extension, and deep lobar and infratentorial (cerebellar) origin. Up to 7% of patients experience a recurrent ICH within 1 year.

Following ICH, only up to 40% of patients can achieve long-term functional independence. The prognosis from anticoagulation-associated ICH is worse than that from spontaneous ICH without anticoagulation, with up to three-quarters of patients with ICH losing their independence or dying.

PATHOPHYSIOLOGY

Primary spontaneous ICH is principally related to HTN or amyloid angiopathy, and accounts for 85% of all patients with ICH. The other 15% of ICH events are secondary to disorders such as bleeding diathesis, vascular malformations, tumors, hemorrhagic conversion of ischemic strokes, or drug abuse.

Of the primary ICH events, 60% are related to HTN, which causes degenerative changes most often in the penetrating arterioles of the pons, basal ganglia, thalamus, and cerebellum. The other 40% are events due to amyloid deposition and angiopathy associated with advanced age, which causes vessel degeneration deeper in the lobes of the cerebrum.

The primary injury related to ICH is from the compressive effects of the initial extravasation of blood on local neurons and support tissues. Secondary injury following ICH occurs from expanding or recurrent hemorrhage, inflammation from blood degradation and iron-mediated free radicals, disruption of the blood-brain barrier, disrupted hemostatic mechanisms, edema, and/or the pathologic increase in ICP.

One-quarter of patients with ICH have significant hematoma growth within 1 hour of the initial bleed, and another 12% will have hematoma expansion within 20 hours.[42] One meta-analysis defined four independent predictors of ICH growth: time from symptom onset to baseline imaging, baseline ICH volume, antiplatelet use, and anticoagulant use.[43] Both 24-hour and 3-month mortality are increased when ICH growth occurs within 6 hours of the ictus.[44]

Intraventricular extension occurs in about two-thirds of patients with primary ICH, which can result in hydrocephalus, exacerbating increased ICP and often requiring mechanical intervention to restore cerebrospinal fluid (CSF) flow and drainage.

APPROACH/THE FOCUSED EXAMINATION

Patients with ICH can present with stroke signs, an alteration in mental status, HTN, headache, syncope, and/or nausea and vomiting. The initial approach must first assess the ABCs and vital signs and treat significant abnormalities emergently. Point-of-care glucose needs to be obtained and hypoglycemia treated.

The general physical examination of such patients must assess for any signs of respiratory distress or aspiration, cardiovascular instability or arrhythmias, vascular abnormalities, peripheral pulses, and evidence of trauma.

The neurologic examination must assess the patient's mental status, including a coma examination, as well as an assessment for any neurologic deficits. A baseline GCS score establishes the patient's initial level of functioning and is useful for monitoring and prognostication. The NIHSS can also be calculated in cases of ICH stroke where the patients are able to cooperate.

Evaluation Tools

Two evaluation tools can be used to assess likely outcomes in patients with ICH: the ICH score and the FUNC score (**Table 15.9**). The ICH score utilizes the GCS score, age, ICH volume,

TABLE 15.9	ICH Outcome Prediction Scores and ICH Volume Formula						
ICH Score: Mortality Rate				**FUNC Score: 90-Day Functional Independence Rate**			
GCS	3-4 +2	5-12 +1	13-15 0		GCS	≥9 +2	≤8 0	
Age ≥ 80	No 0	Yes 1			Age	<70 0	70-79 +1	>80
ICH volume[a] ≥ 30 mL	No 0	Yes 1			[a]ICH volume	<30 cc +4	30-60 cc +2	>60 cc 0
IVH	No 0	Yes 1			ICH location	Lobar +2	Deep +1	Infratentorial 0
Infratentorial location	No 0	Yes 1			Pre-ICH cognitive impairment	No +1	Yes 0	
ICH Score	0	1	2	3	4	5	6	
Mortality (%)	0	13	26	72	94	100	100	
FUNC score	0-4	5-7	8	9-10	11			
% functionally independent 90 days (%)	0	1-20	21-60	61-80	81-100			
[a]ABC/2	ICH volume estimate: multiply A (max length) × B (max width) × C (number of CT slices × slice thickness), divide by 2 for round or ellipsoid ICHs; or 3 for highly irregular ICHs							

FUNC, functional outcome in patients with primary intracerebral hemorrhage score; GCS, Glasgow coma scale; ICH, intracerebral hemorrhage; IVH, intraventricular hemorrhage.

infratentorial origin, and intraventricular hemorrhage (IVH) to estimate mortality.[45] The FUNC score uses the same first four criteria and pre-ICH cognitive impairment to predict functional independence at 90 days.[46] These scores were designed to standardize communication and assist with prognostication, despite some variation across patient populations. A meta-analysis of prognostic ICH tools showed the ICH score to have an overall good performance, and a recent modification, the ICH-grading scale (ICH-GS), to have increased utility.[47] In general, older patients with ICH, those with larger hemorrhage, cerebellar hemorrhage, intraventricular extension, and baseline cognitive impairment have a worse functional outcome and are more likely to die. Regardless of the score used to describe patients with ICH, it is recommended that decisions regarding withholding of therapies not be made solely on the basis of these scores, because no score can discriminate between those who will and will not improve with aggressive management

NEUROIMAGING

A non-contrast brain computed tomography (CT) can be quickly performed to evaluate for hemorrhage, cerebral edema, midline shift, mass effect, hemorrhage size, whether there is hemorrhage related to trauma (subdural, epidural), the presence of subarachnoid blood, and for CNS lesions such as tumors. A CTA may be useful in identifying underlying pathology. There is no need to preferentially perform brain MRI acutely, because hemorrhage can be reliably detected with an NCCT. The ICH volume can easily be calculated using the ABC/2 formula (Table 15.9).[48,49] Two specific CT findings can predict ICH expansion or rebleed. The CT island sign is a collection of blood seen on NCCT that is distinct from the main hemorrhage collection. The CT spot sign on CTA or as a distinct hyperdensity on NCCT is continued extravasation of contrast or blood extravasation into the hematoma.

MANAGEMENT

The most recent comprehensive clinical guidelines that address the management of patients with spontaneous ICH were published in 2015 by the AHA/ASA, and by Canadian collaborators in 2020.[50,51] These guidelines directly address the many therapy issues that are critical for the successful resuscitation of the patient in the ED before transfer or disposition to a critical care bed.

Airway Management and Ventilation

The need for adequate ventilation, oxygenation, and airway control using airway adjuncts, rapid sequence induction, and endotracheal intubation are similar in patients with ICH to any other patients with critical illness or injury. Preoxygenation, prevention of aspiration, and avoiding excessive reaction to airway stimulation all are essential for preventing complications including hematoma growth. The use of nondepolarizing paralytics is indicated. The use of IV lidocaine to prevent ICP spikes during intubation is currently not indicated, because pain management, sedation, and paralytic use minimize reflex coughing and gagging in the setting of rapid sequence intubation (RSI). Oxygenation to a PO_2 >90 mm Hg is essential for maximizing outcome, because hypoxic patients with brain injury have a less favorable outcome. Management of elevated ICP using hyperventilation to decrease PCO_2 and causing vasoconstriction is no longer recommended except as a rescue therapy in extreme situations.

Blood Pressure Management

The goal of BP management in the patient with ICH is to ensure adequate CNS perfusion while minimizing the chance of hematoma expansion and/or increased ICP. Raised ICP occurs when the normal ICP of 7 to 15 mm Hg is elevated above 20 to 25 mm Hg. Normal cerebral perfusion pressure (CPP), which is mean arterial pressure less ICP (MAP − ICP), is in the 50 to 70 mm Hg range. Cerebral ischemia occurs when CPP falls below the 30 to 40 mm Hg range. It is essential to provide adequate perfusion (CPP) by maintaining an adequate MAP with a minimum SBP of 90 mm Hg and by minimizing ICP elevation in this setting.

Elevated BP in the patient with ICH should be lowered to an SBP of 140 to 160 mm Hg range in an attempt to prevent hematoma expansion.[52-54] HTN management can include the use of nitrates (when cardiac ischemia or congestive heart failure [CHF] is present), IV bolus medications such as labetalol (when HTN and tachycardia are present), or the use of continuous infusion medications such as nicardipine. Nicardipine is especially useful when significant persistent SBP elevation above 220 mm Hg complicate the ICH, requiring continuous BP monitoring and control.

Hemostatic Therapy

It is essential to limit the extent of hemorrhage by optimizing the impact of coagulation factors and platelets in providing hemostasis. Factor replacement when deficient and platelet therapy in patients with thrombocytopenia are the initial steps in providing hemostatic support. Although recombinant factor VIIa (rFVIIa) can limit hematoma expansion in patients with ICH, its use in unselected patients is not recommended because of the lack of proven clinical benefit and increased thromboembolic complications.

ICH occurrence in patients taking oral anticoagulants and antiplatelet medications is of special importance because early ICH growth rates are 2 times higher in these patients than in patients not taking these medications.[44] When ICH occurs in the setting of an elevated INR because of vitamin K antagonist use, vitamin K–dependent factors should be used to correct the INR, and IV vitamin K should be provided. Because prothrombin complex concentrates (PCCs) can more rapidly correct the INR with fewer complications compared to fresh frozen plasma (FFP), PCCs are the preferred method of INR correction. rFVIIa is not recommended for vitamin K anticoagulation reversal in patients with ICH.

Patients with ICH taking novel oral anticoagulants (NOACs) such as the thrombin inhibitor dabigatran and the factor Xa inhibitors apixaban and rivaroxaban can be given two FDA-approved reversal therapies: idarucizumab for dabigatran and andexanet alfa for apixaban and rivaroxaban. If these therapies are not available, PCCs can be used to reverse the apixaban and rivaroxaban factor Xa inhibitor effects.[55] Because dabigatran is a small water-soluble molecule with 80% being excreted unchanged in the urine, hemodialysis could be considered for anticoagulation reversal, but may require prolonged dialysis.[56]

Per the AHA/ASA guidelines, the usefulness of platelet transfusion in patients with ICH and a history of antiplatelet use (with low-dose aspirin or other agents) is uncertain and may be associated with untoward complications, such that this therapy is not recommended. Protamine sulfate may be considered to reverse heparin in patients with acute ICH.

Seizure and Other Medical Therapies

Prophylactic therapy with antiepileptic drugs (AEDs) to prevent seizures in patients with ICH is not recommended. Instead, seizures that are evident clinically are treated with the same therapies that are used for all patients with seizures: initial treatment with benzodiazepines followed by second-line therapies for persistent seizures. In patients with ICH having unexplained alterations in mental status or signs of subtle status epilepticus, continuous electroencephalogram (EEG) monitoring may diagnose seizure activity that is not otherwise clinically evident.

Further supportive care should ensure that both glucose and temperature are monitored and maintained at normal levels.

Medical ICP Control Therapies

Elevated ICP from ICH is most often seen in young patients with large, supratentorial hemorrhage and resultant cerebral edema and mass effect, as well as in patients with intraventricular extension with secondary hydrocephalus. Patients with ICH with small, stable hematomas and stable neurologic clinical status do not require ICP management.

Prevention and treatment of elevated intracranial pressure (ICP) is based on the physical examination, CT findings, or measured levels above 20 to 25 mm Hg. Despite a clear rationale for ICP management in patients with ICH, the effects of such treatment remain uncertain. Elevated ICP therapies such as mannitol, hypertonic saline administration, and hyperventilation have not been consistently shown to provide clinical benefit in patients with traumatic brain injury, even those who are comatose with a GCS <9, and are not indicated routinely utilized in patients with ICH.

Elevation of the head of the bed to 30 degrees is one of the simple therapies that can limit ICP elevation, with an understanding that this maneuver might lower CPP. When the decision to treat ICP elevations is made, mannitol can be given at a dose of 0.5 to 1 g/kg while keeping the serum osmolality below 320 mOsms/kg, and hypertonic saline can be titrated to a serum sodium of 145 to 160 mEq/L range. The past practice of hyperventilation to manage elevated ICP is no longer recommended except in the setting of significant patient decline, in which case hyperventilation to a PCO_2 in the range of 25 to 30 mm Hg can be initiated as a potential life-saving measure. Corticosteroids are not indicated for the treatment of elevated ICP in patients with ICH.

Invasive Therapies

Comatose patients with ICH who have IVH, hydrocephalus, or transtentorial herniation will most likely benefit from ICP monitoring and treatment. In patients with ICH and hydrocephalus, ventricular drainage is used to maintain the CPP, especially in those patients with alterations in mental status. The safety and efficacy of intraventricular rt-PA, endoscopic or stereotactic therapies, and minimally invasive clot evacuation for IVH are uncertain.

Operative Intervention

It has been shown that ICH location, size, growth over time, and patient clinical status all predict the need for operative intervention, morbidity, and mortality. Vetting these issues requires neurosurgical consultation, which may not always be available on site and might require transfer to obtain these services.

Operative intervention is indicated for patients with cerebellar hemorrhage that are neurologically unstable, those with evidence of brainstem compression, and those with IVH and hydrocephalus (**Figure 15.10**). Acute surgical intervention is considered for young patients with ICH having supratentorial hemorrhages that are superficial and surgically accessible, and in

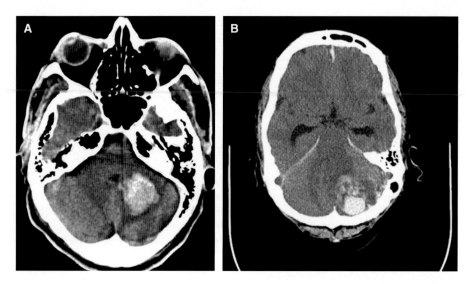

Figure 15.10: Cerebellar hemorrhage on computed tomography (CT) imaging. A, left medial hemorrhage. From Nontraumatic hemorrhage. In: Zamora C, Castillo M, eds. *Neuroradiology Companion*. 5th ed. Wolters Kluwer; 2017:97-106. Figure 9.5. B, Cerebellar hemorrhage with mass effect and fourth ventricle effacement, resulting in obstructive hydrocephalus. From Biller J, Sweis R, Ruland S. The ABCs of neurologic emergencies. In: Biller J, ed. *Practical Neurology*. 5th ed. Wolters Kluwer; 2018. Figure 63.9.

patients who have clinical signs of herniation, especially when associated with a vascular or neoplastic lesion.

Cerebellar hemorrhage occurs in about 10% of patients with ICH, with operative intervention often being required because of the mass effect of the hemorrhage in the limited space of the posterior fossae. Brainstem hemorrhage is a devastating ICH subtype with a mortality rate that approaches 50%. Operative intervention is indicated not only because of the local mass effects that impair normal cardiopulmonary functioning but also because of slow hematoma degradation in the area of the brainstem.

Decompressive craniectomy (with or without hematoma evacuation) might reduce mortality for comatose supratentorial patients with ICH who have large hematomas that cause midline shift or elevated ICP refractory to medical management. When supratentorial hematoma evacuation is performed in such patients who deteriorate, it is considered a life-saving measure. This distinction is made, in part, to provide appropriate context for family members and others who might have expectations following surgery that exceed actual patient outcomes.

The value of routine early surgical intervention for ICH has been controversial since the Surgical Trial in Intracerebral Hemorrhage (STICH) trial in 2005 that compared early operative intervention to initial conservative therapy.[57] Early operative intervention has yet to be definitively proven to provide enhanced patient outcomes when compared to delaying surgery until patients deteriorate. For stable patients with ICH in whom there are no apparent adverse ICP effects, surgical evacuation is not routinely recommended.

OUTCOMES

Among 2801 patients with ICH from three registries, the 3-month mortality was 20% to 28%, and 39% to 48% of patients became severely disabled (mRS 4-5). An analysis of a subpopulation of 288 patients who received antiplatelet therapy to prevent subsequent thromboembolic events showed no added benefit and no additional harm.[58]

Despite the grim prognosis seen following ICH, there is still the need to aggressively treat patients with ICH during the initial hours following the ICH ictus. A 2007 U.S. study demonstrated that independent of other ICH risk factors, an early decision to institute a do-not-resuscitate (DNR) order and the early withdrawal of ongoing care was associated with a worse patient outcome. The authors recommended that DNR orders be delayed until at least the second day of hospitalization to allow the patient the chance to improve before the cessation of treatment efforts.[59]

A subsequent study of the patients with ICH having a median GCS of 7 and a mean hematoma volume of 39 mL who were treated without a DNR showed a 30-day mortality rate 40% less than that predicted by the ICH score. In addition, 30% of such patients had a good outcome at 90 days (mRS 0-3).[60] This data again supports aggressive resuscitation and support of patients with ICH before instituting a DNR order.

The 2015 AHA/ASA guidelines state that the current prognostic models for the patient outcome are biased by the influence of early DNR orders that cause aggressive support to be withdrawn prematurely. They recommended that aggressive care be provided until at least the second full day of hospitalization to maximize the chance for optimal outcomes for patients with ICH. This amplifies the critical role of the emergency medicine specialist in the early care of such patients to optimize patient outcomes.

PEDIATRIC ISSUES

Pediatric strokes occur at a rate of 3 to 25/100,00 children/year in developed countries. They are categorized by age; 28-weeks' gestation to 28 days are considered perinatal strokes, and 28 days to 18 years are considered childhood strokes.

Perinatal stroke occurs in 1:2700-3500 live births. AISs account for 80% of perinatal strokes, and 20% are due to cerebral venous sinus thrombosis (CVST) or hemorrhage. Perinatal AISs are more common in males, and present with seizures (especially focal motor seizures), encephalopathy, delayed motor milestones. or early "handedness." The emergency evaluation includes MRI with MRA and MRV. The primary treatment is supportive care. Because recurrence rates are very low, antiplatelet agents or anticoagulation is rarely used unless indicated by a cardioembolic cause. There is no evidence to use lytics or thrombectomy. Outcomes may include cerebral palsy, impaired cognitive or mental function, speech difficulties, or epilepsy. Motor function impairments are related to basal ganglion involvement.

Perinatal CVST often presents with nonspecific symptoms such as lethargy or seizures. The risk factors include prematurity, emergent C-section, fetal distress, and male sex. Evaluation should include an MRI with an MRA, MRV, and appropriate blood tests. Treatment is directed toward seizure management, correction of dehydration and anemia, as well as addressing any underlying infections. There is no evidence for lytic use or thrombectomy; however, anticoagulation with heparin is safe and likely useful if there is no associated hemorrhage.

Perinatal hemorrhagic stroke occurs in 1 in 6300 live births and presents with seizures and encephalopathy. It can be caused by coagulopathy, thrombocytopenia, trauma, vascular lesion, thrombophilia on heparin, but most are of unknown cause. Family history of bleeding disorders is important to obtain. Imaging is preferably with MRI, MRA, and MRV. Treatment is directed toward the cause, and may include vitamin K deficiency if not given in the newborn period as well as supportive care. Immediate surgical ICH evacuation is rarely indicated, but ventricular drainage and shunting may be indicated; therefore, the neurosurgery service should be consulted.

Childhood strokes (age over 28 days) occur as AIS in 1 to 2 per 100,00 children and ICHs in 1 to 1.7 per 100,00. Risk factors for ischemic stroke include male sex, age younger than 5 years, and Black or Asian race. The risk of ischemic stroke is 200-fold greater in children with SCD. They are caused by cardiac disease with cardioembolism, arterial dissection, SCD, autoimmune disorders, intracranial arteriopathy such as Moya-Moya disease (which causes "silent strokes" and TIAs), thrombophilias, infections (varicella-zoster virus [VZV]), genetic disorders, and, of course, unknown causes. It is unclear if arrhythmias and PFO can cause strokes in children. Most present within 6 hours of onset and have signs and symptoms similar to that of adults, with hemiplegia in 67% to 90%, speech 20% to 25%, visual changes in 10% to 15%; but those younger than 6 years more commonly present with nonspecific symptoms such as seizures (15%-25%), headache (20%-50%), and mental status changes (17%-38%).

Posterior circulation strokes do occur in childhood, typically 7- to 8-year-old males and present with nonlocalizing symptoms such as nausea, vomiting, and headache (in 60%-70%), although they may have symptoms similar to that of adults. These are frequently preceded by minor head or neck trauma, most commonly causing vertebral artery dissection. The danger lies in assuming that children with stroke symptoms have stroke mimics such as Bell palsy or seizures.

The workup is similar to that for a usual stroke/TIA workup presented earlier.

Thrombolysis is considered reasonable treatment in the proper time window. There is some evidence for better clot lysis in children, at the same dose as for adults; however, there are no completed lytic trials in this population. Thrombectomy and IAT are also reasonable, and are supported by numerous case reports.[61] Supportive care is the same as that in adults. Children need an evaluation for long-term secondary prevention (with antiplatelet or anticoagulation agents) because recurrence is 6.8% at 30 days and 12% at 1 year.

Children with SCD can have silent or clinical strokes that occur from thrombosis, hyperviscosity, CVST, or ICH. The preferred evaluation is with MRI/MRA, and MRV, and the treatment is focused on exchange transfusion to a hemoglobin of 11, hydration, correcting hypoxia, and hypotension. Lytic therapy is considered reasonable despite a lack of strong data. The outcome is good in one-third to one-half of children without treatment, especially if the stroke scale on presentation is <6.

ICH in children, including SAH and IVH, is spontaneous in 75% of the cases and from AVMs in 10%: Other causes include bleeding disorders, trauma, and genetic abnormalities.

The initial evaluation is usually with an NCCT and then an MRI/MRA and an EEG. Treatment of childhood ICH includes correcting coagulation abnormalities, isotonic fluids to maintain a normal BP, normalization of glucose and temperature, elevation of the head of bed, AEDs for seizures, and neurosurgical consultation. Outcomes for those younger than 2 years are associated with increased complications such as hydrocephalus, whereas those older than 2 years have a good outcome in 72% of cases.[62]

TIPS AND PEARLS

Stroke

- Only 20% to 25% of stroke-affected patients are eligible for IV t-PA, and only 10% to 12% of such patients have an LVO that is potentially treated by thrombectomy.
- Time matters: For every minute with a large vessel stroke, the average patient loses 1.9 million neurons, 14 billion synapses, and 7.5 miles of axonal fibers.
- Develop systems of care that provide for risk/benefit discussions, team activation, treatment protocols, and transfer protocols.
- The National Institutes of Health (NIH) stroke scale is an important tool for patient evaluation, communication with the stroke team, and decision-making.
- You do not have to wait for laboratory results before treating with IV t-PA unless there is a high suspicion of abnormality.
- IV t-Pa can be administered within 4.5 hours of onset of symptoms, and a thrombectomy for an LVO can be performed within 24 hours; however, the sooner the treatment within a window, the better the outcome. Patients can receive both treatments.
- Patients with stroke and TIA should be kept NPO, even for medications, to prevent aspiration until a swallow screen is performed.
- All patients with acute stroke require meticulous supportive care and should be admitted to an ASU if possible.
- Because of the loss of autoregulation, the BP should not be treated in patients with AIS until it is over 220/120 unless they are receiving IV t-PA, then BP should be 185/110. After IV t-PA, the BP should be maintained at 180/105. IV fluids may decrease the BP in dry patients.

TIA

- The ABCD2 score is commonly used for risk stratification after a TIA so that those with the highest risk can be prioritized for rapid evaluation or admission.
- High-risk patients with TIA have an 8% 2-day risk and a 12% 7-day risk of disabling stroke, and up to 30% to 40% of them will have a lesion on MRI that further increases their risk of subsequent disabling stroke.

ICH

- Patients with TIA need to have an evaluation for the cause of the symptoms within 24 to 48 hours to prevent subsequent disabling stroke.

- ICH outcome is associated with hemorrhage growth. ICH growth is related to time from symptom onset to baseline imaging, initial baseline ICH volume, antiplatelet use, and anti-coagulant use.
- Hemorrhage-specific poor prognostic factors include ICH volume ≥30 mL, intraventricular extension, and deep lobar and infratentorial (cerebellar) origin.
- BP control involves avoiding hypotension to maintain adequate CPP. HTN can be managed by attempting to maintain the SBP at 140 mm Hg.
- Hemostasis is best achieved by providing factor replacement when deficient and platelet therapy in patients with thrombocytopenia. Platelet transfusion in patients with ICH with a history of antiplatelet use (with low-dose aspirin or other agents) is uncertain and is not recommended.
- When ICH occurs in the setting of an elevated INR because of vitamin K antagonist use, vitamin K–dependent factors should be replaced with PCCs, and IV vitamin K provided. Protamine sulfate may be considered to reverse heparin in patients with acute ICH.
- Patients with ICH taking NOACs such as thrombin inhibitor dabigatran; factor Xa inhibitors apixaban and rivaroxaban can be given two FDA-approved reversal therapies; idarucizumab for dabigatran and andexanet alfa for apixaban and rivaroxaban; 4-factor PCC is recommended when these are not available.
- Prophylactic therapy with AEDs to prevent seizures in patients with ICH is not recommended. Instead, seizures that are evident clinically and those noted on EEG in patients with ICH having alterations in mental status are treated with benzodiazepines followed by second-line therapies for persistent seizures.
- Patients with ICH who are comatose and have IVH, hydrocephalus, or transtentorial herniation will most likely benefit from ICP monitoring and treatment. Other minimally invasive therapies are of uncertain benefit.
- Subgroups of patients with ICH who may benefit from early operative intervention include those with cerebellar hemorrhage and are neurologically unstable, have IVH with hydrocephalus, and young patients with superficial supratentorial hemorrhages that are surgically accessible, and in whom there are clinical signs of herniation.
- Even though most patients with ICH have poor reported outcomes, aggressive treatment is still recommended during the initial hours because the current prognostic models for patient outcome are biased by the influence of early DNR orders that cause aggressive support to be withdrawn. It is recommended that aggressive care be provided until at least the second full day of hospitalization to maximize the chance for optimal outcomes for such patients.

EVIDENCE

Can TNK be used instead of t-PA for AIS?

TNK (tenecteplase) is a modification of the t-PA molecule that results in greater fibrin specificity, longer half-life, and can be administered in a single bolus dosing.[63] IV TNK has been studied for AIS in multiple trials compared to IV t-PA that indicate similar safety and efficacy in minor stroke out to 6 hours; however, at present, it is still not considered a proven alternative.[64] The dose of 0.25 mg/kg (maximum dose 25 mg) has been studied before thrombectomy in selected patients and is considered a reasonable use of TNK.[65]

Why is a door-to-needle time of 45 min better than 60 minutes?

Good clinical outcome is related to the time from onset of symptoms to reperfusion with IV t-PA.[66] For every 15-minute increment in decrease of the door-to-needle time, there are improved outcomes with regard to ambulation, discharge to home, sxICH, and mortality.[67] Therefore, it is important to build streamlined systems of care to minimize the duration of brain ischemia and optimize outcomes. Mobile stroke units (MSUs) that are dispatched directly to the patient have been developed in an effort to minimize the time from onset of symptoms to treatment. These are ambulances equipped with CT scanner and trained personnel that can complete the stroke evaluation and administer alteplase in the field. The impact and feasibility of MSUs is under study at this time.[68]

Should minor strokes or those with rapid early improvement be treated?

Yes, minor strokes with disabling symptoms should be treated according to the AHA guidelines. The definition of minor stroke is variable; however, if the patient is likely to suffer disability and not be able to return to all previous activities, even with a stroke scale of 1, they should be treated. The risk of hemorrhage is low at 1.8%,[69] and the efficacy of IV t-PA has been demonstrated to be similar to that in larger strokes.[70] Patients with minor stroke but no disabling symptom at all should not be treated with IV t-PA.[71]

What happens if I treat a patient with a stroke mimic?

There is considerable concern over treating a stroke mimic with IV t-PA. Common mimics such as hypoglycemia or hyperglycemia and seizure can be easily diagnosed during the initial evaluation. The risk of sxICH is extremely low. Tsivgoulis found one case of sxICH among 75 mimics over 5 years in a single center, and meta-analysis of nine centers showed a sxICH rate of 0.5%.[72] Ultimately, the amount of time required for a definitive diagnosis may cause significant harm by delaying the treatment of those with stroke. The current recommendation prefers early treatment over delaying to pursue additional diagnostic studies.[22]

Does early operative intervention in patients with ICH with supratentorial ICH improve outcomes?

Since the publication of the STICH trial, the question of whether operative intervention for patients with ICH should be performed aggressively or only after they fail initial conservative medical management has remained unanswered.[57] The Cochrane Review of 10 trials involving 2059 patients demonstrated a decreased risk of being dead or dependent following surgery (OR = 0.71; $P = 0.001$).[73] However, the result was not sufficiently robust, and further study of which supratentorial patients would benefit from early surgery was recommended. The STICH trial, which allowed crossover to surgery despite being analyzed in the conservative therapy group, may have caused the benefit of surgery to be underestimated in the Cochrane analysis.[74] In the STICH II trial, there was no difference in favorable outcome with early surgery (41% vs. 38%), with the suggestion that early surgery may create a small but clinically relevant survival advantage for patients with spontaneous superficial IVH without intraventricular extension.[75] Both of the guidelines referenced in this chapter, which were developed after these publications, confirm the persistent uncertainty that surrounds the value of early surgical intervention.[50,51]

A recently published retrospective study examined the outcomes of 254 patients with ICH, 27% of whom were in the early surgery group, with a 12-month mortality of 39% and 29% survival without a permanent disability.[76] Using multivariable analysis, early ICH surgery was associated with lower 12-month mortality rates (OR = 0.22) but not with a higher probability of survival without permanent disability (OR = 1.23). An early surgery approach, therefore, improved survival, but with a greater number of patients with ICH who lived with a residual deficit. Still pending is a Chinese clinical trial begun in 2017 that is comparing endoscopic evacuation, stereotactic aspiration, and craniotomy in patients with ICH with a supratentorial ICH >20 mL related to HTN.[77] This and other pending clinical trials are designed to better quantify the value of early surgical intervention in improving outcome in patients with supratentorial ICH.

Does tranexamic acid control hemorrhage and improve outcome in the management of spontaneous patients with ICH?

Hemostatic therapies may be of value in limiting early hematoma growth in patients with spontaneous ICH, which could provide an outcome benefit. Tranexamic acid (TXA) is an antifibrinolytic drug that was studied for its ability to limit death and dependence (mRS 4-6) at 90 days. The TICH-2 (Tranexamic acid for hyperacute primary IntraCerebral Haemorrhage) clinical trial included 2325 patients from 124 hospitals in 12 countries.[78,79] Despite lower 7-day mortality in patients treated with TXA, mortality at 90 days did not differ depending on this treatment. Despite a smaller increase in ICH volume in the TXA subgroup, functional outcome at 90 days did not differ with TXA use. Fewer serious adverse events were noted in TXA-treated patients, and no increase in thromboembolic or seizure events, suggesting that TXA use is safe in patients with ICH. The Cochrane group determined that a larger TXA clinical trial is needed.[43]

References

1. Sacco RL, Kasner SE, Broderick JP, et al. An updated definition of stroke for the 21st century: a statement for healthcare professionals from the American Heart Association/American Stroke Association. *Stroke*. 2013;44(7):2064-2089.

2. Abbott AL, Silvestrini M, Topakian R, et al. Optimizing the definitions of stroke, transient ischemic attack, and infarction for research and application in clinical practice. *Front Neurol*. 2017;8:537.

3. Albers GW, Caplan LR, Easton JD, et al. Transient ischemic attack—proposal for a new definition. *N Engl J Med*. 2002;347(21):1713-1716.

4. Virani SS, Alonso A, Aparicio HJ, et al. Heart disease and stroke statistics—2021 update: a report from the American Heart Association. *Circulation*. 2021;143(8):e254-e743.

5. Centers for Disease Control and Prevention. Stroke Facts. 2021. https://www.cdc.gov/stroke/facts.htm. Accessed on March 22, 2021.

6. Cadilhac DA, Dewey HM, Vos T, Carter R, Thrift AG. The health loss from ischemic stroke and intracerebral hemorrhage: evidence from the North East Melbourne Stroke Incidence Study (NEMESIS). *Health Qual Life Outcomes*. 2010;8:49.

7. World Health organization. The top 10 causes of death. 2021. https://www.who.int/news-room/fact-sheets/detail/the-top-10-causes-of-death. Accessed on March 22, 2021.

8. Feigin VL, Nguyen G, Cercy K, et al. Global, regional, and country-specific lifetime risks of stroke, 1990 and 2016. *N Engl J Med*. 2018;379(25):2429-2437.

9. Easton JD, Saver JL, Albers GW, et al. Definition and evaluation of transient ischemic attack: a scientific statement for healthcare professionals from the American Heart Association/American Stroke Association Stroke Council; Council on Cardiovascular Surgery and Anesthesia; Council on Cardiovascular Radiology and Intervention; Council on Cardiovascular Nursing; and the Interdisciplinary Council on Peripheral Vascular Disease. The American Academy of Neurology affirms the value of this statement as an educational tool for neurologists. *Stroke*. 2009;40(6):2276-2293.

10. Grysiewicz RA, Thomas K, Pandey DK. Epidemiology of ischemic and hemorrhagic stroke: incidence, prevalence, mortality, and risk factors. *Neurol Clin*. 2008;26(4):871-895, vii.

11. Guzik A, Bushnell C. Stroke epidemiology and risk factor management. *Continuum (Minneap Minn)*. 2017;23(1, Cerebrovascular Disease):15-39.

12. Han L, You D, Ma W, et al. National trends in American Heart Association revised Life's Simple 7 metrics associated with risk of mortality among US adults. *JAMA Netw Open*. 2019;2(10):e1913131.

13. Xing CY, Tarumi T, Liu J, et al. Distribution of cardiac output to the brain across the adult lifespan. *J Cereb Blood Flow Metab*. 2017;37(8):2848-2856.

14. Brazzelli M, Chappell FM, Miranda H, et al. Diffusion-weighted imaging and diagnosis of transient ischemic attack. *Ann Neurol*. 2014;75(1):67-76.

15. Adams HP Jr, Bendixen BH, Kappelle LJ, et al. Classification of subtype of acute ischemic stroke. Definitions for use in a multicenter clinical trial. TOAST. Trial of Org 10172 in Acute Stroke Treatment. *Stroke*. 1993;24(1):35-41.

16. Jones TH, Morawetz RB, Crowell RM, et al. Thresholds of focal cerebral ischemia in awake monkeys. *J Neurosurg*. 1981;54(6):773-782.

17. del Zoppo GJ, Sharp FR, Heiss WD, Albers GW. Heterogeneity in the penumbra. *J Cereb Blood Flow Metab*. 2011;31(9):1836-1851.

18. Heiss WD, Graf R. The ischemic penumbra. *Curr Opin Neurol*. 1994;7(1):11-19.

19. Saver JL. Time is brain—quantified. *Stroke*. 2006;37(1):263-266.

20. Rocha M, Jovin TG. Fast versus slow progressors of infarct growth in large vessel occlusion stroke: clinical and research implications. *Stroke*. 2017;48(9):2621-2627.

21. Vagal A, Wintermark M, Nael K, et al. Automated CT perfusion imaging for acute ischemic stroke: pearls and pitfalls for real-world use. *Neurology*. 2019;93(20):888-898.

22. Powers WJ, Rabinstein AA, Ackerson T, et al. Guidelines for the early management of patients with acute ischemic stroke: 2019 update to the 2018 guidelines for the early management of acute ischemic stroke: a guideline for healthcare professionals from the American Heart Association/American Stroke Association. *Stroke*. 2019;50(12):e344-e418.

23. Brandler ES, Sharma M, Sinert RH, Levine SR. Prehospital stroke scales in urban environments: a systematic review. *Neurology*. 2014;82(24):2241-2249.

24. Zhelev Z, Walker G, Henschke N, Fridhandler J, Yip S. Prehospital stroke scales as screening tools for early identification of stroke and transient ischemic attack. *Cochrane Database Syst Rev*. 2019;4(4):CD011427.

25. Jauch EC, Schwamm LH, Panagos PD, et al. Recommendations for regional stroke destination plans in rural, suburban, and urban communities from the prehospital stroke system of care consensus conference: a consensus statement from the American Academy of Neurology, American Heart Association/American Stroke Association, American Society of Neuroradiology, National Association of EMS Physicians, National Association of State EMS Officials, Society of NeuroInterventional Surgery, and Society of Vascular and Interventional Neurology: Endorsed by the Neurocritical Care Society. *Stroke*. 2021;52(5):e133-e152.

26. Nguyen TTM, van den Wijngaard IR, Bosch J, et al. Comparison of prehospital scales for predicting large anterior vessel occlusion in the ambulance setting. *JAMA Neurol*. 2021;78(2):157-164.

27. Kim DG, Kim YJ, Shin SD, et al. Effect of emergency medical service use on time interval from symptom onset to hospital admission for definitive care among patients with intracerebral hemorrhage: a multicenter observational study. *Clin Exp Emerg Med*. 2017;4(3):168-177.

28. Mocco J, Fiorella D, Albuquerque FC. The mission lifeline severity-based stroke treatment algorithm: we need more time. *J Neurointerv Surg*. 2017;9(5):427-428.

29. Lewandowski CA, Libman R. Acute presentation of stroke. *J Stroke Cerebrovasc Dis*. 1999;8(3): 117-26. PMID: 17895154.

30. NINDS rt-PA Stroke Study Group. Tissue plasminogen activator for acute ischemic stroke. *N Engl J Med*. 1995;333(24):1581-1587.

31. Mendelson SJ, Prabhakaran S. Diagnosis and management of transient ischemic attack and acute ischemic stroke: a review. *JAMA*. 2021;325(11):1088-1098.

32. Johnston SC, Rothwell PM, Nguyen-Huynh MN, et al. Validation and refinement of scores to predict very early stroke risk after transient ischaemic attack. *Lancet*. 2007;369(9558):283-292.

33. Tuna MA, Rothwell PM. Diagnosis of non-consensus transient ischaemic attacks with focal, negative, and non-progressive symptoms: population-based validation by investigation and prognosis. *Lancet*. 2021;397(10277):902-912.

34. Lansberg MG, Schrooten M, Bluhmki E, Thijs VN, Saver JL. Treatment time-specific number needed to treat estimates for tissue plasminogen activator therapy in acute stroke based on shifts over the entire range of the modified Rankin Scale. *Stroke*. 2009;40(6):2079-2084.

35. Riedel CH, Zimmermann P, Jensen-Kondering U, Stingele R, Deuschl G, Jansen O. The importance of size: successful recanalization by intravenous thrombolysis in acute anterior stroke depends on thrombus length. *Stroke*. 2011;42(6):1775-1777.

36. Kim YD, Nam HS, Kim SH, et al. Time-dependent thrombus resolution after tissue-type plasminogen activator in patients with stroke and mice. *Stroke*. 2015;46(7):1877-1882.

37. Goyal M, Menon BK, van Zwam WH, et al. Endovascular thrombectomy after large-vessel ischaemic stroke: a meta-analysis of individual patient data from five randomised trials. *Lancet*. 2016;387(10029):1723-1731.

38. Albers GW, Marks MP, Kemp S, et al. Thrombectomy for stroke at 6 to 16 hours with selection by perfusion imaging. *N Engl J Med*. 2018;378(8):708-718.

39. Nogueira RG, Jadhav AP, Haussen DC, et al. Thrombectomy 6 to 24 hours after stroke with a mismatch between deficit and infarct. *N Engl J Med*. 2018;378(1):11-21.

40. Pan Y, Elm JJ, Li H, et al. Outcomes associated with clopidogrel-aspirin use in minor stroke or transient ischemic attack: a pooled analysis of Clopidogrel in High-Risk Patients With Acute Non-Disabling Cerebrovascular Events (CHANCE) and Platelet-Oriented Inhibition in New TIA and Minor Ischemic Stroke (POINT) Trials. *JAMA Neurol*. 2019;76(12):1466-1473.

41. An SJ, Kim TJ, Yoon BW. Epidemiology, risk factors, and clinical features of intracerebral hemorrhage: an update. *J Stroke*. 2017;19(1):3-10.

42. Brott T, Broderick J, Kothari R, et al. Early hemorrhage growth in patients with intracerebral hemorrhage. *Stroke*. 1997;28(1):1-5.

43. Al-Shahi Salman R, Frantzias J, Lee RJ, et al. Absolute risk and predictors of the growth of acute spontaneous intracerebral haemorrhage: a systematic review and meta-analysis of individual patient data. *Lancet Neurol*. 2018;17(10):885-894.

44. Roquer J, Vivanco-Hidalgo RM, Capellades J, et al. Ultra-early hematoma growth in antithrombotic pretreated patients with intracerebral hemorrhage. *Eur J Neurol*. 2018;25(1):83-89.

45. Hemphill JC 3rd, Farrant M, Neill TA Jr. Prospective validation of the ICH Score for 12-month functional outcome. *Neurology*. 2009;73(14):1088-1094.

46. Rost NS, Smith EE, Chang Y, et al. Prediction of functional outcome in patients with primary intracerebral hemorrhage: the FUNC score. *Stroke*. 2008;39(8):2304-2309.

47. Mattishent K, Kwok CS, Ashkir L, Pelpola K, Myint PK, Loke YK. Prognostic tools for early mortality in hemorrhagic stroke: systematic review and meta-analysis. *J Clin Neurol*. 2015;11(4):339-348.

48. Kothari RU, Brott T, Broderick JP, et al. The ABCs of measuring intracerebral hemorrhage volumes. *Stroke*. 1996;27(8):1304-1305.

49. Delcourt C, Carcel C, Zheng D, et al. Comparison of ABC methods with computerized estimates of intracerebral hemorrhage volume: the INTERACT2 study. *Cerebrovasc Dis Extra*. 2019;9(3):148-154.

50. Hemphill JC 3rd, Greenberg SM, Anderson CS, et al. Guidelines for the management of spontaneous intracerebral hemorrhage: a guideline for healthcare professionals from the American Heart Association/American Stroke Association. *Stroke*. 2015;46(7):2032-2060.

51. Shoamanesh A, Patrice Lindsay M, Castellucci LA, et al. Canadian stroke best practice recommendations: *Management of Spontaneous Intracerebral Hemorrhage*, 7th edition update 2020. *Int J Stroke*. 2021;16(3):321-341.

52. Lattanzi S, Cagnetti C, Provinciali L, Silvestrini M. How should we lower blood pressure after cerebral hemorrhage? A systematic review and meta-analysis. *Cerebrovasc Dis*. 2017;43(5-6):207-213.

53. Tsivgoulis G, Katsanos AH, Butcher KS, et al. Intensive blood pressure reduction in acute intracerebral hemorrhage: a meta-analysis. *Neurology*. 2014;83(17):1523-1529.

54. Shi L, Xu S, Zheng J, Xu J, Zhang J. Blood pressure management for acute intracerebral hemorrhage: a meta-analysis. *Sci Rep*. 2017;7(1):14345.

55. Veltkamp R, Horstmann S. Treatment of intracerebral hemorrhage associated with new oral anticoagulant use: the neurologist's view. *Clin Lab Med*. 2014;34(3):587-594.

56. Chai-Adisaksopha C, Hillis C, Lim W, Boonyawat K, Moffat K, Crowther M. Hemodialysis for the treatment of dabigatran-associated bleeding: a case report and systematic review. *J Thromb Haemost*. 2015;13(10):1790-1798.

57. Mendelow AD, Gregson BA, Fernandes HM, et al. Early surgery versus initial conservative treatment in patients with spontaneous supratentorial intracerebral haematomas in the International Surgical Trial in Intracerebral Haemorrhage (STICH): a randomised trial. *Lancet*. 2005;365(9457):387-397.

58. Murthy SB, Biffi A, Falcone GJ, et al. Antiplatelet therapy after spontaneous intracerebral hemorrhage and functional outcomes. *Stroke*. 2019;50(11):3057-3063.

59. Zahuranec DB, Brown DL, Lisabeth LD, et al. Early care limitations independently predict mortality after intracerebral hemorrhage. *Neurology*. 2007;68(20):1651-1657.

60. Morgenstern LB, Zahuranec DB, Sánchez BN, et al. Full medical support for intracerebral hemorrhage. *Neurology*. 2015;84(17):1739-1744.

61. Barry M, Hallam DK, Bernard TJ, Amlie-Lefond C. What is the role of mechanical thrombectomy in childhood stroke? *Pediatr Neurol*. 2019;95:19-25.

62. Ferriero DM, Fullerton HJ, Bernard TJ, et al. Management of stroke in neonates and children: a scientific statement from the American Heart Association/American Stroke Association. *Stroke*. 2019;50(3):e51-e96.

63. Baird AE, Jackson R, Jin W. Tenecteplase for acute ischemic stroke treatment. *Semin Neurol*. 2021;41(1):28-38.

64. Logallo N, Novotny V, Assmus J, et al. Tenecteplase versus alteplase for management of acute ischaemic stroke (NOR-TEST): a phase 3, randomised, open-label, blinded endpoint trial. *Lancet Neurol*. 2017;16(10):781-788.

65. Campbell BCV, Mitchell PJ, Churilov L, et al. Effect of intravenous tenecteplase dose on cerebral reperfusion before thrombectomy in patients with large vessel occlusion ischemic stroke: the EXTEND-IA TNK part 2 randomized clinical trial. *JAMA*. 2020;323(13):1257-1265.

66. Khatri P, Abruzzo T, Yeatts SD, Nichols C, Broderick JP, Tomsick TA. Good clinical outcome after ischemic stroke with successful revascularization is time-dependent. *Neurology*. 2009;73(13):1066-1072.

67. Saver JL, Fonarow GC, Smith EE, et al. Time to treatment with intravenous tissue plasminogen activator and outcome from acute ischemic stroke. *JAMA*. 2013;309(23):2480-2488.

68. Harris J. A review of mobile stroke units. *J Neurol*. 2020. doi:10.1007/s00415-020-09910-4

69. Romano JG, Smith EE, Liang L, et al. Outcomes in mild acute ischemic stroke treated with intravenous thrombolysis: a retrospective analysis of the Get With the Guidelines–Stroke registry. *JAMA Neurol*. 2015;72(4):423-431.

70. Emberson J, Lees KR, Lyden P, et al. Effect of treatment delay, age, and stroke severity on the effects of intravenous thrombolysis with alteplase for acute ischaemic stroke: a meta-analysis of individual patient data from randomised trials. *Lancet*. 2014;384(9958):1929-1935.

71. Khatri P, Kleindorfer DO, Devlin T, et al. Effect of alteplase vs aspirin on functional outcome for patients with acute ischemic stroke and minor nondisabling neurologic deficits: the PRISMS randomized clinical trial. *JAMA*. 2018;320(2):156-166.

72. Tsivgoulis G, Zand R, Katsanos AH, et al. Safety of intravenous thrombolysis in stroke mimics: prospective 5-year study and comprehensive meta-analysis. *Stroke*. 2015;46(5):1281-1287.

73. Prasad K, Mendelow AD, Gregson B. Surgery for primary supratentorial intracerebral haemorrhage. *Cochrane Database Syst Rev*. 2008(4):CD000200.

74. Creutzfeldt C, Tirschwell D. ACP Journal Club. Review: Early surgery improves outcomes in patients with primary supratentorial intracerebral hemorrhage. *Ann Intern Med*. 2009;150(8):JC4-10.

75. Mendelow AD, Gregson BA, Rowan EN, Murray GD, Gholkar A, Mitchell PM. Early surgery versus initial conservative treatment in patients with spontaneous supratentorial lobar intracerebral haematomas (STICH II): a randomised trial. *Lancet*. 2013;382(9890):397-408.

76. Luostarinen T, Satopää J, Skrifvars MB, et al. Early surgery for superficial supratentorial spontaneous intracerebral hemorrhage: a Finnish Intensive Care Consortium study. *Acta Neurochir (Wien)*. 2020;162(12):3153-3160.

77. Xu X, Zheng Y, Chen X, Li F, Zhang H, Ge X. Comparison of endoscopic evacuation, stereotactic aspiration and craniotomy for the treatment of supratentorial hypertensive intracerebral haemorrhage: study protocol for a randomised controlled trial. *Trials*. 2017;18(1):296.

78. Sprigg N, Flaherty K, Appleton JP, et al. Tranexamic acid to improve functional status in adults with spontaneous intracerebral haemorrhage: the TICH-2 RCT. *Health Technol Assess*. 2019;23(35):1-48.

79. Sprigg N, Flaherty K, Appleton JP, et al. Tranexamic acid for hyperacute primary IntraCerebral Haemorrhage (TICH-2): an international randomised, placebo-controlled, phase 3 superiority trial. *Lancet*. 2018;391(10135):2107-2115.

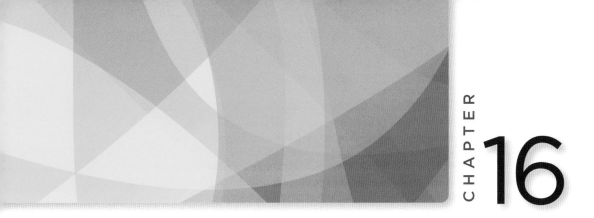

CHAPTER 16

Headache

Steven A. Godwin

Daniel Eraso

THE CLINICAL CHALLENGE

Headache is the fifth most common presenting symptom to the emergency department (ED), which recorded over 4 million visits in 2014, accounting for 3% of ED encounters.[1] Most headaches stem from a benign etiology, and most symptoms are self-limiting, requiring minimal workup and treatment. Such headaches are classified as primary headaches, in contrast to secondary headaches, which are manifestations of underlying disease. The clinical challenge lies in rapidly diagnosing and treating the small minority of deadly secondary headaches masquerading as benign headaches. A focused history and physical, placing emphasis on a thorough neurologic exam, can narrow the differential diagnosis and guide the subsequent workup and treatment (Table 16.1).

TABLE 16.1	Primary versus Secondary Headache
Primary	Migraine
	Tension-type
	Cluster
Secondary	*Vascular:* subarachnoid hemorrhage, giant cell arteritis, cervical artery dissection, cerebral venous thrombosis, reversible cerebral vasospasm syndrome, pituitary apoplexy
	Nonvascular: idiopathic intracranial hypertension, spontaneous intracranial hypotension
	Toxic: carbon monoxide, phosphodiesterase inhibitor induced
	Infectious: bacterial meningitis, viral encephalitis
	Extracranial: acute angle closure glaucoma, sinusitis, temporomandibular joint (TMJ) dysfunction

Adapted from ICHD-3 Headache Classification Committee of the International Headache Society (IHS) The International Classification of Headache Disorders, 3rd edition. *Cephalalgia.* 2018;38(1):1-211.

PATHOPHYSIOLOGY

The parenchyma of the brain lacks pain receptors, and thus the sensation of headache is thought to arise from activation of sensory fibers of the meninges and large blood vessels. Activation of these sensory pathways is poorly localized and can extend to cervical and facial foci. The pathophysiology of migraine headaches has been more closely studied, and symptom activation involves the complex interaction of genetic predisposition, environmental factors, metabolic abnormalities, and hormonal influences, resulting in a cascade of neuropeptide modulation and subsequent central nervous system (CNS) activation.[2] Exact mechanisms for the underlying pathophysiology of migraine have shifted over time, but current theories propose a complex interplay of neurovascular activation and neurochemical feedback loops involving serotonin, calcitonin gene-related peptide (CGRP), and other inflammatory neuropeptides involving the trigeminal nerve, the trigeminal cervical complex in the brainstem, and multiple pathways through the midbrain and cortex. Serotonin functions as both a vasoconstrictor and an inhibitor of CGRP release, whereas CGRP is implicated in vasodilation and the sterile inflammation of the meninges.

PREHOSPITAL CONCERNS

Headache management often starts in the prehospital setting, with approximately 1% of emergency medical service (EMS) transports for a primary complaint of headache; however, treatment is rarely initiated. In one study, most patients transported via EMS for headache did not receive analgesic medications (>90%), and of those who did receive medication the most common analgesic was an opioid, which is incongruent with established guidelines for headache management.[3] Acetaminophen, nonsteroidal anti-inflammatory drugs (NSAIDs), triptans, or antidopaminergic medications may have a role in early symptom control.

EMS systems also play a critical role in destination decisions. For suspicion of headache associated with cerebrovascular accidents, use of a standardized stroke scale such as the Cincinnati Prehospital Stroke Scale should be routinely utilized, and patients with abnormal findings should be transferred to a stroke capable facility. Similarly, headaches secondary to traumatic injury with changes in Glasgow Coma Scale (GCS), pupillary size, or vital sign abnormalities should be transferred to appropriately capable trauma centers, because decreases in mortality have been demonstrated with evaluation at major trauma centers that have neurosurgical capabilities.

APPROACH/THE FOCUSED EXAM

Stabilization

The approach to the patient with headache will be driven largely by the history and physical, which in turn forms the differential diagnosis. Some of these patients will present in extremis, and rapid stabilization and resuscitation may be required. The patient that presents altered and vomiting, with difficulty protecting their airway may require endotracheal intubation to facilitate a safe workup and treatment. The underlying etiologies associated with the initial presentation of headache are diverse and may require both simple and complex stabilization strategies. Addressing the respiratory status and correcting hypoxemia as needed, optimizing hypotension and ensuring adequate cerebral perfusion pressure, or identifying and correcting hypoglycemia or other metabolic derangements all fall within the initial resuscitative pathway.

History

The history may identify red flag findings suggestive of a life-threatening cause of a headache, see **Table 16.2**.

A patient's specific headache history can provide useful information in the workup of undifferentiated headache. Patients may report a prior history of headache similar in character, location, duration, and/or severity.

Clarifying the circumstances surrounding the onset of headache is critical. Patient presentations of severe headaches with acute onset, within seconds to minutes, are considered potentially

TABLE 16.2	**Red Flags by History Onset: Sudden or "Thunderclap," Associated with Trauma**

- Triggers: exertional, positional, cough, coitus
- Quality: change in quality, frequency, or pattern from prior headache
- Radiation to neck
- Severity: "worst headache of life"
- Medications: anticoagulants
- Associated conditions: previous or current malignancy, immunosuppressed state, pregnant, history of connective tissue disorders
- Age > 50

more ominous owing to their "thunderclap" nature and their association with subarachnoid hemorrhage (SAH). Frequently, patients will remember exactly what they were doing at the time of onset. Given the prevalence and high risk of morbidity and mortality, the preponderance of studies involving acute headache have focused mostly on SAH. A headache that develops over hours to days is less concerning for SAH. Other considerations for so-called thunderclap headache presentation include other intracranial hemorrhage, cerebral venous thrombosis (CVT), reversible cerebral vasoconstriction syndrome (RCVS), cervical artery dissection (CeAD), or, less commonly, spontaneous intracranial hypotension (SIH); see **Table 16.3**.

The headache location can likewise narrow the differential. Unilateral headaches with associated phonophobia or photophobia are suggestive of migraine headache, whereas discrete focal head pain can indicate giant cell arteritis (GCA), temporomandibular joint dysfunction, occipital neuralgia, or sinus headaches.

Understanding the duration of the pain can also assist in identifying a diagnosis. Those patients with persistent cephalgia over weeks to months are unlikely to represent an acute process but may have equally concerning underlying pathology, such as chronic subdural hemorrhage, or malignancy.

Clarifying exacerbating or alleviating factors can be helpful. Stress, sleep disorders, food, alcohol, hormonal changes, visual and olfactory stimuli, weather changes, heat, and sexual activity may all be triggers for acute migraines. Positional triggers for the onset of headache may indicate the presence of intracranial hypertension or intracranial hypotension. Geographical headaches can alert the clinician to inquire further to unmask environmental concerns for carbon monoxide poisoning. Visual changes or eye pain can be associated with GCA or acute angle closure glaucoma.

Physical Exam

Vital Signs

The physical exam starts with the evaluation of vital signs, with particular attention paid to temperature and blood pressure. Headaches can develop as a nonspecific manifestation of an acute viral illness with associated fever; however, intracranial infections such as meningitis, encephalitis, and

TABLE 16.3	**Dangerous Causes of Secondary Headache**

- **Thunderclap (sudden severe onset) presentation**
  - Subarachnoid hemorrhage
  - Intracerebral hemorrhage
  - Cerebral venous sinus thrombosis
  - Cervical artery dissection
  - Pituitary apoplexy
  - Spontaneous intracranial hypotension
  - Reversible cerebral vasoconstriction syndrome
- **Giant cell arteritis**
- **Meningitis**
- **Acute angle closure glaucoma**
- **Carbon monoxide toxicity**
- **Preeclampsia**

intracranial abscess must be considered. Posterior reversible encephalopathy syndrome, intracranial hemorrhage, stroke, herniation, and preeclampsia may all present with hypertension. Hypoxia or anemia may also manifest with tachycardia and headache.

Neurologic Exam

The complete neurologic exam is outlined in **Chapter 2: The Neurologic Examination**. The focused neurologic exam in a patient with a complaint of headache should include a mental status exam, motor and sensory exams, gait evaluation, and cranial nerve exam. Nonfocal changes in mental status can be seen in infections or metabolic derangements. Focal neurologic deficits are associated with intracranial pathology such as stroke, intracranial hemorrhage, or more benign etiologies such as hemiplegic migraine. Cranial nerves II to VIII are particularly pertinent to the patient presenting with headache. Evaluation of cranial nerve II includes evaluation of visual fields to localize lesions in the optic tract versus cortical lesions. Fundoscopy is performed to assess for signs of papilledema. Abnormalities in extraocular movements can indicate space occupying lesions that affect cranial nerves III, IV, or VI. Aneurysmal compression of the superficial parasympathetic fibers of cranial nerve III from the posterior communicating artery can cause pupillary dilation manifesting as anisocoria.

Head and Neck

Headache associated with stiff or painful neck movements can reflect inflammation of the meninges and can be seen in meningitis and SAH. Tenderness to palpation along the temporal arteries is concerning for GCA. Palpation lateral to the occipital protuberance may reproduce pain originating from occipital neuralgia. Frontal or maxillary tenderness may represent sinusitis. Acute otitis media can cause headache, and mastoid tenderness is commonly seen in mastoiditis.

Eye

Visual acuity should be checked and documented in all patients presenting with headache and vision changes. In patients presenting with a history consistent with acute angle glaucoma, intraocular pressures should be measured. A fundoscopic exam should be performed to evaluate for papilledema secondary to increased intracranial pressure (ICP), as seen in idiopathic intracranial hypertension (IIH), intracranial hemorrhage, or mass lesions. Alternately, bedside ultrasound has been used to measure optic sheath diameter, with measurements >5 mm concerning for elevated ICP (**Figure 16.1**).

PRIMARY HEADACHES

Primary headaches are biologic disorders of the brain that result in activation of the cerebrovascular pain pathways and include migraine, tension-type, and cluster headache. In contrast, secondary headaches result from underlying medical conditions such as vascular, infectious, anatomic, or metabolic abnormalities.

Migraine headache is the most common headache presentation seen in the ED. More common in females, migraine headaches usually peak in middle age, and then gradually decline in prevalence. The typical presentation is a moderate to severe headache that is unilateral, pulsatile, and often associated with nausea, vomiting, photophobia, and/or phonophobia.[4] A patient may be able to identify migraine triggers such as stress, sleep deprivations, association with menstrual cycle, caffeine, and others. Migraine with aura is a headache preceded by distinct neurologic symptoms that are fully reversible usually after only a few minutes. Typical aura symptoms include visual and/or sensory changes but can also include motor dysfunction or speech abnormalities.

Tension-type headaches account for most headaches in the general population, although symptoms are usually mild enough for home treatment without further workup. Various studies approximate 50% lifetime prevalence, with women affected more than men. Tension-type headaches are usually mild to moderate, bilateral, pressure or bandlike tightening that is not pulsatile or throbbing, and without nausea, vomiting, photophobia, or phonophobia. Tension-type headaches are not typically exacerbated by exertion, whereas migraine headaches usually exhibit this association.

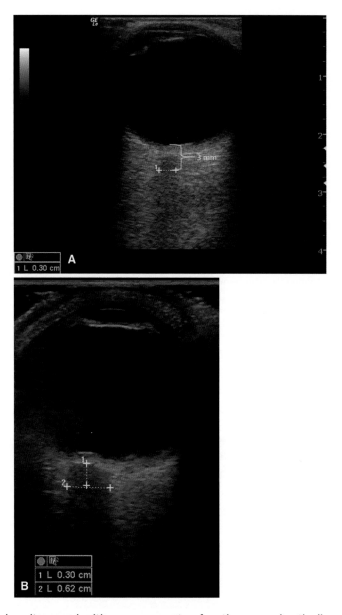

Figure 16.1: Ocular ultrasound with measurements of optic nerve sheath diameter (ONSD) at 3 mm posterior to retina. A, Normal measurement of 3 mm. B, Abnormal measurement of 6.2 mm. Images courtesy of Thomas Cook, MD; and from McAdams BH, Ellis KB. Does this thyroid nodule need to be biopsied? In: Bornemann P, ed. *Ultrasound for Primary Care.* Wolters Kluwer; 2021. Figure 3.5.

Trigeminal autonomic cephalagias are a group of headache disorders that include cluster headaches, paroxysmal hemicrania, and hemicrania continua. Cluster headaches are typically severe, acute in onset, unilateral sharp or stabbing periorbital pain, with associated ipsilateral autonomic symptoms, including lacrimation, ptosis, miosis, eyelid edema, nasal congestion, and/or facial/forehead anhidrosis. These headaches are more common in males in the 20- to 40-year age range and usually last for 15 minutes to 3 hours. They typically recur over weeks to months over a defined period of time. Headaches in paroxysmal hemicrania are similar in character to cluster headaches but shorter in duration. Hemicrania continua is a similar headache that lasts for >3 months. Both paroxysmal hemicrania and hemicrania continua typically respond to indomethacin.

Other primary headache disorders include headaches associated with cough, exercise, sexual activity, cold stimulus ("brain freeze"), as well as primary stabbing headaches, nummular headaches, hypnic headaches, and new daily persistent headaches.

MANAGEMENT

Once a presumptive primary headache disorder is diagnosed and dangerous secondary causes are ruled out, treatment should be administered targeting pain and associated symptoms (**Table 16.4**).[5] As most primary headaches presenting to the ED are accompanied by nausea and vomiting with decreased oral intake, IV fluid replacement is often indicated. Antidopaminergic medications such as prochlorperazine, promethazine, droperidol, and haloperidol are thought to treat the underlying etiology of migraine headaches and have additional antiemetic and sedative effects. Extrapyramidal side effects of antidopaminergic medications, including akathisia and dystonia, occur at rates 10% to 45%, thus coadministration of diphenhydramine is recommended. All of these medications are known to prolong the QT interval, although the clinical significance is less clear. Metoclopramide also has antidopaminergic properties in addition to serotonin reception antagonism.

NSAID medications are frequently given in conjunction with antidopaminergic medications, commonly ketorolac. Acetaminophen can be administered by mouth or intravenously. Sumatriptan or dihydroergotamine can be administered either parenterally or intranasally. Corticosteroids such as dexamethasone have a greater effect on preventing headache recurrence than on the acute management of symptoms and should be considered an adjunct to standard therapy. Regional anesthesia may be useful, such as in sphenopalatine nerve blocks for migraine or occipital nerve blocks for occipital neuralgia.

In patients presenting to the ED with severe migraine, a reasonable initial approach could include intravenous NSAIDs (eg, ketorolac), an antidopaminergic antiemetic (eg, metoclopramide, prochlorperazine), diphenhydramine, and intravenous hydration. An alternate approach administering subcutaneous sumatriptan would circumvent the resource requirements of intravenous access. In view of the ongoing opioid crisis of misuse and abuse, multiple national and

TABLE 16.4	Primary Headache Treatment		
Severity	**Medication**	**Typical Dose**	**Comments**
Mild-Moderate	Acetaminophen	650-1000 mg PO	Caution in liver disease
	Aspirin	900-1000 mg PO	
	Ibuprofen	400-600 mg PO	Caution in renal or peptic ulcer disease
	Naproxen	500-750 mg PO	Caution in renal or peptic ulcer disease
Moderate-Severe	Prochlorperazine	10 mg IV	Potential akathisia
	Metoclopramide	10 mg IV	Potential akathisia
	Sumatriptan (or other triptan)	50-100 mg PO 4-6 mg SQ 10-20 mg IN	Multiple contraindications
	Ketorolac	15 mg IV/IM	Caution in renal or peptic ulcer disease
	Droperidol	2.5-5.0 mg IV	Theoretical risk of QT prolongation
	Dihydroergotamine	2 mg IN 1 mg IV/IM/SQ	Avoid with CYP3A4 inhibitors
Refractory	Ketamine	0.1-0.3 mg/kg	Administer as slow push
Adjunctive	Dexamethasone	4-10 mg IV	Reduces headache recurrence

international organizing committees recommend against the use of opioid medications in favor of the above nonopioid options.[6]

SUBARACHNOID HEMORRHAGE

EPIDEMIOLOGY

With potential mortality >50%, SAH is a condition that requires rapid diagnosis, and even when managed appropriately, up to 50% of survivors have long-term neurologic deficits.[7] SAH accounts for approximately 1% of all patients presenting to the ED with headache; however, this number increases to upward of 10% in those patients presenting with acute onset "thunderclap" headaches.[10] Ruptured aneurysm is the underlying etiology of nontraumatic SAH in 70% to 80% of cases, and other causes include arteriovenous malformations, angiomas, and neoplasm. Risk factors include age (predominantly 40-60 years old), hypertension, smoking history, and sympathomimetic drug use, as well as family histories of aneurysm in first-degree relatives, autosomal dominant polycystic kidney disease, Marfan syndrome, and Ehlers-Danlos syndrome.

PRESENTATION

The classic presentation of SAH is a sudden onset "thunderclap" headache that is often described as the worst in the patient's life and that peaks within seconds or minutes, although a subset of patients may present with worsening headache over an hour. Patients complaining of a headache that is historically different in quality or severity should also prompt investigation of SAH. The headache is often exertional or associated with Valsalva, micturition, or sexual intercourse. Other commonly associated symptoms include nausea and vomiting, neck stiffness, meningismus, focal neurologic deficits, or seizure.

DIAGNOSTICS

The diagnostic modalities for SAH have changed in recent times. Much of the diagnosis relies on risk stratification based on elements of the history and physical. The Ottawa SAH rule has been proposed to rule out SAH and involves certain aspects of the history and physical, including age, neck pain or stiffness, loss of consciousness, exertional component, thunderclap onset, and limited neck flexion on exam.[8] There are a number of specific inclusion and exclusion criteria for utilization. This clinical decision aid has been validated with 100% sensitivity but has a relatively poor specificity, which may result in unnecessary additional testing (**Table 16.5**).

The traditional workup of SAH has included noncontrast head CT (**Figure 16.2**), lumbar puncture (LP), MRI, or angiography. Historically, a negative head CT with a subsequent negative LP was sufficient to rule out SAH. A noncontrast head CT is recommended as the initial diagnostic modality of choice. A negative noncontrast head CT, if obtained within 6 hours of headache onset, is considered sufficient to rule out SAH in the presence of a normal neurologic exam. This is supported by multiple studies, as well as the ACEP Policy on acute headaches. These studies were

TABLE 16.5 Ottawa Subarachnoid Hemorrhage (SAH) Criteria[a]

Symptoms of neck pain or stiffness
Age ≥40 years old
Witnessed loss of consciousness
Onset during exertion
Thunderclap headache
Limited neck flexion on exam

[a]*Inclusion criteria*: alert patients, ≥15 years old, new severe atraumatic headache, maximal intensity within 1 hour. *Exclusion criteria:* patients with new neurologic deficits, prior aneurysm, prior SAH, known brain tumor, history of similar headaches (≥3 episodes for ≥6 months).
SAH can be ruled out if all criteria are negative.

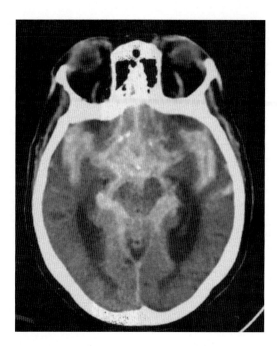

Figure 16.2: Subarachnoid hemorrhage. CT scan at the level of the suprasellar and ambient cisterns shows that the normally low-density *(black)* basal cisterns have been filled with high-density *(white)* material consistent with subarachnoid hemorrhage. From Petrovic B. Brain imaging. In: Farrell TA, ed. *Radiology 101.* 5th ed. Wolters Kluwer; 2020:268-293. Figure 7.11.

predicated on multiple criteria, including the use of newer generation CT scanners, interpretation by neuroradiologists queried for SAH rule out, in patients with a hematocrit >30% and a normal neurologic exam.

In patients presenting 6 hours after the onset of headache, two options for diagnostic pathways are generally recommended. Historically, the first line evaluation has included a nondiagnostic CT head and subsequent LP. On LP, cerebrospinal fluid (CSF) with xanthochromia is diagnostic of SAH. Xanthochromia can last up to 2 weeks but may take up to 12 hours to develop from the degradation of red blood cells (RBCs). The presence of RBCs in CSF can be complicated by a traumatic LP. There are no exact cutoff values to distinguish true SAH from traumatic LP; however, a threshold in tube 4 of <100 RBCs may effectively exclude SAH, and values >10,000 are highly suggestive of SAH.[9] In addition to traumatic taps, other disadvantages of performing LPs include the time-consuming nature of the procedure, difficulties in body habitus, potential bleeding, infection, and post-LP headaches. Despite these drawbacks, the potential benefit in performing an LP lies in evaluating alternate diagnoses. Elevated opening pressures may be consistent with IIH, and CSF studies may demonstrate findings consistent with meningitis or encephalitis.

An alternate diagnostic approach involves CT angiography (CTA) of cerebral vasculature, and current American College of Emergency Physicians (ACEP) clinical policy supports the use of CTA in carefully selected populations. CTA can reliably identify aneurysms as small as 3 mm, as well as diagnose other conditions, including (CeAD).[10] Up to 5% of the general population harbor an incidental aneurysm, and thus the concern with obtaining a CTA for all patients involves the unnecessary downstream evaluation, including neurosurgical consultation with potential intervention in an otherwise healthy patient.

MRI and MRA are additional reliable diagnostic modalities; however, the increased time and resource utilization involved has generally precluded widespread adoption in the ED. MRI is more sensitive in diagnosing alternate conditions such as pituitary apoplexy, neoplasm, acute infarction, or multiple sclerosis.

Multiple factors influence the diagnostic modality of choice, including risk stratification, body habitus, and even patient preference. An informed discussion with the patient regarding relative advantages and disadvantages for each test is useful, with an understanding that "ruling out" SAH after a negative head CT performed within 6 hours' onset carries approximately 0% to 1% miss rate. Each diagnostic modality carries differing risks and benefits.

TREATMENT

Treatment of SAH begins with resuscitation and stabilization. ICP management is paramount, and interventions are focused on prevention of ICP elevations. Patients with a Hunt and Hess grade 3 or higher (**Table 16.6**) are at high risk for clinical decompensation and respiratory depression, often necessitating definitive airway management. Analgesic medications should be administered to prevent pain-associated elevations in blood pressure, as well as antiemetics to prevent transient spikes in ICP associated with emesis and retching.

In order to maintain cerebral perfusion, we recommend that the systolic blood pressure be maintained between 140 and 160 mm Hg. Titratable vasoactive medications such as labetalol or nicardipine are helpful and, whenever possible, should be titrated according to intra-arterial blood pressure monitoring.[11] Simple maneuvers such as elevating the head of bed and avoiding tight-fitting cervical immobilization collars allow for unimpeded venous drainage. Reversal of coagulopathies is indicated and should be undertaken immediately. Assay guided reversal (ie, thromboelastogram [TEG]) may provide additional benefit in some cases through targeted transfusion strategies.[12] For identified aneurysmal SAH, definitive intervention involves neurosurgical clipping or endovascular coiling, with coiling preferred when available. Nimodipine 60 mg PO every 4 hours given within 96 hours, traditionally thought to prevent vasospasm, has been shown to improve outcomes.[13] Admission to an intensive care unit for monitoring is recommended.

OTHER IMPORTANT ETIOLOGIES

Reversible Cerebral Vasoconstriction Syndrome

Reversible cerebral vasoconstriction syndrome (RCVS) is a thunderclap headache variant, often with specific triggers, that can repeat multiple times over a 1- to 2-week period. It is diagnostically characterized by alternating areas of cerebral vasoconstriction and vasodilation. Symptoms usually resolve in <1 month but can last up to 3 months. There is a slight female predilection, with average presentation in the fifth decade of life, whereas males present earlier in the third decade. The exact pathophysiology is unclear; however, the abnormality in cerebral arterial tone is likely in response to sympathetic activation, as indicated by association with exertion, sexual activity, exercise, Valsalva, or emotions. Despite this association, there appears to be a temporal disconnect between symptom manifestation and imaging verified vasoconstriction. Endothelial dysfunction may also play a role.[14]

The typical presentation of RCVS mirrors that of SAH, with severe thunderclap headache with maximal onset within minutes. Headache is more commonly bilateral and often the only presenting symptom but can be associated with nausea, vomiting, photophobia, phonophobia, focal neurologic deficits, or seizure.

The diagnostic process will parallel SAH, with an initial noncontrast CT. The gold standard for diagnosis of RCVS is digital subtraction angiography (DSA); however, it is an invasive test with

TABLE 16.6	**Hunt Hess**	
Grade	Symptoms	Mortality (%)
1	Asymptomatic; or minimal headache, slight nuchal rigidity	<5
2	Moderate to severe headache, nuchal rigidity, no neurologic deficit other than isolated cranial nerve palsy	<10
3	Drowsy, minimal neurologic deficit	15-20
4	Stuporous, moderate to severe hemiparesis, possible decerebrate rigidity	30-40
5	Deep coma, decerebrate rigidity, moribund appearance	50-100

complications that include arterial dissection. A CTA is more likely to be ordered in the ED, but the CTA is ~80% sensitive in diagnosing vasospasm as compared with DSA.[15] Further complicating the diagnosis, vasoconstriction may not manifest at the time of symptom onset, and diagnosis via imaging can thus be problematic. Diagnosis is often clinical, with recurrent thunderclap headache almost pathognomonic for RCVS.

Emergent complications of RCVS include a concomitant reversible posterior leukoencephalopathy syndrome (RPLS) and ischemic or hemorrhagic stroke. Initial CT findings of vasogenic brain edema similar to RPLS may represent differing manifestations of endothelial dysfunction and may be responsive to antihypertensives as indicated. The most common hemorrhagic complication is nonaneurysmal convexity SAH, whereas intraparenchymal and subdural hemorrhage are less common. Ischemic stroke is secondary to vasoconstriction and usually occurs in watershed areas.

Fortunately, most patients recover fully from RCVS without recurrent episodes. Treatment is based largely on symptomatic control and risk factor reduction. Pain can be debilitating and may require multimodal pain control, including narcotic medications as needed. Patients should be counseled to avoid activities that may increase sympathetic activation, as well as medications that are inciting or vasoactive. Treatment options targeting vasospasm, including nimodipine, verapamil, or magnesium sulfate, may reduce the severity of symptoms, but recommendations are based on expert opinion.[15]

Spontaneous Intracranial Hypotension

Spontaneous intracranial hypotension (SIH) is a low-pressure headache associated with a reduction in CSF production or flow. It is clinically similar to a dural puncture (post-LP) headache. Decreased CSF pressure or volume causes increased traction on and activation of pain-sensitive structures in the meninges during orthostatic changes. The SIH headache is classically elicited by postural changes and often throbbing, severe, and occasionally thunderclap; is associated with nausea, vomiting, and neck pain; and can have a range of accompanying neurologic symptoms. Headache resolution is often rapid once recumbent. It affects women more than men, peaking in the fourth decade of life, but is present in a wide range of ages. The pathophysiology was initially thought to arise from low CSF pressure; however, alternate theories describe low CSF volume with subsequent compliance changes of the CSF compartment that explain decreased cushioning of the brain during postural changes.[16] CSF leakage occurs via dural disruption, through either dural tears or fistula. Tears commonly arise from arachnoid diverticula of nerve root sleeves in the thoracic or lumbar spine.[17]

Diagnosis of SIH requires evidence of low CSF pressure or volume, usually via MRI brain with gadolinium contrast as well as MRI of the spine. Typical findings include sagging of brain (effacement of basal cisterns, flattening of the pons, descent of cerebellar tonsils), subdural fluid collections, diffuse meningeal enhancement, or dilated cervical epidural veins.[18] Direct measurement of CSF pressure via LP is not a diagnostic requirement. If LP is performed, a pressure <60 mm water supports the diagnosis.

Treatment of SIH is initially conservative, with bed rest, caffeine (300 mg oral or 500 mg IV), hydration, and nonnarcotic analgesics as needed. For intractable symptoms, an autologous epidural blood patch may be performed; however, multiple patches may have to be performed to control symptoms. For refractory symptoms, advanced imaging, commonly CT myelography, is employed to identify the exact source of CSF leak. A targeted blood patch may be attempted at the level of CSF leak; alternately, surgical revision may be required.

Cervical Artery Dissection

Cervical artery dissections (CeAD) involving the internal carotid or vertebral arteries are a major cause of stroke in patients younger than 50.[19]

Risk factors for CeAD include connective tissue disorders, including Marfan and Ehlers Danlos, along with other inherited arteriopathies, infection, and trauma. Minor trauma, including whiplash or chiropractic manipulation of the neck, can cause CeAD.

Similar to aortic dissections, the underlying pathophysiology of CeAD involves an intimal tear with subsequent hemorrhage and hematoma formation. Subsequent thromboembolic events result in acute ischemic strokes.

Common presentations of carotid dissections include severe unilateral throbbing headache and neck pain, with a partial ipsilateral Horner syndrome (miosis and ptosis, without anhidrosis), and contralateral sensorimotor neurologic deficits. Vertebral artery dissections can present with a unilateral posterior headache with cerebellar findings including ataxia, gait abnormalities, or vertigo. Intracranial dissections are often present as SAH.

Diagnostic workups start with a noncontrast head CT, which is often normal. Vessel imaging, whether CTA, MRA, or traditional angiography, is employed to identify arterial abnormalities. Ultrasound is a rapid bedside tool that can provide immediate information with reasonable specificity; however, its suboptimal sensitivity cannot rule out the disease process.

Treatment for CeAD has traditionally targeted prevention of ischemic complications with the use of anticoagulation or antiplatelet therapy; however, recent trials have not shown any advantage of anticoagulation over antiplatelets.[20] New research is showing promise of endovascular therapy over intravenous thrombolysis for acute ischemic complications of large vessel occlusions with perfusion delay.[21]

Cerebral Venous Thrombosis

Cerebral venous or sinus thrombosis (CVT) is an atypical form of stroke, accounting for <1% of all cerebrovascular accidents, approximately 1.5 cases per 100,000. Typically, patients with CVT are younger than other stroke patients, but the condition has multiple risk factors, including female gender, obesity, oral contraceptive use, pregnancy and puerperium, cancer, neurotrauma, infections, and inherited thrombophilias such as factor V Leiden, or deficiencies in antithrombin III, protein C, or protein S. Prompt treatment is necessary to minimize long-term neurologic disability.

The clinical presentation of CVT is highly variable, largely secondary to the various venous structures at risk for thrombosis; however, headache is the common denominator and is reported in > 90% of cases.[22] Symptoms typically worsen over an extended time frame of days but can also present as thunderclap at onset. Headaches are usually diffuse and associated with other symptoms. Based on additional symptoms, patient presentations can be grouped into phenotypic categories: thrombosis of the superficial venous system with intraparenchymal extension may present with focal neurologic deficits mimicking typical CVA and may be associated with subsequent seizure activity, whereas sagittal sinus thrombosis may precipitate bilateral sensorimotor deficits. Thrombosis of deep central veins with subsequent thalamic or basal ganglia infarcts may present encephalopathic or comatose. Thrombosis of the cavernous sinus may present with predominantly ocular symptoms, including orbital pain, extraocular movement abnormalities, or proptosis. Transverse sinus thrombosis can present with relatively isolated intracranial hypertension.[23] (See **Chapter 1, Figure 1.11**.)

Basic labs (complete blood count [CBC], chemistry, partial thromboplastin time [PTT], international normalized ratio [INR]) can be drawn to evaluate for infection and clotting disorders. Small studies have suggested a negative d-dimer may exclude CVT in low-risk patients. However, prolonged duration of symptoms has been associated with falsely negative d-dimer tests, so caution is advised in these patients.[24]

Definitive diagnosis of CVT involves neuroimaging. Noncontrast CT is commonplace in the initial evaluation of concerning headaches and can identify CVT in a small subset of patients. The addition of CT venography (CTV) has 95% sensitivity as compared to DSA, which has historically been considered the diagnostic gold standard. CT/CTV is readily available in most EDs and is a rapid diagnostic procedure; the benefits generally outweigh the associated risks of radiation and contrast exposure. The classic finding on CTV is the "empty delta sign," or a contrast-outlined triangular filling defect of the superior sagittal sinus (**Figure 16.3**). MRI/MR venography provides added resolution with the disadvantage of time required for scan. Cerebral angiography remains a more invasive option for cases with inconclusive CTV or MRV scans.

Anticoagulation is the primary treatment for CVT to prevent further clot propagation. Current recommendations favor low molecular weight heparin, even in patients with concomitant intracerebral hemorrhage.[25] Unfractionated heparin is preferred when surgical intervention may be required. While direct oral anticoagulants have gained favor in the treatment of other thromboembolic disorders, there is currently insufficient evidence for use in CVT. In patients with worsening clinical conditions despite anticoagulation, or with contraindications to anticoagulation,

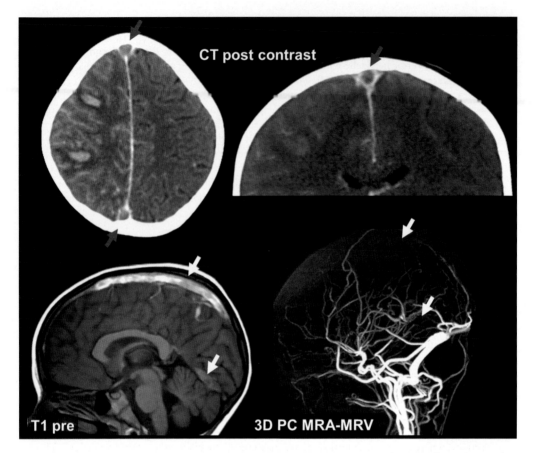

Figure 16.3: "Empty delta sign": CT head with contrast demonstrates a filling defect surrounded by enhancing dura in the sagittal sinus indicative of thrombosis. White arrows demonstrate sagittal sinus thrombosis on CT and red arrows demonstrate sagittal sinus thrombosis on MRI. From Klein J, Vinson EN, Brant WE, Helms CA. *Brant and Helms' Fundamentals of Diagnostic Radiology.* 5th ed. Wolters Kluwer; 2019. Figure 4.30.

endovascular thrombectomy or thrombolysis are options at capable centers. High-quality data is also lacking on definitive outcomes. Antiepileptic medication should be initiated to prevent recurrent seizures, but prophylaxis is not recommended. With no high-quality data available, antiepileptic drug choice will be individualized and institution dependent. For presumptive infectious etiologies of CVT, antibiotics targeting the underlying infection should be initiated, in conjunction with surgical evacuation of infection as indicated. Consultation with neurosurgery and neuro-intensive care should occur, and these patients should be admitted to a stroke unit when feasible.

Idiopathic Intracranial Hypertension

Idiopathic intracranial hypertension (IIH) is a disorder of abnormally elevated ICPs. Most cases involve women and are also associated with obesity or rapid weight gain.[26] Other comorbid conditions, including polycystic ovarian syndrome, and sleep apnea increase the risk of IIH, but this may stem from underlying obesity associated with both disease states. The prevalence has been reported at approximately 2 cases per 100,000, but incidence increases to 12 to 20 per 100,000 in the obese female population. The pathophysiology is not well defined, with 3 possible models suggested: the traditional model of CSF overproduction has not been supported with imaging studies, whereas CSF outflow obstruction across the arachnoid membrane or venous hypertension secondary to sinus stenosis seem more plausible explanations.[27]

Similar to CVT, the clinical presentation of IIH is highly variable. Headache is the primary complaint in most cases and is often described as throbbing, holocephalic, severe, and positional with exacerbation on bending over or while recumbent. The pain will awaken a patient from sleep. However, headache characterization is highly variable. Associated symptoms include visual changes, often transient and recurring visual field defects, likely caused by optic nerve ischemia. Diplopia is common secondary to cranial nerve palsies, which is often called a false localizing sign. Nausea, vomiting, and pulsatile tinnitus are also common. Pulsatile tinnitus may originate from transverse sinus thrombosis and is less prevalent in other headache disorders.

Although elements from the history and physical may strongly suggest elevated ICPs, the diagnosis of IIH is often one of exclusion. Papilledema is a critical feature of IIH and can be identified on fundoscopy, ultrasound, or CT. Despite the high frequency of associated papilledema, IIH can be diagnosed without papilledema in the presence of a sixth nerve palsy or with specific findings on imaging such as papilledema, subarachnoid outpouchings, or sinus stenosis. Advanced neuroimaging is required to rule out other etiologies such as intracerebral hemorrhage or mass, with CT or MR venography employed to rule out sinus thrombosis. In the absence of space occupying lesions, a LP is performed in the lateral decubitus position, with opening pressures >250 mm CSF in adults required for the diagnosis. CSF studies should also rule out infectious etiologies of symptoms.

Treatment of IIH is targeted at both immediate resolution of symptoms and prevention of long-term complications of disease progression. The acute management of symptoms begins with nonopioid analgesics, such as acetaminophen or ketorolac. The LP can be both diagnostic and therapeutic, with frequent resolution of symptoms after CSF drainage to normal pressures. For rapidly progressive vision changes or loss, more invasive measures may be taken to preserve vision function. Placement of a CSF shunt (most commonly, a ventriculoperitoneal shunt) or optic nerve sheath fenestration are interventions made in consultation with neurosurgery or ophthalmology, respectively.[28] Long-term management of symptoms and progression of disease involve weight loss and medications such as acetazolamide 500 mg twice daily, which is considered safe and effective. Weight loss can reduce both the frequency and the severity of symptoms. Therefore, lifestyle modifications (nonsurgical) and surgical bariatric management are both effective options.

Giant Cell Arteritis

Giant cell arteritis is an inflammatory reaction within small- and medium-sized arteries that can occur throughout the body. Involvement of the temporal artery typically presents with headache plus visual changes, fevers, jaw claudication, or proximal muscle weakness (there exists significant overlap with polymyalgia rheumatica). GCA is exceedingly rare before the age of 50 and most common over 70 years, because incidence increases with age. Women are affected more than men.[29]

Among the traditional diagnostic criteria are age >50 years, new onset headache or head pain, temporal artery abnormalities, including tenderness, nodularity, or decreased pulsatility, ESR > 50, and an abnormal temporal artery biopsy. Revised criteria and algorithms include visual disturbances, jaw claudication, polymyalgia rheumatica, and unexplained fever.

Systemic glucocorticoids are the mainstay of treatment. Consensus opinion recommends daily oral glucocorticoids (eg, prednisone 0.5-1 mg/kg, maximum dose 60 mg) for uncomplicated GCA, whereas some recommend intravenous doses for GCA with threatened vision loss (methylprednisolone 500-1000 mg pulse for 3 days, followed by oral regimen).[30] Treatment should begin when the diagnosis of GCA is suspected, rather than waiting for biopsy confirmed disease. Rapid follow-up with ophthalmology and rheumatology are indicated.

Pediatric Issues

Fortunately for both patients and clinicians, most headaches evaluated in the ED are primary in nature, and the same approach and management apply to pediatric patients. If symptoms start at a young age, it is challenging for patients to relay "typical" headache findings, and some patients are less able to clearly elucidate headache quality or triggers. Information obtained from parents can be useful, including the presence of a family history of migraines or of aneurysm. A vaccination history can also be useful if suspicious of an infectious etiology. A thorough social history can reveal multiple stressors that exacerbate headache severity and frequency.[31]

The same red flags of dangerous secondary headache seen in adults also apply to pediatric patients and include sudden severe onset, fevers, nuchal rigidity, focal neurologic abnormalities, or new onset seizure.[32] Historically, the presence of occipital headaches was more concerning for intracranial pathology. This is based on the higher predilection of pediatric posterior fossa tumors or Chiari malformations; however, these patients almost uniformly present with focal neurologic abnormalities as well.

TIPS AND PEARLS

- The use of pain relief as a diagnostic determinant of the severity of underlying pathology causing cephalgia is strongly discouraged. Owing to the common pathway of pain initiated through nociceptors aligning vessels, meninges and muscles, the elicited response is similar across all etiologies. Therefore, pain relief alone should not be used to direct the degree of evaluation required for a presenting headache complaint.
- Opioids are well documented for their association for rebound headaches and should be avoided in the standard management of headache pain.
- GCA is rare prior to the age of 50 years and should be considered for a new onset of constellation of symptoms associated most commonly with a new type of headache. The pain is most commonly temporally located but may be frontal or occipital and associated with generalized fatigue, jaw claudication, visual disturbances, weight loss and/or fever.
- Although hypertension can contribute to cephalgia in the presence of hypertensive emergency, elevated blood pressure alone should not be relied on as the cause of acute cephalgia, and further workup is often warranted.

EVIDENCE

Can a noncontrast CT head performed within 6 hours of symptom onset rule out SAH?

Given the relatively high mortality rate of SAH if untreated, timely diagnosis is critical. A noncontrast CT head has been the initial diagnostic study of choice, which if negative was historically followed by a LP. LP is not without potential hazard, often complicated by postdural headache, potential infection, or a traumatic tap confounding the diagnosis. Perry et al found the sensitivity of CT for diagnosing SAH to be 92.9% for all comers and 100% for those patients presenting within 6 hours of onset.[33] A recent meta-analysis found that CT will miss 1 to 2 cases of SAH per 1000 patients tested.[34] Given the low posttest probability of SAH after a negative CT within 6 hours, the poor specificity of a positive LP may not add meaningful diagnostic information.[35]

Certain limitations of CT can decrease the sensitivity of the test. CT scanners should be newer generation capable of multiple slices per rotation, and images should be read by attending radiologists or neuroradiologists. Patients with marked anemia (hematocrit < 30) may be read as falsely negative.

A negative CT scan performed within 6 hours can safely rule out SAH in patients presenting with acute onset headache and reassuring neurologic exam. Additional testing such as LP or CTA may be pursued in cases of persistently high clinical suspicion, acknowledging the strengths and weakness of those tests. As CT technology advances, the current 6-hour window for adequate sensitivity may extend further.

Is CTA an acceptable alternative to lumbar puncture in patients with suspected SAH?

Lumbar puncture historically followed a negative CT head in patients presenting >6 hours from onset. Inherent disadvantages of LP include pain, potential infection introduction, postdural headache, and unclear results secondary to a traumatic tap. With a sensitivity of 98% to 100% for identifying culprit aneurysms, CTA has emerged as a potential alternative. Unfortunately, the number of high-quality studies directly comparing CTA with LP is lacking, but one small study found CTA to be positive for all 5 cases of SAH.[36]

Identification of aneurysm on CTA is not a definitive diagnosis of SAH with a negative CT head. The incidence of aneurysm in the general population is estimated at 2% and may not represent the underlying pathology of headache. The added benefit of obtaining an LP lies in the evaluation of alternate diagnoses, including meningitis, encephalitis, SIH, or IIH.

Based on the limited data available, current recommendations allow for either CTA or LP, with an understanding of the risks and benefits of both modalities in the context of patient specific factors (eg, patient preference or body habitus).[6]

Can ultrasound reliably identify elevations in intracranial pressure?

ICP management is crucial in certain disease processes such as traumatic elevations, and variations in pressure are diagnostic of other conditions such as SIH and IIH. CT scan is often used to identify ICP changes through abnormalities in ventricle size or structure deviation; however, CT scan exposes the patient to radiation and can be labor intensive for transporting critically ill patients. Neither CT nor findings from physical exam (altered mental status, pupillary changes, posturing) can independently rule out elevations in ICP.[37]

Ultrasound is noninvasive and can be utilized at the bedside. It evaluates for elevations in ICP through measurement of optic nerve sheath diameter (ONSD). Koziarz et al used an optimal cutoff ONSD of 5.0 mm and found a sensitivity of 97% and a specificity of 86% in patients with traumatic head injuries.[38] Sensitivity and specificity for patients with nontraumatic brain injury dropped to 92% and 86%, respectively. Current data suggest that ONSD values <5.0 mm may rule out elevations in ICP, whereas OSND >5.0 mm are suggestive of ICP elevations; confirmatory testing is, however, required.

Are nonopioid analgesics preferred in the treatment of primary headache?

Many therapeutic options for the treatment of primary headaches exist. Although high-quality studies of the direct comparison between medications are scant, a few themes have emerged. A randomized study comparing intravenous prochlorperazine plus diphenhydramine versus IV hydromorphone was halted early secondary to significantly improved symptoms in the prochlorperazine arm.[39] Similar results suggest metoclopramide is as effective.

The American Headache Society recommends that IV prochlorperazine, IV metoclopramide, or subcutaneous sumatriptan should be offered as first line treatments.[5] Intranasal butorphanol has Level A evidence of benefit, and other opioids have Level C evidence of possible effectiveness. However, given the potential for dependence, abuse, and the ongoing opioid crisis, these medications should be avoided as first line therapy.[6,40] The Choosing Wisely Campaign from the American Academy of Neurology recommends only opioids or butalbital as a last resort.[41]

References

1. Burch R, Rizzoli P, Loder E. The prevalence and impact of migraine and severe headache in the United States: figures and trends from government health studies. *Headache*. 2018;58(4):496-505.

2. Charles A. The pathophysiology of migraine: implications for clinical management. *Lancet Neurol*. 2018;17(2):174-182.

3. Jarvis J, Johnson B, Crowe R. Out-of-hospital assessment and treatment of adult with atraumatic headache. *JACEP Open*. 2020;1:17-23.

4. Headache Classification Committee of the International Headache Society (IHS) The International Classification of Headache Disorders, 3rd edition. *Cephalalgia*. 2018;38(1):1-211.

5. Orr SL, Friedman BW, Christie S, et al. Management of adults with acute migraine in the emergency department: the American Headache Society evidence assessment of parenteral pharmacotherapies. *Headache*. 2016;56(6):911-940.

6. Godwin SA, Cherkas DS, Panagos PD, et al. Clinical policy: critical issues in the evaluation and management of adult patients presenting to the emergency department with acute headache. *Ann Emerg Med*. 2019;74(4):e41-e74.

7. Lantigua H, Ortega-Gutierrez S, Schmidt JM, et al. Subarachnoid hemorrhage: who dies, and why? *Crit Care*. 2015;19:309.

8. Perry JJ, Stiell IG, Sivilotti ML, et al. Clinical decision rules to rule out subarachnoid hemorrhage for acute headache. *JAMA*. 2013;310(12):1248-1255.

9. Czuczman AD, Thomas LE, Boulanger AB, et al. Interpreting red blood cells in lumbar puncture: distinguishing true subarachnoid hemorrhage from traumatic tap. *Acad Emerg Med*. 2013;20(3):247-256.

10. Long B, Koyfman A. Controversies in the diagnosis of subarachnoid hemorrhage. *J Emerg Med*. 2016;50(6):839-847.

11. Marcolini E, Hine J. Approach to the diagnosis and management of subarachnoid hemorrhage. *West J Emerg Med*. 2019;20(2):203-211.

12. Salem A, Roh D, Kitagawa R, et al. Assessment and management of coagulopathy in neurocritical care. *J Neurocrit Care*. 2019;12(1):9-19

13. Connolly ES, Rabinstein AA, Carhuapoma JR, et al. Guidelines for the management of aneurysmal subarachnoid hemorrhage: a guideline for healthcare professionals from the American Heart Association/American Stroke Association. *Stroke*. 2012;43(6):1711-1737.

14. Ducros A, Wolff V. The typical thunderclap headache of reversible cerebral vasoconstriction syndrome and its various triggers. *Headache*. 2016;56(4):657-673.

15. Burton TM, Bushnell CD. Reversible cerebral vasoconstriction syndrome. *Stroke*. 2019;50(8):2253-2258.

16. Kranz PG, Gray L, Amrhein TJ. Spontaneous intracranial hypotension: 10 myths and misperceptions. *Headache*. 2018;58(7):948-959.

17. Upadhyaya P, Ailani J. A review of spontaneous intracranial hypotension. *Curr Neurol Neurosci Rep*. 2019;19(5):22.

18. Steenerson K, Halker R. A practical approach to the diagnosis of spontaneous intracranial hypotension. *Curr Pain Headache Rep*. 2015;19(8):35.

19. Debette S, Compter A, Labeyrie MA, et al. Epidemiology, pathophysiology, diagnosis, and management of intracranial artery dissection. *Lancet Neurol*. 2015;14(6):640-654.

20. Markus HS, Hayter E, Levi C, et al. Antiplatelet treatment compared with anticoagulation treatment for cervical artery dissection (CADISS): a randomised trial. *Lancet Neurol*. 2015;14(4):361-367.

21. Lin J, Liang Y. Endovascular therapy versus intravenous thrombolysis in cervical artery dissection-related ischemic stroke: a meta-analysis. *J Neurol*. 2020;267(6):1585-1593.

22. Fam D, Saposnik G, Stroke Outcomes Research Canada Working Group. Critical care management of cerebral venous thrombosis. *Curr Opin Crit Care*. 2016;22(2):113-119.

23. Silvis SM, de Sousa DA, Ferro JM, Coutinho JM. Cerebral venous thrombosis. *Nat Rev Neurol*. 2017;13(9):555-565.

24. Alons IM, Jellema K, Wermer MJ, Algra A. D-dimer for the exclusion of cerebral venous thrombosis: a meta-analysis of low risk patients with isolated headache. *BMC Neurol*. 2015;15:118.

25. Ferro JM, Bousser MG, Canhão P, et al. European Stroke Organization guideline for the diagnosis and treatment of cerebral venous thrombosis: endorsed by the European Academy of Neurology. *Eur J Neurol*. 2017;24(10):1203-1213.

26. Wakerley BR, Tan MH, Ting EY. Idiopathic intracranial hypertension. *Cephalalgia*. 2015;35(3):248-261.

27. Markey KA, Mollan SP, Jensen RH, Sinclair AJ. Understanding idiopathic intracranial hypertension: mechanisms, management, and future directions. *Lancet Neurol*. 2016;15(1):78-91.

28. Stevens SM, Rizk HG, Golnik K, et al. Idiopathic intracranial hypertension: contemporary review and implications for the otolaryngologist. *Laryngoscope*. 2018;128(1):248-256.

29. Hoffman GS. Giant cell arteritis. *Ann Intern Med*. 2016;165(9):ITC65-ITC80.

30. Bienvenu B, Ly KH, Lambert M, et al. Management of giant cell arteritis: recommendations of the French Study Group for Large Vessel Vasculitis (GEFA). *Rev Med Interne*. 2016;37(3):154-165.

31. Blume HK. Childhood headache: a brief review. *Pediatr Ann*. 2017;46(4):e155-e165.

32. Yonker M. Secondary headaches in children and adolescents: what not to miss. *Curr Neurol Neurosci Rep*. 2018;18(9):61.

33. Perry JJ, Stiell IG, Sivilotti ML, et al. Sensitivity of computed tomography performed within six hours of onset of headache for diagnosis of subarachnoid haemorrhage: prospective cohort study. *BMJ*. 2011;343:d4277.

34. Dubosh NM, Bellolio MF, Rabinstein AA, Edlow JA. Sensitivity of early brain computed tomography to exclude aneurysmal subarachnoid hemorrhage: a systematic review and meta-analysis. *Stroke*. 2016;47(3):750-755.

35. Sayer D, Bloom B, Fernando K, et al. An observational study of 2,248 patients presenting with headache, suggestive of subarachnoid hemorrhage, who received lumbar punctures following normal computed tomography of the head. *Acad Emerg Med*. 2015;22(11):1267-1273.

36. Carstairs SD, Tanen DA, Duncan TD, et al. Computed tomographic angiography for the evaluation of aneurysmal subarachnoid hemorrhage. *Acad Emerg Med*. 2006;13(5):486-492.

37. Fernando SM, Tran A, Cheng W, et al. Diagnosis of elevated intracranial pressure in critically ill adults: systematic review and meta-analysis. *BMJ*. 2019;366:l4225.

38. Koziarz A, Sne N, Kegel F, et al. Bedside optic nerve ultrasonography for diagnosing increased intracranial pressure: a systematic review and meta-analysis. *Ann Intern Med*. 2019;171(12):896-905.

39. Friedman BW, Irizarry E, Solorzano C, et al. Randomized study of IV prochlorperazine plus diphenhydramine vs IV hydromorphone for migraine. *Neurology*. 2017;89(20):2075-2082.

40. Marmura MJ, Silberstein SD, Schwedt TJ. The acute treatment of migraine in adults: the American headache society evidence assessment of migraine pharmacotherapies. *Headache*. 2015;55(1):3-20.

41. Langer-Gould AM, Anderson WE, Armstrong MJ, et al. The American Academy of Neurology's top five choosing wisely recommendations. *Neurology*. 2013;81(11):1004-1011.

Seizures and Status Epilepticus

Elaine Rabin

CLINICAL CHALLENGE

Seizures are the clinical manifestations of abnormal, increased, synchronized electrical activity in the brain. An estimated 10% of the population experience at least one seizure in their lifetime, and of those, 3% develop epilepsy, which is a condition of recurrent unprovoked seizures.

Seizures may occur as a result of an acute underlying condition or insult—termed a **provoked** or **acute symptomatic** seizure. A seizure that occurs in the absence of such a condition is termed **unprovoked.** One of the goals in emergency practice is to identify those causative conditions that may lead to further harm and address them if possible (**Table 17.1**). Seizures can also be due to sequelae of a prior intracranial insult such as stroke, trauma, or anoxia, in which case it is referred to as a **remote symptomatic seizure.**

Ictus is often used to refer to the period during which a seizure occurs. Currently used classification systems are summarized in **Table 17.2** and **Figure 17.1.**[1] Seizures can be either **convulsive** or **nonconvulsive**; in the latter case, motor activity is not a key component of the presentation. Seizures may also be classified as **focal** or **generalized**. Focal or partial seizures occur when the abnormal electrical activity is limited to one area of the brain. These may manifest as motor, sensory, autonomic, or behavioral depending on their location. Signs and symptoms can be nonspecific, ranging from jerking of one limb or muscle group, to a strange taste or smell, or a sense of déjà vu or hyper spirituality. In some cases, focal electrical activity can spread to other areas and to the contralateral hemisphere. The symptoms progress in kind until the whole brain and whole body are involved, resulting in a generalized seizure.

Generalized seizures involve both hemispheres of the brain and may also be convulsive (commonly **tonic-clonic**) or nonconvulsive. Some seizures may be preceded by an *aura*, which is itself actually a focal seizure that may help identify the location of an epileptic focus, for example déjà vu points to the temporal lobe. **Status epilepticus** (SE) is a subset of generalized seizures characterized by a single prolonged ictal period or multiple recurrent seizures without return to baseline. This is a true neurologic emergency that is associated with high rates of neurologic injury as well as nonneurologic morbidity and mortality. SE may be convulsive status epilepticus (CSE) or nonconvulsive status epilepticus (NCSE) at the outset. CSE that is undertreated or untreated may progress to NCSE. Historically, SE was defined as a seizure lasting longer than 30 minutes, but current guidelines recommend beginning treatment after only 5 minutes of convulsive activity.[2]

TABLE 17.1	Differential Diagnosis of Provoked Seizures

Tumors
Vascular Event
- Subarachnoid hemorrhage
- Subdural hemorrhage
- Epidural hemorrhage
- Stroke
- Vasculitis

Infection
- Meningitis
- Encephalitis
- Abscess

Metabolic
- Hypoglycemia[a]
- Hyponatremia[b]
- Hypomagnesemia[c]
- Hypocalcemia

Toxic[d]
- Cocaine and sympathomimetics
- Tricyclic antidepressants
- Anticholinergics
- Theophylline
- Isoniazid

Eclampsia

[a]*The most common metabolic cause of seizures.*
[b]*A rare cause of seizures except in infants younger than 6 months old.*
[c]*Rarely an isolated cause of seizures; possibly facilitates seizures, especially in malnourished patients, for example, alcoholics.*
[d]*Consider the following in overdose.*

TABLE 17.2	Seizure Classification

Partial seizures	*Simple partial (without alteration of consciousness)* • Motor • Somatosensory • Autonomic • Psychic *Complex partial* • With focal onset before alteration in consciousness • Without focal onset before alteration in consciousness
Generalized seizures	*Primary generalized nonconvulsive* • Absence *Primary generalized convulsive* • Tonic-clonic • Clonic • Tonic • Myoclonic • Atonic *Secondary generalized* • Convulsive • Nonconvulsive
Status epilepticus	*Convulsive generalized* • Primary generalized • Secondary generalized *Subtle convulsive*[a] *Convulsive focal* *Nonconvulsive* • Primary generalized (absence) • Partial with or without secondary generalization (complex partial)

[a]*Subtle convulsive status epilepticus is sometimes classified as a type of nonconvulsive status epilepticus; however, it is the end stage of a convulsive event and has a very high mortality.*

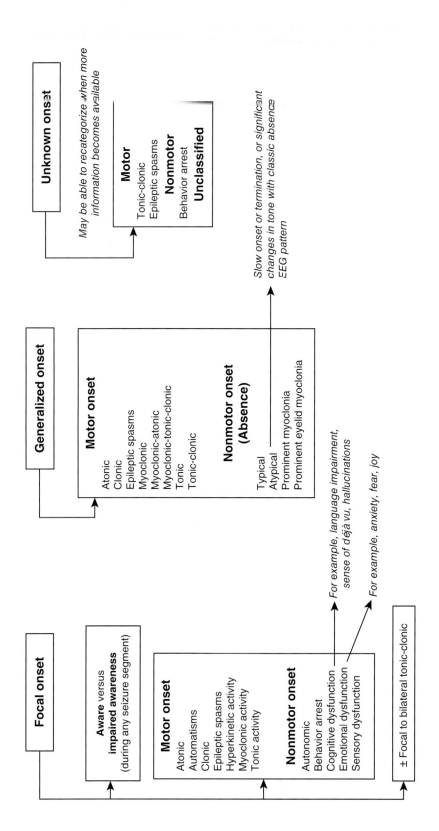

Figure 17.1: International League Against Epilepsy (ILAE) epilepsy classification. EEG, electroencephalogram. Based on Fisher RS, Cross JH, D'Souza CD, et al. Epilepsia2017 instruction manual for 2017 ILEA seizure definitions.pdf. Epilepsia. 2017;58(4):531-542.

TABLE 17.3	Differential Diagnosis of Patient of Altered Mental Status After a Seizure

Postictal state
Nonconvulsive status epilepticus or subtle convulsive status
Hypoglycemia
CNS infection
CNS vascular event
Drug toxicity
Psychiatric disorder

CNS, central nervous system.

Most seizures last under 5 minutes, although they may be followed by a period of confusion or altered mental status termed the ***postictal period***. This is a normal, benign condition that rarely lasts > 1 hour. A prolonged episode of altered mental status following a seizure should prompt investigation of other causes (**Table 17.3**).

The key to seizure diagnosis and management in the emergency department (ED) is gathering as much supporting history as possible and performing a careful neurologic examination to uncover evidence that a seizure took place or is still ongoing. The diagnosis of seizures may not be straightforward; 17% of patients referred to specialty epilepsy centers for "refractory seizures" do not actually have a seizure disorder and may be exposed to unnecessary medications or driving restrictions.[3] More recently, 10% of patients enrolled in a large multicenter study of SE were determined to have been having psychogenic convulsions.[4] Compounding diagnostic error is the failure to consider and or recognize nonconvulsive seizures in patients with altered behavior or are in coma: In one report, 12% of comatose patients in intensive care units (ICUs) were found to be in NCSE.[5]

PATHOPHYSIOLOGY

Brain function requires communication among organized networks of neurons. This communication is driven by electrical activity created by changes in sodium and potassium gradients across neuronal membranes. Neurotransmitters such as glutamate cause excitatory states in nearby neurons, leading to increased electrical activity. Other neurotransmitters, such as gamma aminobutyric acid (GABA) are inhibitory, suppressing electrical activity.

Under normal circumstances, equilibrium between excitation and inhibition keeps electrical activity at normal levels; seizures are initiated when excitatory activity is abnormally high and organized in rhythmic pulses. In generalized seizures, this activity is thought to start in the cortex, and then recruits subcortical structures, with the rhythmic activity possibly coordinated by the thalamus. Perpetuation of the excitatory activity occurs when the high levels of potassium exiting the cells interfere with the usual inhibitory mechanisms of the neuronal networks. Abnormal electrical activity usually terminates spontaneously, possibly due to depletion of excitatory substances or reflex activation of inhibitory substances. GABA-mediated inhibition among certain neuronal networks may contribute to both initiation and cessation of seizures.[6,7]

Genetic abnormalities that regulate neurotransmitters, and control the sodium-potassium pump, have been associated with epilepsy. Brain tissue may become "epileptogenic" after an insult, for example, trauma, stroke, or infection; a process termed ***epileptogenesis***. Identification and removal of epileptogenic foci is the basis of some epilepsy surgeries. In addition, a seizure may be incited by a change in the neuronal homeostatic environment because of a wide variety of pathologies including drug toxicity, withdrawal, infection, and electrolyte abnormalities.

Pathophysiologic consequences of a seizure may include a period of transient apnea and hypoxia. There may be autonomic dysfunction, with fluctuations in blood pressure. Serum lactate and serum glucose levels may increase, and there is often an increase in the white blood cell (WBC) count (but with no increase in bands). Body temperature is frequently elevated after a generalized convulsion. Acidosis due to elevated lactate occurs within 60 seconds of a convulsive event, but should normalize within 1 hour of ictus. A transient cerebrospinal fluid (CSF) pleocytosis of up to 20 WBCs/mm^3 has been reported to occur in 2% to 23% of patients with seizures.

After 30 minutes of seizure activity, many of the body's homeostatic regulating mechanisms fail. Cerebral blood flow autoregulation may be lost and, combined with alterations in blood pressure, cerebral perfusion may be compromised; combined, these factors contribute to the high mortality seen in CSE. The addition of increased neuronal metabolism to this picture may result in neuronal damage. Even if systemic factors such as acidosis and hypoxia are controlled, prolonged SE results in neuronal damage secondary to the release of neurotoxic excitatory amino acids and influx of calcium into cells.

PREHOSPITAL CONSIDERATIONS

Seizures are a common reason patients activate emergency medical services (EMS). Although most patients evaluated by prehospital providers will have stopped seizing by the time of first contact, a small but important minority will have persistent convulsions and should generally be presumed to be in SE. Multiple trials have demonstrated that treatment of seizures by prehospital providers is safe, efficacious, and results in improved patient outcome.[6] EMS protocols for managing prehospital SE vary by region, but must take into account the feasibility of drug storage and challenges to parenteral administration in the prehospital environment. Management begins with a blood glucose determination, whereas intramuscular (IM) midazolam or intravenous (IV) lorazepam are recommended first-line abortive therapies. Rectal diazepam is not first line because absorption and onset are variable. Other commonly performed interventions include provision of supplemental oxygen and continuous monitoring of SpO_2 and end-tidal CO_2.

For patients who have had a witnessed seizure but are not actively seizing, no specific therapy is indicated. Routine supportive care should be provided, and the patient should be placed in a position of comfort to facilitate maintenance of a patent airway and to prevent hypoxia. Routine IV placement may be considered, but is not mandatory. Precautions should be taken to prevent patient and provider injury in the case of recurrent seizure.

APPROACH/THE FOCUSED EXAMINATION

Approach to the patient who has had a seizure requires a careful history to characterize circumstances surrounding the event and to identify potential precipitants. Patients who are actively seizing or postictal may present challenges to obtaining a history, and the focus is on stabilization and treatment. All patients with a seizure history are at risk for another event, and at all times need to be in a safe environment, that is, guard rails up on the stretcher and never allowed to ambulate or go into the bathroom alone. **Figure 17.2** outlines a possible approach to the patient with suspected seizure.

History

In the case of a patient who is actively seizing, assessment and stabilization must occur simultaneously. EMS should be queried as to the circumstances under which the patient was found, and specific questions should be asked regarding evidence of trauma or paraphernalia suggestive of alcohol or drug use, as well as any medications found. Family or friends, if available, should be asked about preceding events, especially trauma, or any recent complaints such as headache, fever, confusion, or other systemic signs. They should be asked to supply known past medical and surgical history with particular attention to any history of seizure disorder or current use of antiepileptic drugs (AEDs). Additional sources of collateral history should be sought, including seeking out the patient's primary or specialist physicians and additional bystanders not present in the ED.

If the patient is not actively convulsing, has returned to baseline, and has a known history of seizures, the provider should determine whether the event was a typical seizure for them and whether it fits within the usual pattern of recurrence. An atypical episode should not automatically be presumed to have been a seizure, and other etiologies must be considered. History of specific triggers for a seizure should be investigated including sleep deprivation, medication nonadherence,

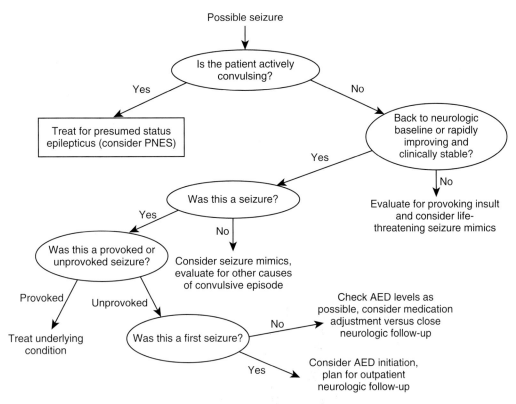

Figure 17.2: Approach to the patient with a suspected seizure. AED, antiepileptic drug; PNES, psychogenic nonepileptic seizure.

new medications, or trauma. A history of drug or alcohol use, or sudden abstinence thereof, and any signs or symptoms of a systemic insult such as infection or ischemia should be sought.

For the patient who has no history of prior seizure, the emergency clinician's first goal must be to determine whether this is, in fact, the diagnosis. Typically, the challenge is to differentiate between seizure and other causes of transient loss of consciousness such as syncope, and psychogenic events. The provider should enquire into the circumstances surrounding the event such as the presence of an aura, palpitations, light-headedness, blurred vision, or chest pain. Obtaining a history from witnesses can often provide the key to the diagnosis. Witnesses are better at recalling some aspects of the event such as muscle tone or eye deviation. Medical and social history should be obtained, with specific attention to risk factors for seizure such as prior intracranial injury, lesion, or surgery; current medication use that might lower the seizure threshold such as bupropion; and recent drug and alcohol use. Risk factors for syncope such as prior cardiac disease, personal or family history of dysrhythmias, and family history of sudden cardiac death should also be sought. Specific historic factors that may assist in distinguishing between seizure and syncope are discussed in the **Evidence** section.

Many patients who present with an apparent first-time seizure will, on careful questioning, have had prior seizures that were either unrecognized or for which medical attention was not sought. Open-ended questioning about prior "spells" or episodes may prompt recall. Enquiring about signs of nocturnal seizures such as waking to find a bitten tongue, enuresis, or other injuries, and evidence of nonconvulsive seizures such as spells of unresponsiveness, myoclonic jerking, or sensory experiences suggestive of an aura, may also stimulate recollection of prior events. Identification of these prior episodes allows for a better determination of the risk of seizure recurrence and can inform decisions regarding therapy.

The Focused Examination

The examination should begin with an accurate and complete set of vital signs. Tachycardia, hypertension, and transient hypoxia may be encountered during active convulsions, but generally recover rapidly following their termination. Etiologies of persistent vital sign abnormalities should be investigated. If the patient is actively convulsing at the time of examination, specific note should be made of the body parts involved and the type of movements. Note should be made of abnormalities in tone such as head turning and gaze deviation. If the onset of the episode is witnessed, attention should be paid to the order in which differing body parts become involved.

In the patient who has had a seizure but has returned to baseline, a more thorough examination can be obtained with the patient's cooperation. A general physical examination should be undertaken to evaluate for complications of seizures such as aspiration or trauma; tongue injury may be noted. Posterior shoulder dislocations are rare, but possible.

The neurologic examination should begin with assessment of the patient's level of consciousness, attention, and orientation. Comparison to baseline should be made. Altered behavior including subtle changes only appreciated by the family may be the result of an NCSE. A full examination of the cranial nerves and extremity strength and sensation will reveal focal motor or sensory deficits, if present. Signs of upper motor neuron lesions such as hyperreflexia and abnormal Babinski reflex should be sought; these are often present in the postictal period and resolve quickly. Gait testing should be performed, and assessment of balance and coordination made. Specific testing for cerebellar function such as finger-to-nose, heel-to-shin, and rapid alternating movements should be performed as well. Visual fields should be assessed. Funduscopic examination may reveal evidence of papilledema if there is increased intracranial pressure from a mass lesion or edema.

Diagnostic Testing

Laboratory Studies

For patients presenting after a first-time seizure who are alert, oriented, and have no clinical findings, appropriate laboratory studies include a serum glucose level, electrolytes, and a pregnancy test in women of child-bearing age. A drug-of-abuse screen should be considered. Other tests are of very low yield in this group of patients. Those who are on dialysis, malnourished, taking diuretics, or who have underlying significant medical disorders usually require more extensive testing including a complete blood count (CBC), blood urea nitrogen (BUN), creatinine, calcium, phosphate, and magnesium, as well as a urinalysis.

Rhabdomyolysis is a rare consequence of a seizure and is diagnosed if the urine tests positive for blood in the absence of red blood cells on the microscopic examination. Serum creatine phosphokinase (CPK) levels are not useful in differentiating seizures from other causes of loss of consciousness.

Patients with a known seizure disorder who have a "typical" event but who are asymptomatic, alert, and oriented in the ED do not routinely require serum chemistries aside from an AED level, if available. Those with other underlying disease such as diabetes that could result in a metabolic derangement may warrant more extensive evaluation. It is important to consider potential precipitants such as infections or new medications that might have contributed to the event.

Patients in CSE, and patients who are not actively convulsing but are persistently altered, require comprehensive diagnostic testing, which may include serum glucose, electrolytes, urea nitrogen, creatinine, magnesium, phosphate, calcium, CBC, pregnancy test in women of child-bearing age, AED levels, liver function tests, and a drug-of-abuse screen. An arterial blood gas (ABG) analysis obtained in a convulsing patient will show an anion gap metabolic acidosis that is usually secondary to lactic acidosis. The anion gap acidosis should resolve within 1 hour of the seizure ending; persistence after 1 hour suggests the presence of one of the other causes of an anion gap acidosis.

Lumbar Puncture

In the immunocompetent patient, Lumbar puncture should strongly be considered in the immune-competent patient with SE of unknown etiology, a prolonged post-ictal period or persistently-altered mental status, or with signs or symptoms of meningitis such as fever, headache, or neck stiffness. Prospective data do not support routine LP in other immunocompetent patients with a first-time seizure.[8] Patients with human immunodeficiency virus (HIV) and new-onset seizure have historically demonstrated a high prevalence of central nervous system (CNS) infection—in particular, cryptococcal meningitis—with some manifesting no additional signs of infection. LP in the absence of other signs of infection may be considered in this population.

Neuroimaging

Up to 40% of patients with a first-time seizure have an abnormal head computed tomography (CT).[9] An estimated 20% of patients with a first-time seizure and an abnormal CT have a normal neurologic examination. A head CT should be performed in the ED whenever a patient with seizure has a suspected acute intracranial process, a history of acute head trauma, malignancy, immunocompromised state, fever, persistent headache, anticoagulation, or a new focal neurologic examination[10]: In those cases where the patient has a normal neurologic examination, has returned to a normal baseline, and has no concerning comorbidities, a neuroimaging study can be deferred if the patient has access to timely follow-up. In these cases, a magnetic resonance imaging (MRI) would be the preferred imaging.

Electroencephalography

An electroencephalogram (EEG) in the ED may be useful for those patients with persistently altered mental status in whom subtle CSE or NCSE is suspected (see subsequent text). An EEG may also be useful when a patient's motor activity has been suppressed by either paralysis or barbiturate coma and there is a need to assess ongoing seizure activity.

MANAGEMENT

Management priorities will vary depending on whether the patient is suspected to be in SE or has returned to baseline. The presence or absence of a history of prior seizures and risk factors such as immune compromise and drug or alcohol use will also influence decision-making.

Status Epilepticus

Seizures lasting longer than 5 minutes should be considered SE and treated with AEDs to terminate convulsions and EEG ictal activity. Benzodiazepines are the most effective first-line therapy for SE and should be administered expeditiously and in appropriate doses once the diagnosis is established.[11] Delay in initiation of therapy beyond 10 minutes and inadequate initial dose of benzodiazepines are associated with worse outcomes.[12] See **Table 17.4** for a treatment pathway for SE. An in-depth discussion of particular medication choices is presented in the **Evidence** section.

After maximum dosing with a benzodiazepine, second-line therapy with another AED should follow regardless of whether the seizure terminated after benzodiazepine administration.[13] The goal of the second-line medications is to rapidly achieve therapeutic serum levels for maintenance therapy to prevent recurrence in all patients with SE.[13]

Second-line drugs commonly used in the treatment of benzodiazepine refractory SE include levetiracetam, valproic acid, and phenytoin or fosphenytoin. No one drug is clearly superior to others in benzodiazepine-refractory SE.[3] The choice of optimal agent may depend on ease of administration in a particular clinical setting, the patient's home drug regimen if known, and local clinical policies.

Refractory SE occurs in patients whose seizures persist despite treatment with adequate benzodiazepines and one other AED. Patients with refractory SE and the subset of patients with super-refractory SE (those who fail to respond to both second- and third-line agents) suffer high morbidity and mortality. With increasing seizure duration, the likelihood of response to GABAergic medications decreases and control of seizure activity becomes more difficult to obtain. For this reason, current guidelines recommend early progression to a continuous infusion of AED in those patients with refractory SE.[11] The goal of treatment should be complete termination of clinical and electrographic seizures within 60 minutes of onset. Options for continuous infusions include midazolam, propofol, or pentobarbital. Continuous EEG monitoring of patients with refractory SE is recommended to titrate AED dosing to elimination of electrographic seizure activity.

Good supportive care, in addition to therapy aimed at terminating seizure activity, will prevent secondary brain injury from hypotension or hypoxia that may complicate SE. Administration

TABLE 17.4	Management of Active Convulsion and Status Epilepticus (SE)
0-5 min	Supportive care Supplemental oxygen, airway repositioning if necessary Obtain IV access if able to Check blood glucose
5-10 min	First-line therapy—Benzodiazepine • Midazolam (10 mg IM if >40 kg or 5 mg IM if 13-40 kg) • Lorazepam (0.1 mg/kg IV up to 4 mg) • Diazepam (0.2 mg/kg up to 10 mg)

20-40 min	Second-line therapy
	• Consider repeat dose of lorazepam or diazepam 5-10 min after initial administration if convulsions persist
	• Administer urgent control AED
	  • Levetiracetam (20-60 mg/kg IV)
	  • Phenytoin/fosphenytoin (20 mg/kg IV; 20 mg PE/kg of fosphenytoin)
	  • Valproate (20 - 40 mg/kg)

40-60 min	Third-line therapy— Refractory SE
	• Airway protection—consider intubation for airway protection in anticipation of continuous AED infusion
	• EEG monitoring—consider continuous EEG monitoring to titrate AED therapy
	• Medications for refractory SE:
	  Consider repeat dose of another second-line AED
	Phenobarbital—15 mg/kg
	  Continuous anesthetic infusion—titrated to EEG
	    • Propofol (20-200 mcg/kg/min [max 65 mcg/kg/min in children])
	    • Midazolam (0.05-2 mg/kg/hr)
	    • Pentobarbital (0.5-5 mg/kg/hr)

AED, antiepileptic drug; EEG, electroencephalogram; IM, intramuscular; IV, intravenous.
Data from Kapur J, Elm J, Chamberlain JM, et al. Randomized trial of three anticonvulsant medications for status epilepticus. N Engl J Med. 2019;381(22):2103-2113; Glauser T, Shinnar S, Gloss D, et al. Evidence-based guideline: treatment of convulsive status epilepticus in children and adults: report of the guideline committee of the American Epilepsy Society. Epilepsy Curr. 2016;16(1):48-61; and Brophy GM, Bell R, Claassen J, et al. Guidelines for the evaluation and management of status epilepticus. Neurocrit Care. 2012;17(1):3-23.

of the agents used to terminate refractory SE can cause sedation and loss of airway reflexes and respiratory drive; the clinical assessment of airway patency and protection as well as oxygenation and maintenance of eucapnia are factors in deciding when to intubate and how to ventilate.

Caution must be exercised during intubation. Convulsive activity is metabolically demanding, and may lead to metabolic acidosis and increased oxygen extraction such that prolonged apnea during a difficult intubation will be poorly tolerated. All efforts should be made to ensure first-pass success in the procedure; the use of neuromuscular blocking agents (NMBAs) to facilitate intubation should not be avoided out of a fear of masking ongoing seizure activity. The half-life of typical agents is either short (in the case of succinylcholine) or the effect may be pharmacologically reversed (in the case of rocuronium). In addition, upward of 40% of patients with SE who remain altered after cessation of clinically apparent convulsive activity will have ongoing epileptic activity on EEG, suggesting that clinical observation alone will be insufficient for determination of treatment success whether or not NMBAs are employed.[14]

Resolved Seizure

In the case of a patient who has had a seizure but returned to their baseline, clinical decision-making includes if and when to obtain neuroimaging, EEG, and whether to initiate or adjust an AED.

Established Seizure History

For patients with an established seizure disorder, the evaluation centers on ascertaining treatment compliance and identifying potential precipitants. Obtaining serum levels of the patient's AED may be helpful; many patients are well controlled on a low level as long as they avoid situations that provoke their seizure, for example, sleep deprivation, photic stimulation, and stimulant use. If serum AED levels return in the subtherapeutic to zero range, this may prompt administration of a loading dose of the patient's medications in the ED to rapidly achieve therapeutic serum concentrations and prevent seizure recurrence. Consideration may also be given to administering a dose of a patient's home AEDs if a history of nonadherence to medical therapy is obtained and serum levels of the agent are not readily available. Oral and IV routes, when available, are both reasonable options for administering a loading dose of medications; there is no literature that a patient must be at a therapeutic level before discharge as long as proper instructions are provided and discharged into a safe environment.[15]

First-Time Seizure

The management of patients with an apparently unprovoked first-time seizure raises specific questions including determining which routine studies should be performed to exclude occult symptomatic causes and whether initiation of AED therapy is appropriate. These questions are addressed in the **Evidence** section.

Acute Symptomatic Seizures

Patients with a History of Alcohol Use

Abrupt cessation of alcohol use can precipitate alcohol withdrawal seizures (AWSs). These typically occur 6 to 48 hours after the last drink, are brief generalized tonic-clonic convulsions, and may occur before the serum alcohol level falls to zero. AWSs frequently occur in the absence of other signs and symptoms of withdrawal, which may complicate the diagnosis. Recurrence of seizures is common, typically within 6 to 12 hours of the first episode. Treatment with lorazepam even in the absence of active convulsions or signs of withdrawal significantly reduces this risk.[16] In addition to withdrawal, patients with a history of chronic alcohol use are at risk for occult trauma, electrolyte abnormalities, and other CNS insults that may precipitate seizures. In the absence of a clearly established history of recurrent seizures, a thorough investigation to evaluate for acute or remote symptomatic etiologies including neuroimaging and laboratory testing is warranted. In patients with a history of chronic alcohol use, we recommend treating empirically for AWS if suspicion is high, although it should be considered a diagnosis of exclusion until other acute symptomatic etiologies have been ruled out.

Suspected Toxic Ingestions

Toxins may cause seizures through a variety of mechanisms. Isoniazid, for example, depletes concentrations of the inhibitory neurotransmitter GABA, and medications that function by increasing effectiveness of GABA such as benzodiazepines and barbiturates may be ineffective. Early administration of pyridoxine (5 g IV, 70 mg/kg) should be undertaken if isoniazid ingestion is suspected. Sympathomimetic drugs such as cocaine and methamphetamine may precipitate seizures due to excess sympathetic activity. These tend to respond best to sedative hypnotics such as benzodiazepines, barbiturates, or propofol. If the offending agent is unknown, or there is suspicion for a sodium channel–blocking drug such as a tricyclic antidepressant, local anesthetics, diphenhydramine, or cocaine, then phenytoin should be avoided.

Hyponatremia

Hyponatremia may cause seizures in both adults and children. These are usually generalized tonic-clonic events, but may be partial or focal. In acute hyponatremia, the risk of neurologic complications increases as the sodium level falls below 120 to 125 mEq/L; in chronic hyponatremia, these symptoms tend to manifest as the level approaches 110 mEq/L. In cases of severe hyponatremia complicated by seizures or severe neurologic disturbances, the serum sodium concentration should be raised emergently by about 4 to 6 mEq/L, which is generally sufficient to resolve convulsions. This can be accomplished by infusion of 3% hypertonic saline bolus, either 100 mL over 10 minutes or 150 mL over 20 minutes, repeated as necessary to a maximum of 300 mL with serum sodium levels checked in between. Care must be taken to avoid overly rapid correction because this may result in the neurologically devastating complication of osmotic demyelination syndrome.

Patients with chronic alcoholism and those with chronic hyponatremia and initial serum sodium level less than 105 mEq/L for ODS.

SPECIAL POPULATIONS

Pediatric Consideration

The most common cause of seizures in children younger than 5 years old is febrile seizures. These are generalized tonic-clonic convulsive episodes that occur in the context of a fever $\geq$38 °C in the absence of CNS infection. Febrile seizures are divided into simple and complex; this distinction has implications for prognosis and need for subsequent evaluation. Simple febrile seizures are those that occur in children aged 6 to 60 months, are primarily generalized, last fewer than 15 minutes, do not recur within 24 hours, and are associated with complete recovery to neurologic baseline. Episodes that are focal, secondarily generalized, of longer duration, or recurrent are regarded as complex.

Simple febrile seizures are benign self-limited events that carry little risk of future sequelae. The occurrence of a simple febrile seizure is associated with only a small increase in the lifetime incidence of epilepsy. Risk factors for recurrence of simple febrile seizures include a lower degree of fever at presentation, shorter interval between onset of fever and convulsion, and a family history of simple febrile seizure. Complex febrile seizures, on the other hand, are associated with an increased risk of nonfebrile seizure; these are more common in children with low APGAR scores at birth, a history of abnormal development, and a family history of epilepsy.

The ED evaluation of a child with a suspected febrile seizure who has returned to neurologic baseline should focus on identification of fever source. A careful history and physical may readily identify the cause, with ancillary studies such as chest x-ray, urinalysis and culture, and respiratory virus testing employed as necessary. Children with simple febrile seizures do not appear to be at an increased risk for bacteremia as compared to those with fever alone. Viral illnesses are commonly identified in children with febrile seizures, with human herpesvirus-6 (HHV-6), adenovirus, respiratory syncytial virus (RSV), cytomegalovirus (CMV), and influenza A being the most common.

The main immediate challenge for the emergency clinician evaluating a child with a febrile seizure is to rule out a CNS infection. The majority of children with bacterial meningitis who present with seizure will have other signs or symptoms of this disease. In one retrospective cohort study of 503 children presenting with meningitis before the advent of multivalent pneumococcal vaccine, 115 had seizures as the main presenting symptom.[17] Of those presenting with seizures, 105 (91%) had a persistently altered level of consciousness following convulsions. The remainder had either a viral etiology or other signs or symptoms of meningitis such as nuchal rigidity, prolonged focal seizure, or recurrent seizures with a petechial rash. Therefore, LP is not routinely indicated in children with a simple febrile seizure who have returned to baseline and have neither signs nor symptoms of meningitis.[18] However, LP in the absence of other signs of meningitis may be considered in children younger than 12 months of age with an incomplete immunization or those pretreated with antibiotics because this may mask signs of meningitis such as nuchal rigidity. Simple febrile seizures, by definition, do not occur in children younger than 6 months of age.

Because of the benign prognosis of simple febrile seizures, there is no indication for routine evaluation with immediate or elective neuroimaging, EEG, serum chemistries, or blood counts. In general, children with simple febrile seizures who are neurologically normal and well appearing without a serious cause of fever or meningitis suspected after a careful evaluation may be discharged home after a period of observation in the ED. Follow-up with a primary care physician or in the ED for reevaluation within 24 to 48 hours is appropriate. Caregivers should be reliable to return for follow-up and should be cautioned to re-present to the ED immediately if seizures recur or if any signs of meningitis develop.

Seizures in Pregnancy

Faced with a pregnant patient having a seizure, physicians must determine whether the seizure is associated with an existing disorder, is of new onset, or is due to eclampsia. Patients with seizures due to eclampsia are treated with magnesium sulfate, which has been shown to be superior to phenytoin and diazepam in eclamptic seizures.[19] Once eclampsia has been ruled out, precipitating etiologies such as sleep deprivation, infections, and drug toxicities should be considered. In patients with a history of seizures, compliance with therapy should be explored. Pregnancy changes the "free" AED level of those AEDs that are protein bound. "Free AED levels" are required to accurately assess the true serum drug level. Fetal monitoring is a consideration in patients in the second half of pregnancy, and an obstetrics consultation should be obtained.

EVIDENCE

What historic and examination findings can help distinguish seizures from syncope?

A clinical decision rule with reported sensitivity and specificity of 94% for the diagnosis of seizure was derived and validated from a cohort of 102 patients with EEG-proven seizures, and 539 with syncope of a defined etiology (**Table 17.5**).[20] Tongue lacerations, head turning during the episode, and unusual posturing were found to have the highest positive likelihood ratios (16.5, 12.5, and 12.9, respectively) for the diagnosis of seizure.

Should patients with first-time seizure be started on AEDs in the ED?

Two unprovoked seizures at least 24 hours apart meet the definition of epilepsy. At that point, the chance that an adult will seize again is 60% to 90% at 4 years and increases with subsequent seizures.[21] Consensus exists that epilepsy should be treated with AEDs, which reduce or eliminate seizure recurrence. Thus, the emergency clinician should perform detailed questioning regarding whether a "first" seizure was truly a first episode; up to 50% of patients referred to epilepsy clinics for "first" unprovoked seizures had previous episodes, meeting criteria for AED initiation.[22]

The new definition of epilepsy includes first unprovoked seizures with "a probability of further seizures similar to the general recurrence risk (at least 60%) after two unprovoked seizures, occurring over the next 10 years."[23] Factors that increase the likelihood that a patient will develop epilepsy include abnormal findings on neuroimaging or EEG, nocturnal seizures, and focal seizures. A history of prior CNS insult also increases this risk; a landmark study found the risk of recurrent seizure to be 71% for patients presenting with first unprovoked seizure and history of stroke, 47% for history of traumatic brain injury (TBI), and 64% for history of CNS infection.[24] However, overall, the evidence on recurrence is sparse, inconsistent, and unclear regarding whether effects are additive.

Whether AEDs should be initiated after an apparent first unprovoked seizure is less clear. It is often impossible to confirm in the ED that a seizure occurred. Furthermore, only 21% to 45% of adults who have a single unprovoked seizure will have another, with the likelihood dropping if they remain seizure-free for 2 years.[23]

TABLE 17.5 Clinical Decision Rule to Differentiate Seizure and Syncope		
Clinical Feature	Point Value	+LR Seizure
Tongue laceration	2	16.46
Head turning to one side	1	13.48
Associated with emotional stress	1	3.7
Prodromal déjà vu or jamais vu	1	3.34
Postictal confusion	1	3.03
Abnormal behavior noted	1	2.8
Any presyncope	−2	0.273
Preceding diaphoresis	−2	0.169
Associated with prolonged sitting or standing	−2	0.049
Total score of ≥1 suggestive of seizure		

LR, likelihood ratio
From Sheldon R, Rose S, Ritchie D, et al. Historical criteria that distinguish syncope from seizures. J Am Coll Cardiol. 2002;40(1):142-148.

Starting AEDs before a second seizure renders unknowable whether a seizure-free patient would have seized without the AED. Once started on AEDs, patients are often afraid to discontinue them, and may continue AEDs for years or decades longer than necessary. Also, indirectly labeling patients as epileptics has consequences for their ability to drive legally and purchase life or medical insurance, and so on.

What is the diagnostic yield of routine serum chemistries or imaging studies in the healthy patient with an apparent first-time seizure without evidence of provoking factors identified on history or physical examination?

Laboratory Testing

Biomarkers: Some serum biomarkers have been shown to rise transiently in patients after a seizure including lactate, prolactin, and CPK. Prolactin's utility is limited by the number of other processes that can increase it, notably syncope.[24]

Lactate, if drawn within 2 hours of an event, was found to have a sensitivity of 0.88 and specificity of 0.87 in distinguishing generalized seizure from other forms of syncope or nonepileptic convulsions.[25] The Denver score, created in 2011 and since validated, revealed that bicarbonate and anion gap levels can be used to distinguish seizure from syncope with solid reliability.[26] However, this score was based on levels drawn within 30 minutes of an event. A more recent comparative study using samples drawn within 2 hours found lactate to be a more reliable discriminator than those markers.[27]

CPK rises in a minority of patients with seizures, and the rise may be delayed for several hours and not peak for 48 hours.[28] One systematic review found the specificity of elevated CPK to be 100% in distinguishing epileptic versus nonepileptic psychogenic seizure, but it was insensitive and cannot be used to exclude seizure from the differential.[29]

Serum Chemistries: In 2004, the American College of Emergency Physicians (ACEP) Clinical Policy Committee emphasized that broad serum testing is not indicated in patients with a first-time seizure who return to baseline, and that only a serum glucose and pregnancy test in women of childbearing age were indicated.[9] The current update to this policy did not make any recommendations.

Others suggest testing electrolytes and kidney and liver function after a first seizure to rule out easily identified metabolic processes as an underlying cause, although there is no supporting evidence to limited supporting evidence, especially when a patient has no predisposing comorbidities. For example, in a 2014 study of 439 patients with a first-time seizure presenting to an ED in Doha, Qatar, no patient was found to have electrolyte abnormalities.[28] Myocardial infarction, rhabdomyolysis, and other dangerous sequelae are rare after brief seizures. For patients in whom the diagnosis of seizure is uncertain, a concomitant evaluation for other potential etiologies of transient loss of consciousness or abnormal movement may involve more intensive laboratory evaluation.

Imaging

In a 2004 Clinical Policy, ACEP issued two Level B recommendations regarding neuroimaging in the ED of patients with a first-time seizure who have returned to baseline mental status.[9]

1. When feasible, perform neuroimaging of the brain in the ED on patients with a first-time seizure.
2. Deferred outpatient neuroimaging may be used when reliable follow-up is available.

(By the 2014 update to the policy, the issue was considered settled and was not revisited.) In 2007, a panel appointed by the Therapeutics and Technology Association of the American Academy of Neurology was even less committal on the issue, stating, "Immediate noncontrast CT is possibly useful for emergency patients presenting with seizure to guide appropriate acute management especially where there is an abnormal neurologic examination, predisposing history, or focal seizure onset."[10] Recent studies still report wide-ranging yields of positive findings on head CT after a seizure: from 4.8% in a single-hospital Turkish study,[30] to 35.3% in a Qatari study of their population where neurocysticercosis is common,[28] to 53% in a Finnish study.[31] The portion of findings requiring emergent intervention was smaller but still nontrivial, 12%[32] and 14.7%. As such, authors of newer reviews continue to endorse use of CT in the ED for patients with a first-time seizure.[33]

In general, MRI detects a greater number of intracranial lesions that can cause seizures than does CT. However, CT head without contrast is the most common imaging available immediately in the ED setting, and can be performed on many patients who have contraindications to MRI. Thus, CT is the widely recommended initial test in the ED.

Is there evidence to recommend one benzodiazepine over another in the treatment of SE?

Despite a number of large, well-designed studies examining the issue, there is no evidence to establish definitive superiority of one benzodiazepine over another as first-line therapy for CSE. Timeliness of administration and adequacy of dosing probably have a greater impact on outcome than does drug choice alone.

Much of the data on benzodiazepine selection comes from studies performed in the prehospital environment. Alderidge et al. randomized patients with SE to receive either IV lorazepam (2 mg), IV diazepam (5 mg), or placebo by EMS.[34] They found that any treatment with benzodiazepines was superior to placebo in terms of the primary endpoint of seizure termination at ED arrival. Lorazepam was more effective than was diazepam in the study cohort, but the difference did not achieve statistical significance. Adverse events were similar between the study groups, and lower than those in the placebo group. This study clearly demonstrated the utility and safety of prehospital benzodiazepine therapy in SE.

The most ambitious study of prehospital SE treatment, the Rapid Anticonvulsant Medication Prior to Arrival Trial ?(RAMPART) trial, compared IM midazolam (10 mg if >40 kg or 5 mg if 13-40 kg) to IV lorazepam (4 mg if >40 kg or 2 mg if 13-40 kg) in prehospital SE.[35] Almost 900 patients including adults and children over 13 kg were randomized. IM midazolam was superior with regard to the primary outcome of termination of seizure activity without administration of rescue medication before ED arrival. The groups were similar with regard to frequency of adverse events including respiratory depression requiring immediate intubation. IM midazolam was associated with a decreased risk of hospitalization. Among those subjects who met the primary endpoint, the total time to cessation of seizure activity was similar between the groups. Time to drug administration was faster in the IM midazolam group, although time from drug administration to seizure termination was shorter in the lorazepam group, reflecting the faster onset of IV administration and real-world challenges of placing an IV in an actively seizing patient.

With regard to hospitalized patients, the Veterans Administration (VA) Cooperative Study conducted a four-arm randomized trial of therapy for patients with SE, randomizing 384 patients to receive either lorazepam (0.1 mg/kg), diazepam (0.15 mg/kg) plus phenytoin, phenobarbital (15 mg/kg), or phenytoin alone.[36] In the subgroup of patients with confirmed overt generalized tonic-clonic SE, lorazepam was the most effective therapy for achieving the primary endpoint of termination of electrographic and clinical seizures within 20 minutes of initiation of therapy without recurrence in the next 60 minutes. This was followed, in order of descending efficacy, by the phenobarbital group, diazepam/phenytoin group, and the phenytoin group. In head-to-head comparison, the difference between lorazepam and diazepam plus phenytoin did not achieve statistical significance.

Is there evidence to support one agent over another in benzodiazepine-refractory SE?

The optimal second-line therapy for SE remains unclear. Phenytoin was a standard second treatment, but carries risks of hemodynamic compromise and extravasation injury. These risks are reduced by the use of the prodrug fosphenytoin. Levetiracetam and valproate have emerged as potential alternatives.

In 2015, a prospective randomized study compared treatment of lorazepam combined with phenytoin versus valproate versus levetiracetam. No differences were found among groups, and 71.3% overall terminated with one of the regimens. One of the drugs not used was then administered in refractory cases, followed by the other if needed: 86.7% terminated after the second drug in addition to lorazepam, and 92% after all were given.[37]

More recently, three large, well-designed trials came out in 2019 and have added to the evidence for therapeutic equipoise. Two multicenter, open-label randomized trials compared phenytoin to levetiracetam in pediatric populations. Lyttle et al. studied patients between 6 months and 18 years. In their sample of 286 patients, SE was terminated in 70% of the levetiracetam group versus 64% of the phenytoin group with a median time of 35 minutes after randomization.[38] Dalziel et al. studied patients 3 months to 16 years and found that seizure activity terminated within 5 minutes of administration of levetiracetam in 60% and after phenytoin in 50%.[29] Both sets of authors concluded that levetiracetam was not superior to phenytoin.

Kapur et al. performed a multicenter randomized double-blinded trial comparing levetiracetam, fosphenytoin, and valproate in patients 2 years or older, with the primary outcome of "absence of clinically-evident seizures and improvement in level of consciousness by 60 minutes after the start of drug infusion."[4] The trial was stopped early due to clinical futility. In the 384 patients enrolled, there was no evidence of superiority of any single therapy. Seizure activity was deemed to have ceased in 47% of the levetiracetam group, 45% of the phenytoin and fosphenytoin groups, and 46% of the valproate group. Nonsignificantly greater episodes of hypotension and intubation occurred in the fosphenytoin group and deaths in the levetiracetam group.

What is the utility of portable EEG performed in the ED to rule out NCSE?

Obtaining an emergent EEG in the ED is uncommonly done, but in theory may detect clinically occult seizure activity. In one center, emergent EEG facilitated a diagnosis in 51% of cases and changed management in 4%.[29] In another study utilizing a four-channel EEG montage on patients in the ED, seizure activity was identified in 12% of the 227 enrolled.[39] No follow-up with full montage electrocardiogram (ECG) was provided, so sensitivity and specificity of the limited EEG could not be ascertained. In this study, clinicians were blinded to the EEG results; the fact that they discharged 9 of the 24 patients who had a seizure focus identified suggests that availability of EEG data might have had significant impact on management. In another retrospective review of eight-channel emergent EEGs performed in the ED and inpatient wards at a single center, NCSE was diagnosed in 33% of patients in the cohort; when compared to full montage EEG, they found the emergent EEG had a sensitivity of 92.1% and specificity of 97.2%.[39]

Emergent EEG is available full time at only a minority of centers in the United States. Efforts have been made to develop EEG apparatuses that are easier to apply, and automated EEG interpretation also to reduce the need for expert technicians or interpreters. Three studies have compared four-channel EEG montages to standard EEG in patients admitted to the ICU or epilepsy monitoring unit. The limited montage has a sensitivity of 54% to 72% compared to full EEG, thereby limiting its usefulness to rule out seizure.[40] Similarly, commercially available computerized seizure detection has not demonstrated sensitivity adequate to rule out seizure activity in the ED. In a study of 1478 EEGs, computerized interpretation was only 53% sensitive when compared with expert interpretation.[41] On the basis of the best available evidence, bedside EEG has potential and is helpful when positive, but cannot be used alone to rule out a diagnosis of NCSE.

TIPS AND PEARLS

- Nonconvulsive seizures present with altered mental status or changed behavior, and should be considered especially when the presentation is stereotypical or associated with automatisms.
- Twenty percent to 40% of patients treated for CSE remain in nonconvulsive status after termination of motor activity; the diagnosis is made with an EEG.
- Many patients with a "first-time" seizure will have evidence of past similar events upon targeted and detailed questioning.
- The goal of therapy in SE is termination of clinical and electrographic seizures within 60 minutes. Therapy should be rapidly escalated to continuous infusion of AEDs if necessary.
- Phenytoin has a pH of 13, and is associated with a high incidence of phlebitis; it should not be administered through a small vein. Fosphenytoin is safer and an equally effective choice.
- AEDs may be administered by oral or parenteral routes; in the patient with a low serum level who has seized, neither is superior in the awake and cooperative patient.
- Lorazepam 2 mg administered to patients with suspected alcohol withdrawal syndrome—even if not actively seizing—prevents recurrence and may facilitate a safe disposition.

- Simple febrile seizures are generally benign self-limited events, and the clinician should focus on identifying the cause of fever. In infants who are young, incompletely vaccinated, or on antibiotics, a higher index of suspicion for meningitis should be had.
- A high index of suspicion should be had for eclampsia in pregnant patients presenting with seizure. Treatment is IV or IM magnesium.
- Midazolam is the best benzodiazepine for IM administration to terminate seizures; lorazepam is preferred with there is IV access because it is longer acting.
- Initially, maximal doses of benzodiazepines (ie, lorazepam 4 mg IV for an adult) should be given to actively seizing patients because GABA receptors downregulate quickly.

References

1. Fisher RS, Cross JH, D'Souza CD, et al. Instruction manual for the ILAE 2017 operational classification of seizure types. *Epilepsia*. 2017;58(4):531-542.

2. Trinka E, Cock H, Hesdorffer D, et al. A definition and classification of status epilepticus—report of the ILAE task force on classification of status epilepticus. *Epilepsia*. 2015;56(10):1515-1523. doi:10.1111/epi.13121

3. Labate A, Mumoli L, Curcio A, et al. Value of clinical features to differentiate refractory epilepsy from mimics: a prospective longitudinal cohort study. *Eur J Neurol*. 2018;25(5):711-717. doi:10.1111/ene.13579

4. Kapur J, Elm J, Chamberlain JM, et al. Randomized trial of three anticonvulsant medications for status epilepticus. *N Engl J Med*. 2019;381(22):2103-2113. doi:10.1056/NEJMoa1905795

5. Varelas PN, Hacein-Bey L, Hether T, Terranova B, Spanaki MV. Emergent electroencephalogram in the intensive care unit: indications and diagnostic yield. *Clin EEG Neurosci*. 2004;35(4):173-180. doi:10.1177/155005940403500406

6. Chang M, Dian JA, Dufour S, et al. Brief activation of GABAergic interneurons initiates the transition to ictal events through post-inhibitory rebound excitation. *Neurobiol Dis*. 2018;109:102-116. doi:10.1016/j.nbd.2017.10.007

7. Krumholz A, Wiebe S, Gronseth G, et al. Practice parameter: evaluating an apparent unprovoked first seizure in adults (an evidence-based review): report of the quality standards subcommittee of the American Academy of Neurology and the American Epilepsy Society. *Neurology*. 2007;69:1996-2007.

8. Sempere AP, Villaverde FJ, Martinez-Menéndez B, Cabeza C, Peña P, Tejerina JA. First seizure in adults: a prospective study from the emergency department. *Acta Neurol Scand*. 1992;86(2):134-138. doi:10.1111/j.1600-0404.1992.tb05054.x

9. American College of Emergency Physicians. Clinical policy: critical issues in the evaluation and management of adult patients presenting to the emergency department with seizures. *Ann Emerg Med*. 2004;43(5):605-625. doi:10.1016/j.annemergmed.2004.01.017

10. Harden CL, Huff JS, Schwartz TH, et al. Reassessment: neuroimaging in the emergency patient presenting with seizure (an evidence-based review): report of the therapeutics and technology assessment subcommittee of the American Academy of Neurology. *Neurology*. 2007;69(18):1772-1780. doi:10.1212/01.wnl.0000285083.25882.0e

11. Glauser T, Shinnar S, Gloss D, et al. Evidence-based guideline: treatment of convulsive status epilepticus in children and adults: report of the guideline committee of the American Epilepsy Society. *Epilepsy Curr*. 2016;16(1):48-61. doi:10.5698/1535-7597-16.1.48

12. Gaínza-Lein M, Fernández IS, Jackson M, et al. Association of time to treatment with short-term outcomes for pediatric patients with refractory convulsive status epilepticus. *JAMA Neurol*. 2018;75(4):410-418. doi:10.1001/jamaneurol.2017.4382

13. Brophy GM, Bell R, Claassen J, et al. Guidelines for the evaluation and management of status epilepticus. *Neurocrit Care*. 2012;17(1):3-23.

14. DeLorenzo RJ, Waterhouse EJ, Towne AR, et al. Persistent nonconvulsive status epilepticus after the control of convulsive status epilepticus. *Epilepsia*. 1998;39(8):833-840. doi:10.1111/j.1528-1157.1998. tb01177.x

15. Huff JS, Melnick ER, Tomaszewski CA, Thiessen MEW, Jagoda AS, Fesmire FM. Clinical policy: critical issues in the evaluation and management of adult patients presenting to the emergency department with seizures. *Ann Emerg Med*. 2014;63(4):437-447.e15. doi:10.1016/j. annemergmed.2014.01.018

16. D'Onofrio G, Rathlev NK, Ulrich AS, Fish SS, Freedland ES. Lorazepam for the prevention of recurrent seizures related to alcohol. *N Engl J Med*. 1999;340(12):915-919. doi:10.1056/ NEJM199903253401203

17. Green SM, Rothrock SG, Clem KJ, Zurcher RF, Mellick L. Can seizures be the sole manifestation of meningitis in febrile children? *Pediatrics*. 1993;92(4):527-534. doi:10.1016/s0196-0644(94)80410-9

18. Duffner PK, Berman PH, Baumann RJ, et al. Clinical practice guideline—neurodiagnostic evaluation of the child with a simple febrile seizure. *Pediatrics*. 2011;127(2):389-394. doi:10.1542/ peds.2010-3318

19. Lucas MJ, Leveno KJ, Cunningham FG. A comparison of magnesium sulfate with phenytoin for the prevention of eclampsia. *N Engl J Med*. 1995;335(4):201-205. doi:10.1056/NEJM199507273330401

20. Sheldon R, Rose S, Ritchie D, et al. Historical criteria that distinguish syncope from seizures. *J Am Coll Cardiol*. 2002;40(1):142-148. doi:10.1016/S0735-1097(02)01940-X

21. Fisher RS, Acevedo C, Arzimanoglou A, et al. ILAE official report: a practical clinical definition of epilepsy. *Epilepsia*. 2014;55(4):475-482. doi:10.1111/epi.12550

22. Rizvi S, Ladino LD, Hernandez-Ronquillo L, Téllez-Zenteno JF. Epidemiology of early stages of epilepsy: risk of seizure recurrence after a first seizure. *Seizure*. 2017;49:46-53. doi:10.1016/j. seizure.2017.02.006

23. Krumholz A, Wiebe S, Gronseth GS, et al. Evidence-based guideline: management of an unprovoked first seizure in adults: report of the guideline development subcommittee of the American Academy of Neurology and the American Epilepsy Society. *Neurology*. 2015;85(17):1525. doi:10.1212/ WNL.0000000000002093

24. Nass RD, Sassen R, Elger CE, Surges R. The role of postictal laboratory blood analyses in the diagnosis and prognosis of seizures. *Seizure*. 2017;47:51-65. doi:10.1016/j.seizure.2017.02.013

25. Matz O, Zdebik C, Zechbauer S, et al. Lactate as a diagnostic marker in transient loss of consciousness. *Seizure*. 2016;40:71-75. doi:10.1016/j.seizure.2016.06.014

26. Bakes KM, Faragher J, Markovchick VJ, Donahoe K, Haukoos JS. The Denver Seizure Score: anion gap metabolic acidosis predicts generalized seizure. *Am J Emerg Med*. 2011;29(9):1097-1102. doi:10.1016/j.ajem.2010.07.014

27. Brigo F, Igwe SC, Erro R, et al. Postictal serum creatine kinase for the differential diagnosis of epileptic seizures and psychogenic non-epileptic seizures: a systematic review. *J Neurol*. 2015;262(2):251-257. doi:10.1007/s00415-014-7369-9

28. Pathan SA, Abosalah S, Nadeem S, et al. Computed tomography abnormalities and epidemiology of adult patients presenting with first seizure to the emergency department in qatar. *Acad Emerg Med*. 2014;21(11):1264-1268. doi:10.1111/acem.12508

29. Ziai WC, Schlattman D, Llinas R, et al. Emergent EEG in the emergency department in patients with altered mental states. *Clin Neurophysiol*. 2012;123(5):910-917. doi:10.1016/j.clinph.2011.07.053

30. Ozturk K, Soylu E, Bilgin C, Hakyemez B, Parlak M. Neuroimaging of first seizure in the adult emergency patients. *Acta Neurol Belg*. 2018;(0123456789):1-6. doi:10.1007/s13760-018-0894-z

31. Kotisaari K, Virtanen P, Forss N, Strbian D, Scheperjans F. Emergency computed tomography in patients with first seizure. *Seizure*. 2017;48:89-93. doi:10.1016/j.seizure.2017.04.009

32. Kotisaari K, Virtanen P, Forss N. Emergency computed tomography in patients with first seizure. *Seizure*. 2017;48:89-93.

33. Tranvinh E, Lanzman B, Provenzale J, Wintermark M. Imaging evaluation of the adult presenting with new-onset seizure. *Am J Roentgenol*. 2019;212(1):15-25. doi:10.2214/AJR.18.20202

34. Alldredge BK, Gelb AM, Isaacs SM, et al. A comparison of lorazepam, diazepam, and placebo for the treatment of out-of-hospital status epilepticus. *N Engl J Med*. 2001;345(9):631-637. doi:10.1056/NEJMoa002141

35. Silbergleit R, Durkalski V, Lowenstein D, et al. Intramuscular versus intravenous therapy for prehospital status epilepticus. *N Engl J Med*. 2012;366(7):591-600. doi:10.1056/NEJMoa1107494

36. Treiman DM, Meyers PD, Walton NY, et al. A comparison of four treatments for generalized convulsive status epilepticus. *N Engl J Med*. 1998;339(12):792-798. doi:10.1056/NEJM199809173391202

37. Mundlamuri RC, Sinha S, Subbakrishna DK, et al. Management of generalised convulsive status epilepticus (SE): a prospective randomised controlled study of combined treatment with intravenous lorazepam with either phenytoin, sodium valproate or levetiracetam—pilot study. *Epilepsy Res*. 2015;114:52-58. doi:10.1016/j.eplepsyres.2015.04.013

38. Lyttle MD, Rainford NEA, Gamble C, et al. Levetiracetam versus phenytoin for second-line treatment of paediatric convulsive status epilepticus (EcLiPSE): a multicentre, open-label, randomised trial. *Lancet*. 2019;393(10186):2125-2134. doi:10.1016/S0140-6736(19)30724-X

39. Bastani A, Young E, Shaqiri B, et al. Screening electroencephalograms are feasible in the emergency department. *J Telemed Telecare*. 2014;20(5):259-262. doi:10.1177/1357633X14537775

40. Máñez Miró JU, Díaz de Terán FJ, Alonso Singer P, Aguilar-Amat Prior MJ. Emergency electroencephalogram: usefulness in the diagnosis of nonconvulsive status epilepticus by the on-call neurologist. *Neurolgia (English Ed)*. 2018;33(2):71-77. doi:10.1016/j.nrleng.2016h

41. González Otárula KA, Mikhaeil-Demo Y, Bachman EM, Balaguera P, Schuele S. Automated seizure detection accuracy for ambulatory EEG recordings. *Neurology*. 2019;92(14):E1540-E1546. doi:10.1212/WNL.0000000000007237

18

Central Nervous System Infections

Benjamin H. Schnapp

Corlin Jewell

THE CLINICAL CHALLENGE

Infections of the central nervous system (CNS) can be rapidly fatal and require prompt intervention in order to maximize good outcomes. Providers are forced to act quickly to provide treatment, often without knowing the exact underlying pathology. Many patients will have a nonspecific presentation with a wide differential diagnosis. Although fever is common in pathologies such as meningitis (inflammation of the meninges) or encephalitis (inflammation of the brain), it may not be present in other types of CNS infections, such as neurocysticercosis or opportunistic fungal infections in immunocompromised patients.

More than half of cases of bacterial meningitis in the United States are caused by *Streptococcus pneumoniae*.[1] However, *Neisseria meningitidis, Escherichia coli, Haemophilus influenzae,* and *Listeria monocytogenes* also represent frequently isolated bacterial species. Even with treatment, mortality is as high as 16%.[2] *Mycobacterium tuberculosis* also represents a common cause of meningitis worldwide, with as many as 1% to 2% of patients with active tuberculosis (TB) being affected by CNS infection. As with many CNS infections, meningitis secondary to *M tuberculosis* is more frequently seen in patients with compromised immune systems, such as those afflicted by human immunodeficiency virus (HIV).

Viral meningitis is the most common CNS infection; it is generally associated with lower morbidity and mortality than bacterial meningitis. Enteroviruses are the most common infectious pathogens, particularly in warmer seasons. However, other important pathogens include herpes simplex virus (HSV), varicella-zoster virus (VZV), cytomegalovirus (CMV), Epstein-Barr virus (EBV), and HIV. Often, the exact pathogen is not identified. Owing to modern vaccination practices, rates of certain previously common etiologies of viral meningoencephalitis, such as measles and mumps, have decreased. Although viral infections are typically less severe and often have excellent outcomes, many features of bacterial and viral meningitis overlap, making the distinction between them difficult, especially at the onset of disease.

Certain fungal species can also invade the CNS. The most common being *Cryptococcus neoformans,* followed by *Coccidioides immitis*. Mucormycosis can also spread to the CNS; diabetic patients are at higher risk for this severe invasive infection. Other common invasive fungal species, such as *Aspergillus* and *Candida,* only rarely cause meningitis. Fungal CNS infections were previously found mainly in patients with HIV/acquired immunodeficiency syndrome (AIDS), but the incidence has been increasing because of the greater numbers of patients on chronic immunosuppression for transplanted organs and autoimmune conditions.

The most common parasitic CNS infection worldwide is neurocysticercosis, mostly occurring in lower income countries.[2] This is caused by ingestion of the larva of the tapeworm *Taenia solium*, classically from eating undercooked infected pork products. Another common CNS parasite is *Toxoplasma gondii*; Although widely prevalent in the population, it generally causes no symptoms but can cause active infection in patients with decreased immunity. Infrequently, other species of worms, such as *Strongyloides*, can also cause meningitis.

Infectious encephalitis, a more severe infection, can caused by bacterial, viral, fungal, or parasitic infections and will commonly present with focal neurologic symptoms, behavioral change, cognitive deficits, or even seizures.[3] The most common causes of meningoencephalitis are summarized in **Table 18.1**.

Intracranial abscesses are distinct from the granulomas that form secondary to parasitic and TB infections and most often occur in those with immune disorders or recent surgery. Rarely, they can occur in healthy individuals with normal immune systems. Infections are most commonly caused by *Streptococcus* species, followed by *Staphylococcus* (predominantly *S aureus*) and gram-negative bacteria (*Proteus, E coli,* etc.). Mortality rate, although still relatively high, has declined to as low as 10% in recent years, likely secondary to advanced diagnostic and treatment modalities.[4]

The epidural space represents another site where CNS abscesses can occur. Unlike many of the other types of CNS infections discussed in this chapter, the incidence of epidural abscess has been increasing in recent years, likely caused by an increase in spinal procedures, increasing numbers of immunocompromised patients, and high numbers of intravenous (IV) drug users. *S aureus* is the most common pathogen involved in epidural abscesses, with a high proportion of methicillin-resistant *S aureus* (MRSA). Although rare, mycobacteria and fungi also can cause spinal epidural abscesses.

Finally, prions represent an unusual form of CNS infection. They are transmissible misfolded proteins that, once acquired, induce progressive, fatal CNS disease. They induce a group

TABLE 18.1	Common Etiologies of Meningoencephalitis in Adults
Bacterial	
	S pneumoniae
	N meningitidis
	L monocytogenes (older individuals)
	H influenzae
	M tuberculosis
Viral	
	Enterovirus
	HSV
	VZV
	CMV/EBV
	HIV
Fungal	
	C neoformans
	C immitis
	Aspergillus
	Candida

CMV, cytomegalovirus; EBV, Epstein-Barr virus; HIV, human immunodeficiency virus; HSV, herpes simplex virus; VZV, varicella-zoster virus.

of disorders known as transmissible spongiform encephalopathies (TSEs). TSEs are very rare, but include Kuru, Creutzfeldt-Jakob disease (CJD), and fatal familial insomnia (FFI), with CJD being the most common.[9]

PATHOPHYSIOLOGY

Normally, the cerebrospinal fluid (CSF) is a sterile liquid bathing the structures of the CNS. In order for microorganisms to enter this space, they must pass through the blood-brain barrier (BBB), a collection of endothelial cells whose primary function is to protect the brain from harmful substances in the blood. The simplest way for pathogens to pass through the BBB and gain access to the CNS is through direct contiguous spread from an infection in an adjoining structure. Common points of entry include the mouth, sinuses, or ear. Another potential direct entry point is through penetrating traumatic injury to the skull or a neurosurgical procedure. Pathogens may gain access to the CNS via hematogenous spread as well.

In bacterial meningitis, the presence of bacteria in this normally sterile space elicits an inflammatory response, leading to the characteristic symptoms of the disease. This inflammatory response can lead to the release of inflammatory cytokines to such a degree that cerebral edema results, as proteins and fluid leak through the altered BBB. In some cases of tuberculous meningitis, granuloma formation can also occur, causing mass effects. If these granulomas rupture, severe vasculitis may result and cerebral blood flow can be threatened, resulting in stroke.

Some viruses, such as HSV, herpes zoster virus (HZV), and rabies, have a unique way of entering CNS tissue not seen in other pathogens. In addition to hematogenous spread, these viral pathogens can travel along the axons of peripheral nerves backward until they reach the CNS. The virus can lie dormant within the host, potentially for years, until the immune system is compromised, allowing viral reactivation to occur. The virus then spreads via retrograde passage into the CNS, leading to the development of meningitis or encephalitis. Fungal CNS infections typically occur when a previously existing systemic fungal infection penetrates the BBB in an immunocompromised patient. CNS infection with mucormycosis, for example, is caused by direct spread from an existing sinus infection.

The development of an abscess within the brain can occur via different mechanisms, similar to other forms of CNS infection. Most brain abscesses are thought to occur through contiguous spread, with a smaller proportion caused by hematogenous seeding from infections present elsewhere. Typically, these abscesses are found near their inciting infection, such as otitis or mastoiditis. They can also result from neurosurgical procedures that require direct access to the CNS. The expected pathogen is based on the mechanism of entry into the CNS, but *Streptococcus* and *Staphylococcus* species are common. Just as with other infections of the CNS space, the resultant inflammation of the surrounding tissue can result in severe edema of the surrounding brain tissue, which can result in permanent neurologic deficits.

Epidural abscesses can occur along any portion of the spinal cord but are most commonly found in the posterior portion of the thoracolumbar spine. Most occur via hematogenous spread, followed by contiguous spread from adjacent infection, including osteomyelitis and psoas abscesses. Direct inoculation from spinal operations can also occur. This can lead to focal neurologic deficits from compression of the cord or the cauda equina.

Parasitic CNS infections also occur via hematogenous spread. The parasite *T solium* enters its host once its eggs are ingested via contaminated food. Once inside the human gastrointestinal (GI) tract, the eggs hatch and the larvae pass through the intestinal mucosa. They are distributed throughout the body and encyst. Those that pass through the BBB to form cysts within the CNS are thought to survive via protection from the host immune system by the BBB itself. Eventually, these cysts are discovered by the immune system and the resultant response will cause the cyst to become granulomatous and then finally clear into a calcified scar within the brain. Symptoms in the human host are caused by the inflammatory reaction of degenerating cysts or via mass effect if significant clusters build up within the parenchyma. **Figure 18.1** shows the characteristic cysts of neurocysticercosis. Toxoplasmosis is acquired from ingestion of meat contaminated with animal feces, or transplacental. Following primary infection, the parasite forms cysts in various structures, including the CNS. These can persist in a lifelong dormant state but can become reactivated if the host becomes immunocompromised, leading to active symptoms of encephalitis.

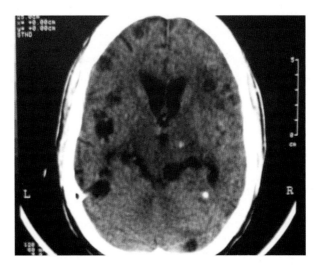

Figure 18.1: Multiple cystic lesions in a patient with neurocysticercosis as seen on CT scan. By Indmanu-aba (Creative Commons Attribution-ShareAlike License), via Wikicommons. CT, computed tomography.

In prion disease, the abnormal proteins are present in their normal configurations in healthy individuals but become misfolded and therefore resistant to protease activity. It is unknown what initially causes the abnormal folding of these proteins, but it appears to develop sporadically, through inheritance, or acquired by contact with affected brain tissue. Once present, the proteins spread the misfolded state to healthy proteins and eventually accumulate and form vacuoles that destroy neurons.

PREHOSPITAL CONCERNS

The focus for prehospital providers is on recognizing critical patients and transporting them to the closest appropriate hospital. Given that many CNS pathologies can result in altered mental status and loss of protective airway mechanisms, an assessment of the patient's airway and ability to oxygenate should be completed first following local emergency medical service (EMS) protocols. If there is a concern for bacterial meningitis (eg, a febrile patient with a headache and altered mental status), the patient and crew should maintain droplet precautions by using personal protective equipment to prevent the spread of the disease. If possible, IV access should be obtained and crystalloid fluid resuscitation started.

If seizures occur prior to arrival at the emergency department (ED), abortive therapy with intramuscular (IM) midazolam or lorazepam, or IV lorazepam is recommended. There is no evidence supporting the use of prehospital antibiotics; sepsis studies on prehospital antibiotics have not demonstrated improved mortality, and we currently do not recommend prehospital antibiotic treatment. If bacterial meningitis from meningococcus is confirmed, providers in close contact with the patient's respiratory secretions (eg, the provider who intubated) should receive antibiotic prophylaxis (see discussion below and **Table 18.2**).[5]

APPROACH

Meningitis

Classically, bacterial meningitis presents with fever, nuchal rigidity, and headache from the systemic and localized inflammatory responses. The majority of patients will present with at least one of these classic signs.[1] However, relatively few patients present with all three components of this triad. Other common symptoms include nausea, vomiting, fatigue, and body aches. Viral meningitis presents similarly, but symptoms are typically less severe and more subacute in onset.

Risk factors for meningitis include immunocompromise (including diabetes), malignancy, pulmonary disease, and residence in a group home.[6] All patients with suspected meningitis should have a focused history taken with attention to the symptoms and risk factors above, along with a full neurologic examination. Although patients with meningitis may initially appear altered because of lethargy

TABLE 18.2 Recommended Chemoprophylaxis for Contacts of Those with CNS Infections, by Infective organism

	Population	Medication	Dose	Frequency
N meningitidis	Those in prolonged close contact (roommates, partners, daycare workers), health care workers exposed to secretions	Rifampin	600 mg	Every 12 hours for 4 doses
		Ciprofloxacin	500 mg	Single dose
		Ceftriaxone	250 mg	Once (preferred in pregnancy)
H influenzae	Immunocompromised children <4 years old (including unvaccinated) or those living with these individuals	Rifampin	20 mg/kg	Daily for 4 days
Other causes	Prophylaxis for other forms of bacterial, viral, or parasitic CNS infections is not recommended in any population	None	None	None

CNS, central nervous system.

or severe headache, they generally do not exhibit focal neurologic deficits. If these signs are present, then infection of the brain parenchyma itself, that is, encephalitis, should be considered. In addition to the comprehensive neuro examination, jolt accentuation (worsening of the headache in response to rapid horizontal movements of the head) as well as the Kernig and Brudzinski maneuvers can be performed. A positive Kernig sign refers to an inability of the examiner to fully extend the knee secondary to resistance and hamstring pain when the patient is lying supine with their hip flexed to a right angle. Brudzinski sign is considered positive if attempts to passively flex the neck are accompanied by unintentional flexion of the hips. If Kernig and Brudzinski signs are negative, it should not be taken as evidence against CNS infection; these signs have been found to have very poor sensitivity (<5%) though are highly specific (>95%) for CSF pleocytosis (an elevation in leukocytes strongly suggestive of meningitis).[7]

Unless there are complicating factors such as suspected spinal epidural abscess, bleeding tendency (including anticoagulated status), findings suggestive of increased intracranial pressure, or overlying skin infection, patients with suspected meningitis should have a lumbar puncture (LP) performed. Prior to the LP, computed tomography (CT) without contrast of the head should be considered in certain situations (see **Table 18.3**).[8] CSF cultures, in addition to blood cultures, should be obtained to determine bacterial species and provide susceptibility information.

An opening pressure should be measured with the patient in a supine position, and ideally three to four vials containing at least 1 mL of CSF obtained for analysis. In addition to cultures, CSF cell counts, glucose, and protein should be sent on all patients at a minimum. Serum glucose should be obtained as well to allow for interpretation of the CSF level (normal CSF glucose reading is approximately two-thirds of serum glucose in a normoglycemic individual). **Table 18.4** shows common CSF profiles of various etiologies of meningoencephalitis. Additional testing, including further viral polymerase chain reaction (PCR) (eg, HSV, VZV) studies, and fungal testing can be ordered on those in whom specific additional diseases are suspected when it will alter management,

TABLE 18.3 Indications for Noncontrast Head CT before LP

Underlying immunocompromised state
History of CNS disease
Seizure activity without known seizure disorder
Papilledema on examination
Recent head trauma
Abnormal level of consciousness
Focal neurologic deficit

CNS, central nervous system; CT, computed tomography; LP, lumbar puncture.

TABLE 18.4	Common CSF Characteristics of CNS Infections with Bacterial, Viral, or Fungal Etiologies, along with Normal CSF Characteristics			
	Normal	**Bacterial**	**Viral**	**Fungal**
Opening pressure	<25 cm H$_2$O	Elevated	Normal	Normal or slightly elevated
Cell count	<5 WBC, 0 PMNs	>1000 WBC	<1000 WBC	<500 WBC
Cell predominance	None	Neutrophils	Lymphocytes	Lymphocytes
CSF glucose (mg/dL)	>2/3 serum glucose	Decreased	Normal	Decreased
CSF protein (mg/dL)	<45	Elevated	Normal	Elevated

CNS, central nervous system; CSF, cerebrospinal fluid; PMN, polymorphonuclear; WBC, white blood cells.
Adapted from Dorsett M, Liang SY. Diagnosis and treatment of central nervous system infections in the emergency department. *Emerg Med Clin North Am*. 2016;34:917-942.

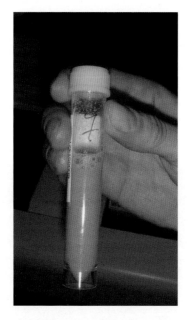

Figure 18.2: A purulent-appearing sample of cerebrospinal fluid, suggestive of bacterial meningitis. By Whein (GNU Free Documentation License), via Wikicommons.

such as in immunocompromised individuals. **Figure 18.2** shows a purulent CSF sample, a highly abnormal finding concerning bacterial meningitis. Serum procalcitonin, CSF lactate, erythrocyte sedimentation rate (ESR), and C-reactive protein (CRP) may also have a role as adjunct means to differentiate bacterial from viral meningitis (see Evidence section).

Encephalitis

When patients with signs of meningeal infection are also exhibiting neurologic deficits such as altered mentation, seizures, personality changes, cranial nerve deficits, or radiculopathies, encephalitis should be strongly considered. These signs may be subtle; meningitis and encephalitis exist along a continuum and, in many cases, are best referred to as meningoencephalitis. Symptoms correlate with the function of the brain parenchyma involved. HSV encephalitis, for example, classically involves the frontotemporal lobes, which can result in abnormal behavior and dysarthria that could be confused with psychosis. It is essential to consider viral encephalitis in all immunocompromised patients presenting with altered mental status because they may not have other classic signs of a CNS infection.

Rapid neuroimaging is the priority in patients with suspected encephalitis; a head CT aids in ruling out other emergent causes of encephalopathy including hemorrhage and mass lesions. All patients should also undergo LP and CSF analysis to evaluate for infectious causes if encephalitis is suspected. Magnetic resonance imaging (MRI) can help detect the changes associated with viral encephalitis if the diagnosis is unclear and can reveal alternative causes of the patient's symptoms, if present (**Figure 18.3**). Although many viral etiologies of encephalitis have PCR testing available, most require only supportive care, and therefore only HSV and VZV (as these can be treated with antiviral medications) should be sent routinely. Serum HIV testing may also be valuable in those at increased risk.

Brain Abscess

The onset of symptoms in intracranial abscesses is typically more gradual than in bacterial meningitis. Symptoms are dependent on the location of the abscess and can include hemiparesis, abnormal gait, and symptoms of increased intracranial pressure. Fever is only present in about half of patients and, in many cases, the only presenting symptom is headache, requiring clinicians to keep the diagnosis on their differential, especially in immunocompromised patients.[4] Imaging allows detection of the abscess and can provide information on the extent of the disease. Suspected brain abscess is one of the few indications for a CT of the head with IV contrast, which will reveal a ring-enhancing lesion, though MRI is more sensitive if available (see **Figure 18.4**).

Laboratory testing is not diagnostic for CNS abscesses, and white blood cell counts can be normal. However, an elevated ESR and/or CRP may be suggestive, and blood cultures should be drawn to allow early identification of the causative organism as up to 60% of patients have associated bacteremia. LP is typically not useful because the CSF is usually sterile.

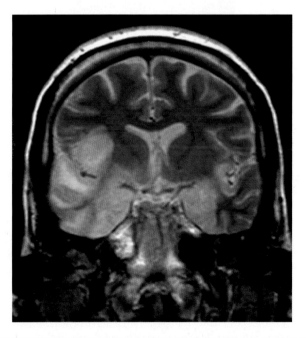

Figure 18.3: MRI of the brain showing temporal lobe enhancement suggestive of HSV encephalitis. HSV, herpes simplex virus; MRI, magnetic resonance imaging. By Dr. Laughlin Dawes (Creative Commons Attribution 3.0 Unported), via Wikicommons.

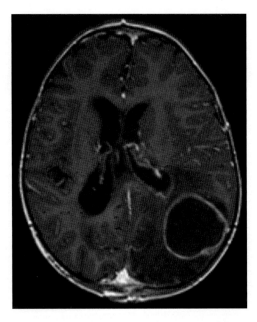

Figure 18.4: Large ring-enhancing lesion in the occipital region on MRI of the brain, consistent with a brain abscess. MRI, magnetic resonance imaging. From Jamjoom AA, Waliuddin AR, Jamjoom AB. Brain abscess formation as a CSF shunt complication: a case report. *Cases J.* 2009;2:110. Figure 1.

Spinal Epidural Abscess

As with other CNS infections, the sensitivity of the classic symptoms associated with spinal epidural abscess is poor (<33%).[9] Back pain is common, but many patients will not have fever, especially early in the disease course. Symptoms are often consistent with compression of the spinal cord, including focal weakness or bowel/bladder incontinence, but these may be absent early in the disease process. Risk factors include alcohol abuse, IV drug use, and compromised immunity. Patient with suspected epidural abscess should undergo a full neurologic examination including reflexes and sensory examination.

MRI with contrast is the most sensitive imaging modality; it typically shows involvement of one or two vertebral levels, though *skip* lesions can be present and therefore total spine imaging is recommended (**Figure 18.5**). A CT myelogram is less sensitive but can be used if MRI cannot be performed.

Serum inflammatory markers are typically elevated, and, like other CNS abscesses, blood cultures can provide bacterial speciation and sensitivity information to guide treatment. LP is contraindicated, given the risk of spreading the disease.

CNS Shunt Infection

CNS shunt infections manifest with signs of increased intracranial pressure and hydrocephalus (eg, headache, altered mental status, nausea, vomiting). They most often occur within 6 months of shunt placement and are typically the result of skin flora being introduced into the CSF space. Evaluation should include neuroimaging (either CT or rapid MRI protocol) as well as neurosurgical consultation.[15]

Prion Disease

Diagnosis for CJD is typically done through electroencephalogram (EEG) testing (showing a biphasic or triphasic sharp wave pattern), MRI (showing increased intensity in the basal ganglia and thalamus; **Figure 18.6**), and CSF testing for elevated CSF protein 14-3-3 levels (highly sensitive and specific for CJD).

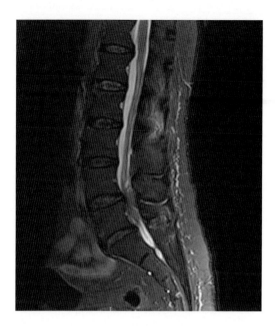

Figure 18.5: MRI of the lumbar spine showing an epidural abscess. MRI, magnetic resonance imaging. From Chan J, Oh JJ. A rare case of multiple spinal epidural abscesses and cauda equina syndrome presenting to the emergency department following acupuncture. *Int J Emerg Med.* 2016;9:22. Figure 3.

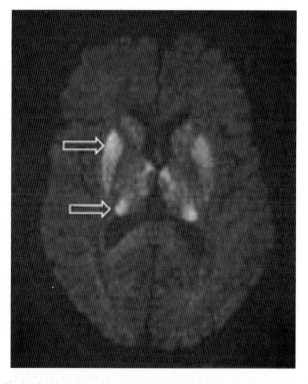

Figure 18.6: MRI of the brain showing characteristic changes of prion disease, including enhancement (*arrows*) in the basal ganglia and thalamus. MRI, magnetic resonance imaging. From Rudge P, Jaunmuktane Z, Adlard P, et al. Iatrogenic CJD due to pituitary-derived growth hormone with genetically determined incubation times of up to 40 years. *Brain.* 2015;138(11):3386-3399. Figure 2.

PEDIATRICS

Infants with CNS infections represent a great clinical challenge as they do not present with classic symptoms. Meningitis may manifest in many different ways, including fussiness, sleepiness, decreased feeding, or poor tone. Temperature instability is also common, and patients can present with either fever or hypothermia, though these are not always present. In children who still have an open anterior fontanelle, physical examination may reveal a bulging anterior fontanelle as a result of increased intracranial pressure. However, their presentation begins to normalize toward more classic adult symptoms as they age. The most common microorganisms that cause meningitis differ greatly based on the age of the patient. In neonates, group B streptococcus (GBS) and *E coli* are common etiologies that are not typically seen in other age groups. *L monocytogenes* is also common in this group.[6] The evaluation for CNS infections is essentially unchanged in pediatric patients, however, including serum and CSF studies, and neuroimaging. If available, radiation-sparing imaging modalities can be considered as preferred options in this population.

MANAGEMENT

The first step in the management of patients with potential CNS infections is to ensure brain oxygenation and perfusion. Patients with concern for airway compromise, such as those with prolonged seizure activity or profoundly altered mental status, should be intubated. Those showing evidence of shock physiology should be fluid resuscitated with crystalloid solution, as septic shock is usually the underlying cause. Once initial stabilization is completed, further definitive testing and treatment can be initiated.

Meningitis

For adults, empiric therapy should cover the most common pathogens (*S pneumoniae, N meningitidis*). We recommend ceftriaxone (2 g every 12 hours) plus vancomycin (15-20 mg/kg every 8 hours) due to increased resistance of *S pneumoniae* in many areas. In infants, ceftriaxone should be exchanged for cefotaxime (50 mg/kg every 6-12 hours depending on age) because ceftriaxone can result in hyperbilirubinemia by displacing bilirubin from albumin-binding sites. Adults older than age 50 should also receive coverage with ampicillin (2 g IV every 4 hours) as well as infants, 1 month old (50 mg/kg every 8 hours), given the risk of *Listeria* and gram-negative bacilli.[10] High-risk patients, such as those who are immunocompromised or those who acquired meningitis from head trauma, may be infected with less typical bacteria (eg, *Staphylococcus, Pseudomonas,* and *Salmonella*) and benefit from broader coverage with the addition of cefepime (2 g IV every 8 hours) or meropenem (1 g IV every 8 hours), as well as consideration of acyclovir (10 mg/kg IV every 8 hours) to cover for HSV.[11]

In children, treatment consists of IV cefotaxime (50 mg/kg every 8 hours) along with ampicillin (50 mg/kg every 8 hours) for *Listeria* coverage. Ceftriaxone should be avoided in infants as cited previously.

Patients with suspected bacterial meningitis should also be given steroids (0.4 mg/kg; max dose 10 mg IV dexamethasone every 6 hours for 4 days) when antibiotics are administered. Use of adjunctive steroids for *H influenzae* bacterial meningitis is associated with a decrease in hearing loss in pediatric cases (see Evidence section that follows).

Patients receiving IV antibiotics should be admitted to the hospital to continue therapy and await the results of the CSF culture; well-appearing patients in whom viral meningitis is clearly established may be considered for discharge home if symptoms are well-controlled and support systems are in place.

Meningitis Prophylaxis

Those in close contact (including health care workers) with patients with *N meningitidis* meningitis should receive oral rifampin (600 mg every 12 hours for four doses) or a single dose of ciprofloxacin (500 mg) for prophylaxis. Rifampin prophylaxis (20 mg/kg once daily for 4 days) for patients with *H influenzae* meningitis is also recommended for the patient's household contacts if they reside with immunocompromised children or children <5 years who have not completed their vaccinations.[12] Prophylaxis for *H influenzae* meningitis contacts is recommended in childcare facilities caring for immunocompromised or unvaccinated children only in instances where two confirmed cases have occurred. See Table 18.2 for summarized recommendations.

Encephalitis

Antimicrobial management of encephalitis essentially mirrors that of meningitis. Patients with suspicion for viral infection (eg, lymphocyte predominance in CSF, cutaneous vesicles) should be given empiric acyclovir (10 mg/kg every 8 hours) to cover for the possibility of HSV, as this is a frequent cause of encephalitis; the care for other viral etiologies is supportive.[13] Encephalitis can also cause complications such as increased intracranial pressure and seizures that may require aggressive medical management. Because of the need for close neurologic and hemodynamic monitoring in these patients, disposition will likely be to intensive care. A flowchart summarizing recommended management appears in **Figure 18.7**.

CNS Abscess

Empiric antimicrobial treatment for brain abscesses is dependent on the condition that predisposed the patient to the abscess. If the source is not known, empiric coverage should be directed at skin flora, including *S aureus* and *Streptococcus*, as well as MRSA and *Pseudomonas*. For example, for abscesses secondary to otitis or mastoiditis, ceftriaxone (2 g IV every 12 hours) plus metronidazole (500 mg every 8 hours) would be recommended. For epidural abscesses, vancomycin (15-20 mg/kg IV every 8 hours) and ceftriaxone (2 g IV every 12 hours) are recommended. If the patient is at

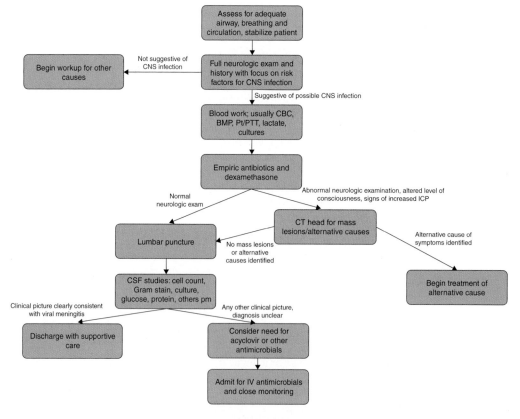

Figure 18.7: A summary of management recommendations for patients with potential meningo-encephalitis, from initial evaluation to disposition. BMP, basic metabolic panel; CBC, complete blood count; CNS, central nervous system; CSF, cerebrospinal fluid; CT, computed tomography; ICP, intracranial pressure; Pt/PTT, prothrombin time/partial thromboplastin time.

risk for infection with *Pseudomonas* (recent admission or neurosurgical procedure), then cefepime should be initiated (2 g IV every 8 hours) along with vancomycin (15-20 mg/kg every 8 hours). Neurosurgical consultation for drainage is warranted for potential source control and culture, either through aspiration or through excision depending on clinical factors such as the size and location of the lesion.

Other Infections

Treatment of CNS infections not due to viruses or bacteria is highly dependent on the causative agent. Parasitic infections such as toxoplasmosis and neurocysticercosis are managed with antiparasitics, antiepileptics, surgery, or merely observation depending on the presentation. Fungal

TIPS AND PEARLS

- Ideally, CSF and bacterial cultures should be obtained prior to the initiation of antibiotics. However, when bacterial meningitis is suspected, antibiotics should not be delayed. If it is not possible to obtain an LP immediately (eg, difficulty with LP, need for head CT prior to the procedure).[14] However, culture data rapidly become unreliable 4 hours after initiation of antibiotic therapy, sometimes within 1 hour.[15]
- When obtaining an LP, the sitting position may increase interspinous distance more than the lateral decubitus position and increase the success rate. However, a valid opening pressure can only be obtained in the lateral decubitus position. Use of ultrasound has also been shown to increase the odds of success for LP in both adults and children.[16,17] In properly chosen patients, minimal sedation with a low-dose opiate and/or benzodiazepine may also increase success rate by improving patient compliance during what can be an uncomfortable procedure.
- Post-LP headache is a common complication of LP. Although many patients being evaluated for possible CNS infection are already experiencing headaches, a post-LP headache can prolong symptoms. These headaches are postulated to arise from ongoing CSF leak after the procedure; use of atraumatic (pencil tip) and smaller bore needles are highly effective at preventing this complication.[18] There is no need for patients to remain in the supine position after LP, as this has not been associated with post-LP headache or other complications.
- If a case of meningococcal meningitis is identified, close contacts such as household members and health care providers in contact with the patient's respiratory secretions should be treated prophylactically with antibiotics to prevent additional cases. Vaccination can also be considered as a supplemental prevention strategy in these contacts (see Table 18.2).

infections require systemic fungicidal agents, often alongside steroids to treat associated inflammation. Mycobacterial infections such as TB can be treated with standard TB therapies, often paired with steroids. These treatments are not commonly started empirically in the ED setting without input from an infectious disease specialist. There are no known effective therapies for prion disease or rabies once they have reached the CNS, and treatment is palliative as these diseases are nearly uniformly fatal.

EVIDENCE

What role do inflammatory markers, procalcitonin, and CSF lactate play in distinguishing bacterial from viral or fungal infection?

Multiple studies have shown that serum procalcitonin can be useful for differentiating bacterial from viral meningitis. A recent meta-analysis showed that an elevation in procalcitonin had a 90% sensitivity, 98% specificity, and a positive likelihood ratio (LR) of 27.3 for bacterial meningitis.[19] Although an elevation in procalcitonin may be suggestive, the sensitivity is insufficient to allow it to be used to rule out bacterial meningitis. CSF lactate measurements have also been proposed as an adjunct means to differentiate bacterial from viral meningitis with an elevated level suggestive of bacterial meningitis.[20] When multiple clinical variables were studied, including CSF lactate, cell count, glucose, and protein, elevations in CSF lactate had the greatest accuracy for differentiating bacterial and viral meningitis. There is no evidence describing lactate levels in fungal CNS infections. Some evidence also suggests that elevated ESR and CRP may be indicative of a bacterial etiology.[21]

Multiple studies have shown that fungal meningitis typically is associated with decreased CSF glucose (ie, hypoglycorrhachia) with a lymphocytic predominance, whereas the glucose is typically normal in viral cases of meningitis. Protein can be elevated in all causes of meningitis, especially when HSV is the cause of viral meningitis, so this finding is less specific.

Overall, these tests have not proven sufficiently reliable to rule out bacterial meningitis. If clinical suspicion for bacterial meningoencephalitis remains after initial testing, these patients should be admitted for ongoing antimicrobials until cultures result. Although these tests should not currently be considered a routine part of the evaluation for suspected CNS infections, they may be useful adjuncts to support a diagnosis of bacterial meningitis in patients in whom the CSF is otherwise inconclusive, or, in the case of ESR/CRP or procalcitonin, the LP could not be obtained.

Are steroids indicated in all patients with suspected CNS infection?

In patients with suspected CNS infection, no benefits in mortality or severe neurologic sequelae have been shown when adding steroids to traditional antimicrobials. However, there are significantly lower rates of hearing loss among survivors in patients that receive steroids and no significant harmful effects.[22] An earlier review showed similar benefits for hearing loss in both children and adults, as well as an improvement in neurologic sequelae, but this effect was seen only in high-income countries. Although there is some evidence to suggest that the beneficial effects of steroids are seen only in *S pneumoniae* infections, the causative organism is unlikely to be known at the time when treatment is needed.[23] At this time, the evidence favors treating all patients with suspected CNS infection with steroids (0.4 mg/kg; max dose 10 mg IV every 6 hours for 4 days), given immediately prior to or concurrently with the first dose of antibiotics.

Should vancomycin be given to all patients with suspected bacterial CNS infection?

For patients in areas of low *S pneumoniae* resistance to penicillins, the evidence supports treating with a third-generation cephalosporin alone. Unfortunately, in many areas, such as the United States, Asia, and southern and western Europe, high resistance rates of *S pneumoniae* make the addition of empiric vancomycin necessary. Interestingly, new pneumococcal vaccines that protect against additional subtypes may be causing susceptibility to ceftriaxone to increase. This suggests that vancomycin could be dropped as a recommendation in the future, as the number needed to treat (NNT) with empiric vancomycin for a single case of ceftriaxone-resistant pneumococcus is estimated to be 12,500.[24] For now, it is prudent to give vancomycin to all patients with suspected bacterial CNS infection if in an area of elevated antibiotic resistance.

Is acyclovir indicated in all patients with suspected meningoencephalitis?

It can be difficult to determine the etiology of a CNS infection at presentation; as a result, some clinicians empirically cover all of their patients with suspected meningoencephalitis with acyclovir (10 mg/kg IV every 8 hours) on arrival. Immunocompromised patients do show improved neurologic outcomes when their HSV meningitis is treated with acyclovir,[25] and we recommend to cover immunocompromised patients with IV acyclovir on arrival. HSV encephalitis has also been shown to have improved outcomes with antiviral treatment, so all cases of even potential encephalitis on arrival to the ED should be given acyclovir. However, acyclovir has not shown a clear benefit in HSV meningitis in immunocompetent patients.[26,27] There are no meaningful data to support or refute acyclovir treatment in VZV CNS infections, but based on extrapolation from other VZV-associated conditions, acyclovir is generally given in VZV encephalitis and considered in VZV meningitis.[28] There is no evidence to support the efficacy of acyclovir for any other viral cause of meningoencephalitis.

Do all patients with HIV/AIDS and new headache require a CSF analysis?

Clinicians should have a low threshold to pursue a diagnostic workup, including imaging and CSF analysis, in any HIV-positive patient presenting with a headache and a CD4 count <200 cells/μL, given their higher risk of developing opportunistic infections such as TB, toxoplasmosis, or CMV.[29] Evidence suggests that patients with HIV who are well-controlled on antiretroviral therapy (ART) with undetectable viral loads do not automatically necessitate CSF analysis and that the degree of immunosuppression along with clinical suspicion can be used to guide the need for workup.[30]

Is a CSF analysis required in pediatric patients with a first-time complex febrile seizure?

It is well established that CSF analysis is not indicated in children with a simple febrile seizure. In a large multicenter study of patients presenting with complex febrile seizures (ie, multiple seizures, focal seizures), only 0.7% of cases represented bacterial meningitis and no cases of HSV meningoencephalitis were discovered.[31] All cases of bacterial meningitis or HSV occurred in patients with an abnormal examination. This is in concordance with a previous meta-analysis and other studies showing that severe CNS infection was uncommon in those with complex febrile seizures.[32] Patients with complex febrile seizures who remain altered, have signs of meningitis, focal seizures, or neurologic deficits may be at increased risk for bacterial infection and require an LP. In all other children with complex febrile seizures, CSF analysis can be omitted as evidence suggests that yield is extremely low.

Is PCR testing indicated in patients with suspected CSF analysis?

Multiple studies have shown PCR to be a valuable diagnostic tool in the workup of select patients with CNS infections. PCR testing has been shown to be 70% sensitive 1 week following antibiotic treatment and may be beneficial in providing the diagnosis in patients who have already started treatment.[15] The utility of PCR has also been seen in viral and tuberculous meningitis.[33,34] However, the utility of these tests should be weighed against the need for the additional quantity of CSF required to run the test, as well as cost. Therefore, we do not recommend routinely obtaining PCR testing in patients with suspected meningoencephalitis.

References

1. van de Beek D, Cabellos C, Dzupova O, et al. ESCMID guideline: diagnosis and treatment of acute bacterial meningitis. *Clin Microbiol Infect*. 2016;22(suppl 3):S37-S62.

2. Robertson FC, Lepard JR, Mekary RA, et al. Epidemiology of central nervous system infectious diseases: a meta-analysis and systematic review with implications for neurosurgeons worldwide. *J Neurosurg*. 2018:1-20.

3. McGill F, Griffiths MJ, Bonnett LJ, et al. Incidence, aetiology, and sequelae of viral meningitis in UK adults: a multicentre prospective observational cohort study. *Lancet Infect Dis*. 2018;18:992-1003.

4. Brouwer MC, Coutinho JM, van de Beek D. Clinical characteristics and outcome of brain abscess: systematic review and meta-analysis. *Neurology*. 2014;82:806-813.

5. Telisinghe L, Waite TD, Gobin M, et al. Chemoprophylaxis and vaccination in preventing subsequent cases of meningococcal disease in household contacts of a case of meningococcal disease: a systematic review. *Epidemiol Infect*. 2015;143:2259-2268.

6. Davis LE. Acute bacterial meningitis. *Continuum (Minneap Minn)*. 2018;24:1264-1283.

7. Nakao JH, Jafri FN, Shah K, Newman DH. Jolt accentuation of headache and other clinical signs: poor predictors of meningitis in adults. *Am J Emerg Med*. 2014;32:24-28.

8. Salazar L, Hasbun R. Cranial imaging before lumbar puncture in adults with community-acquired meningitis: clinical utility and adherence to the Infectious Diseases Society of America Guidelines. *Clin Infect Dis*. 2017;64:1657-1662.

9. Chow F. Brain and spinal epidural abscess. *Continuum (Minn Minn)*. 2018;24:1327-1348.

10. McGill F, Heyderman RS, Panagiotou S, Tunkel AR, Solomon T. Acute bacterial meningitis in adults. *Lancet*. 2016;388:3036-3047.

11. van de Beek D, Brouwer MC, Thwaites GE, Tunkel AR. Advances in treatment of bacterial meningitis. *Lancet*. 2012;380:1693-1702.

12. Briere EC, Rubin L, Moro PL, et al. Prevention and control of Haemophilus influenzae type b disease: recommendations of the advisory committee on immunization practices (ACIP). *MMWR Recomm Rep*. 2014;63:1-14.

13. Gaieski DF, O'Brien NF, Hernandez R. Emergency neurologic life support: meningitis and encephalitis. *Neurocrit Care*. 2017;27:124-133.

14. Michael B, Menezes BF, Cunniffe J, et al. Effect of delayed lumbar punctures on the diagnosis of acute bacterial meningitis in adults. *Emerg Med J*. 2010;27:433-438.

15. Brink M, Welinder-Olsson C, Hagberg L. Time window for positive cerebrospinal fluid broad-range bacterial PCR and Streptococcus pneumoniae immunochromatographic test in acute bacterial meningitis. *Infect Dis (Lond)*. 2015;47(12):869-877.

16. Millington SJ, Silva Restrepo M, Koenig S. Better with ultrasound: lumbar puncture. *Chest*. 2018;154:1223-1229.

17. Neal JT, Kaplan SL, Woodford AL, Desai K, Zorc JJ, Chen AE. The effect of bedside ultrasonographic skin marking on infant lumbar puncture success: a randomized controlled trial. *Ann Emerg Med*. 2017;69:610-619.e1.

18. Xu H, Liu Y, Song W, et al. Comparison of cutting and pencil-point spinal needle in spinal anesthesia regarding postdural puncture headache: a meta-analysis. *Medicine (Baltimore)*. 2017;96:e6527.

19. Vikse J, Henry BM, Roy J, Ramakrishnan PK, Tomaszewski KA, Walocha JA. The role of serum procalcitonin in the diagnosis of bacterial meningitis in adults: a systematic review and meta-analysis. *Int J Infect Dis*. 2015;38:68-76.

20. Giulieri S, Chapuis-Taillard C, Jaton K, et al. CSF lactate for accurate diagnosis of community-acquired bacterial meningitis. *Eur J Clin Microbiol Infect Dis*. 2015;34:2049-2055.

21. Sanaei Dashti A, Alizadeh S, Karimi A, Khalifeh M, Shoja SA. Diagnostic value of lactate, procalcitonin, ferritin, serum-C-reactive protein, and other biomarkers in bacterial and viral meningitis: a cross-sectional study. *Medicine (Baltimore)*. 2017;96:e7637.

22. Shao M, Xu P, Liu J, Liu W, Wu X. The role of adjunctive dexamethasone in the treatment of bacterial meningitis: an updated systematic meta-analysis. *Patient Prefer Adherence*. 2016;10:1243-1249.

23. Brouwer MC, McIntyre P, Prasad K, van de Beek D. Corticosteroids for acute bacterial meningitis. *Cochrane Database Syst Rev*. 2015:CD004405.

24. Jhaveri R. The time has come to stop using vancomycin as part of empiric therapy for meningitis. *J Pediatric Infect Dis Soc*. 2019;8(1):92-93.

25. Noska A, Kyrillos R, Hansen G, Hirigoyen D, Williams DN. The role of antiviral therapy in immunocompromised patients with herpes simplex virus meningitis. *Clin Infect Dis*. 2015;60:237-242.

26. Miller S, Mateen FJ, Aksamit AJ Jr. Herpes simplex virus 2 meningitis: a retrospective cohort study. *J Neurovirol*. 2013;19:166-171.

27. Kaewpoowat Q, Salazar L, Aguilera E, Wootton SH, Hasbun R. Herpes simplex and varicella zoster CNS infections: clinical presentations, treatments and outcomes. *Infection*. 2016;44:337-345.

28. Grahn A, Studahl M. Varicella-zoster virus infections of the central nervous system: prognosis, diagnostics and treatment. *J Infect*. 2015;71:281-293.

29. Tan IL, Smith BR, von Geldern G, Mateen FJ, McArthur JC. HIV-associated opportunistic infections of the CNS. *Lancet Neurol*. 2012;11:605-617.

30. Kirkland KE, Kirkland K, Many WJ Jr, Smitherman TA. Headache among patients with HIV disease: prevalence, characteristics, and associations. *Headache*. 2012;52:455-466.

31. Guedj R, Chappuy H, Titomanlio L, et al. Do all children who present with a complex febrile seizure need a lumbar puncture? *Ann Emerg Med*. 2017;70:52-62.e6.

32. Fletcher EM, Sharieff G. Necessity of lumbar puncture in patients presenting with new onset complex febrile seizures. *West J Emerg Med*. 2013;14:206-211.

33. Bradshaw MJ, Venkatesan A. Herpes simplex virus-1 encephalitis in adults: pathophysiology, diagnosis, and management. *Neurotherapeutics*. 2016;13:493-508.

34. Bahr NC, Nuwagira E, Evans EE, et al. Diagnostic accuracy of Xpert MTB/RIF ultra for tuberculous meningitis in HIV-infected adults: a prospective cohort study. *Lancet Infect Dis*. 2018;18:68-75.

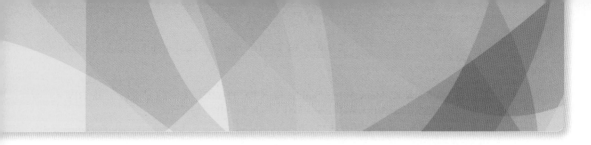

Index

Note: Page numbers followed by *f* and *t* denote figures and tables respectively.